TEXT BOOK
OF
DRAVYAGUNA

THE
CHAUKHAMBA AYURVEDA STUDIES
7

TEXT BOOK
OF
DRAVYAGUNA

[According to the Syllabus of CCIM, New Delhi]

By
Dr. K. Nishteswar
M.D. Ph.D. DAFE
Professor & Head
Department of Dravyaguna
Dr. NRS Govt. Ayurvedic College
Vijayawada (A.P.)

CHAUKHAMBA SURBHARATI PRAKASHAN
VARANASI (INDIA)

Text Book of Dravyaguna – K. Nishteswar

ISBN : 978-93-85005-01-5

Published by :
CHAUKHAMBA SURBHARATI PRAKASHAN
(*Oriental Publishers or Distributors*)
K 37/117, Gopal Mandir Lane
Post Box No. 1129
Varanasi 221001 (India)
Tel. : +91 542 2335263, 2335264
e-mail : csp_naveen@yahoo.co.in
website : www.chaukhamba.co.in
@chaukhambabooks
@chaukhambabooks

Edition : 2023
₹ 595.00

Distributor :
CHAUKHAMBA PUBLISHING HOUSE
4697/2, Ground Floor, Street No. 21-A
Ansari Road, Daryaganj
New Delhi 110002
Tel : +91 11 23286537, 41530947 (Mob.) +91 9811104365
e-mail : chaukhambapublishinghouse@gmail.com

*

Also can be had from :
CHAUKHAMBA SANSKRIT PRATISHTHAN
4360/4, Ansari Road, Daryaganj, New Delhi - 110002

*

CHOWKHAMBA VIDYABHAWAN
Chowk (Behind Bank of Baroda Building)
Post Box No. 1069, Varanasi 221001

Printed by : A. K. Lithographer Delhi

DEDICATION

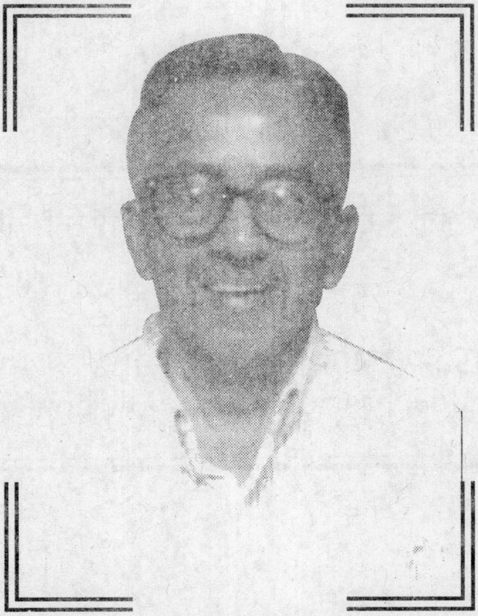

To my beloved Preceptor

Dr. A.P. Deshpande, Ph.D.,

Professor (Retd.),

Tilak Ayurved Mahavidyalaya,

Pune

नानौषधीभूतं जगति किञ्चिद् द्रव्यमुपलभ्यते तां तां युक्तिमर्थं च तं तमभिप्रेत्य । (CS Su 26:12)

There is no substance in the universe that has no medicinal value, provided you know how to use it.

PREFACE

Dravyaguna is interpreted as clinical pharmacology since the most of the Ayurvedic drugs were initially evaluated only in human beings. Seers of Ayurveda have collected the information regarding the clinical usage of several herbs from cowherds, shepherds, tribals and other forest dwellers and they never felt the necessity of evaluating their activity in animals.

Dravyaguna encompasses the information of all other allied fields of pharmacology like:

- *Namarupa Vijnanam*—Pharmacognosy (the science of identification of drugs).
- *Gunakarma Vijnanam*—Pharmacodynamics (mechanism of drugs action) & Pharmacokinetics (study of absorption, distribution, metabolims and excretion of drugs).
- *Amayikaprayoga Vijnanam*—Therapeutics (branch of medicine concerned with cure of disease or relief of symptoms).
- *Kalpana Vijnanam*—Pharmacy (science of selection, preservation & compounding of drug).

The major object of teaching Dravyaguna to the medical students of Ayurveda is to provide a rational basis for choosing or using drugs skillfully to relieve ailments of the patient population. The modern pharmacology is traditionally associated with the study of drugs in different animals like dogs, monkeys, cats, rabbits, rats etc. Whereas the clinial pharmacology involves the study of various aspects of drug action and metabolism in humans, both in health and disease. The ultimate aim of pharmacological studies in animals is to find out a therapeutic agent suitable for clinical evalutation in man. The animal models (cat, rat etc.) cannot act as an ideal model of human being. The drug has to be carefully evaluated in human being for its safety and efficacy before it is accepted for therapeutic use.

Majority of the drugs that are currently used in modern medicine are synthetic where as the Ayurvedic therapeutics mainly employ plant-based medicines (*oudbhija*) along with metals & minerals (*parthiva*) and animal products (*jagama dravya*). Among the plant products, the important pharmacologically active principles (*utkrishta guna-sampanna dravyamsha*) are—

(a) alkaloids (basic substances containing cyclic nitrogen) (b) glycosides (a combination of sugars with other organic structures) (c) glucosides (glycoside which yields glucose on acid hydrolysis) (d) oils (fixed or volatile) (e) resins (formed by oxidation of volatile oils which are insoluble in water but soluble in alcohal) (f) gums (dispersible in water) (g) tannins (precipitate proteins from the cells and are non-nitrogenous).

Scientists of modern pharmacy generally argue that plant based medicines should be processed in the medium of alcohal as the majority of active principles (mainly alkaloids) are made available and according to them water extracts of plants are useless as they are devoid of maximum alkaloid content. The review of various *bheshaja-kalpanas* (pharmaceutical processes), namely *kwatha, phanta, hima, taila, ghrita, arishta* except *asava-kalpana* clearly indicates that water was suggested as the medium of extraction. Some of the scholars of Ayurveda following the concept of modern pharmaceutical scientists suggest to prefer *kanjikam* (contains self generated alcohal) as the medium for extracting the active portion of the drugs. But a careful review of different formulations indicates that *kanjikam* was not mentioned for majority of formulations. To achieve the maximum therapeutic action it is always preferable to administer the *swarasa* (fresh juice) or *kalka* (paste) or *churna* (powder) of fresh herb or dried herb. The human gut, which is highly sophisticated, and also the selective chemical laboratory can synthesize the required portion of the active principle and makes in available to various bodily organs and tissues. Ayurvedic pharmacology delineates five important principles namely *rasa, guna, virya, vipaka* and *prabhava* (*Rasapanchaka*) which are responsible for any drug action. Many times the terms 'action' and 'effects' of a drug are being used as synonyms. However, it is useful to term the initial consequences of drug-cell interactions as the action (*karma*) of the drug, the remaining events that follow are called drug effects (*phala*). In practice, no drug produces only a single effect but has spectrum of effects or actions. Further, a drug may be selective in one respect but non-selective in another. With this view only the most of the Ayurvedic Nighantus attributed a spectrum of actions and therapeutic indications to the majority of drugs. Most of the actions of drugs are attributed to the potent *gunas* which are given *virya* status. Most of the actions of drugs are attributed to the potent *gunas* which are given *virya* status. Ayurvedic classics firmly established the relationship between the various pharmacological actions and the principles of drug action like *rasa, vipaka* and *guna/virya.* In my view *rasa,* which is identified, by *nipata* (contact with the tongue) and *vipaka* by *nishtha karma* (final action) serve as indices of *guna* at the tongue level and at the stage of biotransformation (alteration of drug within living organism) respectively. After absorption, drugs could undergo three possible fates, namely, that could be metabolized by enzymes (*dhatwagni paka*), they could change into other substances without intervention of enzymes (it happens in the case of *vyavayi* drugs) or they could be excreted unchanged and in the case of *samana pratyayarabdha dravyas.* In the case of *samana pratyayarabdha dravyas* through *rasa,* it becomes easy to draw the profiles of other principles of drug action and in the case of *vichitra pratyayarabdha dravyas* the pharmacological principles barring *rasa* (which is perceivable) are identified by inference basing on pharmacological action/therapeutic (*karma* & *phala*). The drugs metabolized by enzymes (*vipaka*) result in their activation, inactivation or modification. *Vipaka* alone engenders *virya* (activated drug energy) and it alone—

(i) activates the *gunas* like *ushna* to become *ushnatara/ushnatama* or

(ii) inactivates the action of gunas like *sheeta* which is unable to produce *vata vriddhi* (as in the case of *ksheera* (milk)

(iii) modifies *gunas* originally attributed to *rasa* eg. *sheeta virya* of *madhura rasa* becomes *ushna virya* after *vipaka* (such drugs are categorized as *vichitra pratyayarabdha dravyas*).

It is generally observed that most of the Ayurvedic scholars are inclined to interpret *virya* of a *dravya* as the active principle. Acharya Priyavrat Sharma has disagreed with this concept and rightly suggested that active principle is the *adhisthana* of *virya, Sushruta* alone initiated a debate to discuss the relative importance of all the principles of drug action and finally concluded that *dravya* is the only prime one among all the principles. If the active principle or active drug molecule (*drayva*) is attributed with drug action, it can also be safely interpreted that *rasa* (taste) serves as one of the indices to identify pharmacological behaviour of active principle and *vipaka* indicates the metabolic process to synthesize the active drug molecules and *virya* indicates the release of energy from the active drug molecule (active principle).

Drayvaguna in some respects as a bridge between basic medical sciences on one hand and clinical medicine on the other. An attempt is made in this book to give all the relevant details of the entire Dravyaguna subject in accordance with CCIM curriculum and students will get all the necessary information by reading this book. Students should not 'cram' this book to get through the examination successfully but I expect them to learn the basic pharmacology of drugs in common clinical use and their rational application in therapeutics. The CCIM syllabus in the subject of Dravyaguna consists of two papers—first paper contains the fundamental principles of Dravyaguna and second paper deals with the details of 365 herbs and the subject of modern pharmacology in brief. I wish to acknowledge the help taken form the works of great scholars of Dravyguna late Acharya Yadavji Trikamji, late Acharya Bapalal Vaidya, late C. Dwarakanath, Acharya Priyavrata Sharma and Achrya K.C. Chunekar, which have rendered important guidelines in the preparation of this hand book. My heartfelt thanks are due to Sri K. Arunee Kumar, Lecturer in Botany, P.R. Govt. College, Kakinada for his ablest guidance in all my academic pursuits. I specially thank Mr. Naveen Gupta, Chaukhamba Surbharati Prakashan for taking up the task of publication.

Vijaya Dashami, **K. Nishteswar**

Dt. 12-10-2005

CONTENTS

First Paper

Part - A

INTRODUCTION 1
DRAVYA 5
DRAVYA VARGIKARANA 9
GUNA VIJNANA 18
RASA VIJNANA 29
VIPAKA 45
VIRYA 53
PRABHAVA 68

Part - B

DRAVYAGATA PADARTHAS AND PARASPARIKA SAMBANDHA 73
KARMA 76
MODERN PHARMACOLOGICAL ACTIONS 91
AUDBHIDADI GANA 96
DRAVYA SAMGRAHANA AND SAMRAKSHANA 103
DRAVYA SHODHANA 118
BHESAJA PRAYOGA VIJNANA 123
HISTORY OF DRAVYAGUNA 139

Second Paper

Part - A (I)

VATSANĀBHA 151
ATIVIṢĀ 152
GUḌŪCĪ 153
PĀṬHĀ 155
DĀRUHARIDRĀ 156
AHIPHENA 158
VARUṆA 159
TUVARAKA 160
NĀGAKEŚARA 161
ŚĀLA 162
BALĀ 163
NĀGABALĀ 165
ŚĀLMALĪ 167
GOKṢURA 168
CĀṄGERĪ 170
NIMBŪKA 171
BILVA 172
GUGGULU 173
TEJOHVA 176
NIMBA 177
JYOTIṢMATĪ 179
KARKAṬAŚṚṄGĪ 180
BHALLĀTAKA 182
ŚIGRU 184
PALĀŚA 186
APARĀJITĀ 188
MADHUYAṢṬI 189
YAVĀSA 191
ŚĀLAPARṆĪ 192
PṚŚNIPARṆĪ 194
KARAÑJA 195
LATĀKARAÑJA 197
KAPIKACCHŪ 199
ŚARAPUṄKHĀ 201
BĀKUCĪ 203
KĀÑCANĀRA 205
AŚOKA 207
ŚIRĪṢA 209
ĀRAGWADHA 211
KHADIRA 213
HARĪTAKĪ 215
VIBHĪTAKA 217
ĀMALAKĪ 219
LAVAṄGA 221
JAMBŪ 222
DĀḌIMA 224
DHĀTAKĪ 226
INDRAVĀRUṆĪ 227
KŪṢMĀṆḌA 229
MAṆḌŪKAPARṆĪ 231
PAṬOLA 233
HIṄGU 234
ŚATAPUṢPĀ 235
MIŚREYA 236
DHĀNYAKA 237
AJAMODĀ 239
YAVĀNĪ 240
JĪRAKA 242
KṚṢṆAJĪRAKA 244
MAÑJIṢṬHĀ 245
MADANAPHALA 247
GANDHAPRASĀRIṆĪ 249
JAṬĀMĀṀSĪ 250
BHṚṄGARĀJA 252
PUṢKARAMŪLA 253
KUṢṬHA 254
CITRAKA 256
VIḌAṄGA 258
LODHRA 259
SAPTAPARṆA 260
KUṬAJA 261
SARPAGANDHĀ 263
KARAVĪRA 264
ARKA 266
SĀRIVĀ 268
KŪPĪLU 270
KIRĀTATIKTA 272
ŚAṄKHAPUṢPĪ 274

TRIVṚT 275
KAṆṬAKĀRĪ 276
BṚHATĪ 278
AŚWAGANDHĀ 279
DHATTŪRĀ 281
PĀRASĪKA YAVĀNĪ 282
KAṬUKĪ 283
BRĀHMĪ 285
ŚYONĀKA 287
PĀṬALĀ 289
VĀSĀ 291
NIRGUṆḌĪ 293
AGNIMANTHA 295
BHĀRṄGĪ 297
GAMBHĀRĪ 298
TULASĪ 300
DROṆAPUṢPĪ 302
PUNARNAVĀ 303
APĀMĀRGA 305
MARICA 306
PIPPALĪ 307
JĀTIPHALA 309
TWAK 311
KARPŪRA 312
AGURU 313
CANDANA 314
ERAṆḌA 316
DANTĪ 318
ARJUNA 320
UDUMBARA 322
BHAṄGĀ 323
DEVADĀRU 325
TĀLĪŚAPATRA 327
HARIDRĀ 328
ĀRDRAKA 330
ELĀ 332
RASONA 334
KUMĀRĪ 336
ŚATĀVARĪ 338
VACĀ 340
MUSTĀ 342
UŚĪRA 344
PIPPALĪMŪLA 345
PALĀṆḌU 346

Part - A (II)

MAMĪRĀ 349
NIRVIṢĀ 350
UPAKUÑCIKĀ 351
KĀNDĪRA 352
CAVYA 353
CAMPAKA 354
SĪTĀPHALA 355
KĀṢṬHADĀRU 356
PĀTĀLAGARUḌĪ 357
GIRI PARPAṬA 358
KAMALA (SACRED LOTUS) 359
KUMUDA (WATER LILY) 361
SATYĀNĀŚĪ 362
MAKHĀNNA 363
PARPAṬAKA 364
SARṢAPA 365
RĀJIKĀ 366
CANDRAŚŪRA 367
KHŪBAKALĀ 368
TODARĪ 369
MŪLAKA 370
TILAPARṆĪ 371
HIṀSRĀ 372
VYĀGHRANAKHĪ 373
KARĪRA 374
BANAPHŚĀ 375
VIKAṄKATA 376
PUNNĀGA 377
SURAPUNNĀGA 378
TAMĀLA 379
SARJA 380
VṚKṢĀMLA 381
AŚWAKARṆA 382
LATĀKASTŪRĪ 383
PĀRĪṢA 384
KHATMĪ 385
KĀRPĀSA 386
MUCAKUNDA 387
PIŚĀCA KĀRPĀSA 388
ĀVARTANĪ 389
PARŪṢAKA 390
GĀṄGERUKĪ 391
GUḌAŚARKARĀ 392
DHANWANA 393
ATASĪ 394
CAÑCU 395
KARMARAṄGA 396
BĪJAPŪRA 397
SUDDĀVA 398
HARAMALA 399
AMLAVETASA 400
ARALU 401
IṄGUDĪ 402
BOLA 403
ŚALLAKĪ 404
KUṄDURU (ŚALLAKĪ) 405
MĀṀSAROHIṆĪ 406
BADARA 407
UNNĀVA 408
DRĀKṢĀ 409
ASTHISAṀHĀRAKA 410
ARIṢṬAKA 411
KOŚĀMRA 412
ĀMRA 413
TINTIḌĪKA 415
PRIYĀLA 416
AṄKOṬA 417
RUMĪMASTAGĪ 418
GUÑJĀ 419
AGASTYA 420
JAYANTĪ 421
NĪLĪ 422
AŚMANTAKA 423
GORAKṢA 424
MUDGAPARṆĪ 425

MĀṢAPARṆĪ	426
BĪJAKA	427
ŚIṀŚAPĀ	428
PĀRIBHADRA	429
VĪRATARU	430
AMLIKĀ	431
ŚAMĪ	432
PATRĀṄGA	433
CAKRAMARDA	434
KĀSAMARDA	435
METHIKĀ	436
RAKTACANDANA	437
VIDĀRĪ	438
CAKṢUṢYA	439
KULATTHA	440
TINIŚA	441
IRIMEDA	442
MĀRKAṆḌIKĀ	443
ĀVARTAKĪ	444
BABBŪLA	445
LAJJĀLU	446
TARUṆĪ	447
VĀTĀDA	448
PADMAKA	449
PĀṢĀṆABHEDA	450
PARṆABĪJA	451
SILHAKA	452
DHAVA	453
TILAPARṆA	454
HIJJALA	455
MADAYANTIKĀ	456
SṚṄGĀṬAKA	457
SAPTACAKRĀ	458
ERAṆḌAKARKAṬĪ	459
TRAPUṢA	460
KAṬUTUMBĪ (IKṢVĀKU)	461
KOŚĀTAKĪ	462
JĪMŪTAKA	463
DHĀMĀRGAVA	464
BIMBĪ	465
KĀRAVELLAKA	466
GARJARA	467
CORAKA	468
NĀḌĪHIṄGU	469
KADAMBA	470
HARIDRĀ	471
TAGARA	472
DAMANAKA	473
CAUHĀRA	474
SAHADEVĪ	475
MUṆḌĪ	476
ĀKĀRAKARABHA	477
ARAṆYAJĪRAKA	478
KUKUNDARA	479
JHAṆḌU	480
ĀYĀPĀNA	481
DUGDHAPHENĪ	482
CHIKKIKĀ	483
KĀSANĪ	484
RĀSNĀ	485
MADHŪKA	486
BAKULA	487
PĀRIJĀTA	488
JĀTĪ	489
YŪTHIKĀ	490
TINDUKA	491
PĪLU	492
KARAMARDA	493
JĪVANTĪ	494
MEṢAŚṚṄGĪ	495
MŪRVĀ	496
KATAKA	497
TRĀYAMĀṆĀ	498
SLEṢMĀTAKA	499
GOJIHWĀ	500
ADHAḤPUṢPĪ	501
VṚDDHADĀRUKA	502
KṚṢṆABĪJA	503
ĀKHUPARṆĪ	504
AMARAVALLĪ	505
KĀKAMĀCĪ	506
KAṬUVĪRA	507
TĀMRAPARṆA	508
HṚTPATRĪ	509
ROHITAKA	510
TILA	511
SAIREYAKA	512
KOKILĀKṢA	513
KĀLAMEGHA	514
UṬAṄGANA	515
BHĀṆḌĪRA	516
PRIYAṄGU	517
PŪTIHĀ	518
JŪPHĀ	519
PARṆAYAVĀNĪ	520
AŚVAGOLA	521
GORAKṢAGUÑJĀ	522
CUKRIKĀ (CUKRA)	523
PĪTAMULĪ	524
ĪŚWARĪ	525
KĪṬAMĀRĪ	526
SUGANDHA-VĀSTUKA	527
KAṄKOLA	528
PATRAKA (TEJAPATRA)	529
MEDĀSAKA	530
BANDĀKA	531
SNUHĪ	532
KAMPILLAKA	533
PUTRAJĪVAKA	534
BHŪMYĀMA-LAKĪ	535
SWARṆĀKṢĪRĪ	536
KAṄKUṢṬHA	537
JAYAPĀLA	538
NĀGADANTĪ	539
VAṬA	540
AŚWATTHA	541
PLAKṢA	542
TŪDA	543
KĀKODUMBARA	544
CIRABILWA	545
PANASA	546

AKṢOṬA 547
KAṬPHALA 548
MĀYĀPHALA 549
BHŪRJAPATRA 550
SOMA 551
SARALA 552
HAPUṢĀ 553
ŚAṬĪ 554
TAVAKṢĪRA 555
ĀMRAGANDHĪ HARIDRĀ 556
NĀGADAMANĪ 557
MAHĀBHARĪ VACĀ 558
KEBUKA 559
KADALĪ 560
ANĀNĀSA 561
SUDARŚANA 562
KUṄKUMA 563
TĀLAMŪLĪ 564
VĀRĀHĪKANDA 565
VANAPALĀṆḌU 566
DWIPĀNTARA VACĀ 567
UŚAVA 568
LĀṄGALĪ 569
SURAÑJĀNA 570
MŪSALĪ 571
NĀRIKELA 572
PŪGA 573
TĀLA 574
KHARJŪRA 575
RAKTANIRYĀSA 576
KETAKĪ 577
SŪRAṆA 578
MĀNAKANDA 579
KUMBHIKĀ 580
KAŚERUKA 581
VAṀŚA 582
KUŚA 583
ŚARA 584
KĀŚA 585
NALA 586
DŪRVĀ 587
ROHIṢA 588
HAṀSARĀJA 589
MAYŪRAŚIKHĀ 590
ŚAILEYA 591
ŚAIVĀLA 592
CHATRAKA 593
ŚAṆAPUṢPĪ 594
SŪCĪ 595
DUGDHIKĀ 596

Part - B (I)

AṄGARASA 599
AGNIJĀRA 600
KASTŪRĪ 601
GOROCANA 602
PRAVĀLA 603
PŪTI (KHATTĀŚĪ) 604
MUKTĀ 605
ŚAṄKHA 606
ŚAṂBŪKA 607
ŚUKTI 608
VARĀṬIKĀ 609
MṚGAŚṚṄGA (STAG'S HORN) 610

Part - B (II)

IKṢU VARGA 611
DUGDHA VARGA 613
MŪTRA VARGA 615
TAILA VARGA 616
MADYA VARGA 617
MADHU VARGA 619
VĀRI VARGA 621
MĀṀSA VARGA 623
ŚŪKADHĀNYA VARGA 624
ŚIMBĪDHĀNYA VARGA 625
LAVAṆA VARGA 627
ĀHĀROPAYOGĪ VARGA 628

Part - B (III)

GUḌŪCĪ 629
MAÑJIṢṬHĀ 632
KUṬAJA 634
DHATTŪRA 636
VĀSĀ 639
PIPPALĪ 641
ARJUNA 643
SĀRIBĀ 644
AŚWAGANDHĀ 645
ŚATĀVARĪ 647

Part - B (IV)

MODERN PHARMACOLOGY 649
Index of Latin Names of Dravyas 660

FIRST PAPER

Part - A (Chapters 1-8)

Part - B (Chapters 9-16)

1

INTRODUCTION

- Dravyaguna Shastra Lakshana (Characteristics of Dravyaguna)
- Samanya Parichaya of Sapta Padarthas (General information about Dravya, Rasa, Guna, Virya, Vipaka, Prabhava and Karma)

Dravyaguna Shastra Lakshana
(Characteristics of Dravyaguna)

The importance of Dravyaguna is well reflected in its being given a place among Ashtangas of Ayurveda by the author of Raja-nighantu.

The science which deals with the Guna (principles/qualities), Karma (action) and Prayoga (therapeutic profiles) of the Dravya (food substances/drug) is called Dravyaguna.[1]

Dravya is the chief component of Dravyaguna Shastra. This Dravya contains Rasa, Guna, Virya, Vipaka and Shakti (Prabhava) which perform their own actions.[2]

The subject of Dravyaguna is divided into 4 branches:

a. Pharmacognosy (Namarupa Vijnana)
b. Pharamacology (Guna-karma Vijnana)
c. Therapeutics (Prayoga Vijnana)
d. Pharmacy (Bheshaja Kalpana)

Samanya Parichaya of Saptapadarthas
(General Information about Dravya, Rasa, Guna, Virya, Vipaka, Prabhava and Karma)

Dravya:

The one which is substratum of the qualities (Guna) and action (Karma) and which is a concomitant cause (Samavayi karana) is known as 'Dravya' (matter).[3] By definition, matter happens to be substratum of Guna and Karma and it is also the concomitant cause of another matter, qualities and actions. The capacity to produce something out of its own rests only in matter but not either in quality or action.

Eg: Guduchi, Arjuna etc.

Rasa:

The principle which is identified by the tongue is known as 'Rasa'. The quality which makes a gustatory appeal i.e., Rasa is considered as one of the principles of drug action.[4]

Guna:

Guna is the inherent principle of a Dravya which acts as the causative principle for generating similar type of Gunas and remains as devoid of action.[5]

Virya:

The power which performs work or action is 'Virya'.[6]

Eg: Sheeta, Ushna etc.

Vipaka:

The change in the taste (of substances) that occurs at the end of digestion by the association of the Jatharagni is called as 'Vipaka'.

The factors which is the final out come of biotransformation of Rasa through the action of Jatharagni is 'Vipaka'.[7]

Eg: Madhura, Amla & Katu vipakas.

Prabhava:

The principle responsible for a specific action which may not be explained in terms of known principles viz., Rasa, Virya, Guna and Vipaka is knoun as prabhava.[8]

The inexplicable energy (Achintya shakti or Virya) is named as 'Prabhava'.

Eg: Antitoxic effect of Shirisha.

Karma:

'Karma' (action) is defined as the causative factor of Samyoga (combination) and Vibhaga (seperation/dissociation) which resides in the Dravya.[9] Action is the performance of what is to be done. It depends on nothing. Prof. B.N. Seal interprets that the term Karma connotes different aspects of physico-chemical reactions, viz., decomposition, dissociation, displacement, double decomposition, substitution, hydrolysis, addition etc.

Eg: Chedana, Lekhana etc.

The Rasas are percieved by the gustatory sense organs, their compostition is inferred by their effects on the Doshas (Vata, pitta, kapha) of the body. Six Rasas either pacify or aggravate the Doshas. In course of observation, the ancient scholars noted dissimilar effects in case of several drugs which are not according to Rasa of the respective Dravya. For instance, pippali, which is Katu in Rasa should have ketabolic effect but, on the contrary, it posses rasayana effect. Similar is the result in cases of Haritaki, Amalaki etc. This observation has made them to formulate another concept termed as Vipaka. Vipaka can be inferred by the effect of one drugs on Doshas, Dhatus and Malas. It was also conceived that there is a principle in the drug which is responsible for its action. This was confirmed by the law of agreement in presence and absence (Anvayavyatireka). It is seen that some particular part of the plant is used and not all at random. The drug also loses its action over a period of time. All these observations lead to the promulgation of Virya (potency) concept for explaining the drug action. The drug actions which can not be interpreted in a most rational way are grouped as empirical action and the principle responsible for it is designated as Prabhava.

●

References

1. यतश्चायुष्यानायुष्याणि च द्रव्यगुणकर्माणि वेदयत्यतोऽप्यायुर्वेदः। (च. सू.-30.23)
द्रव्याणां गुणकर्माणि प्रयोगा विविधास्तथा।
सर्वशो यत्र वर्ण्यन्ते शास्त्रं द्रव्यगुणं हि तत्।। (प्रियव्रत शर्मा)
2. द्रव्ये रसो गुणो वीर्यं विपाकः शक्तिरेव च पदार्थाः पञ्च तिष्ठन्ति स्वं स्वं कुर्वन्ति कपि च। (भा.प्र.)
3. यत्राश्रिताः कर्मगुणाः कारणं समवायि यत्, तत् द्रव्यम्। (च.सू. 1)
गुणशब्देन चेह धर्मवाचिना रसवीर्यविपाकप्रभावाः सर्व एव गृह्यन्ते।
(च. सू.-1.51 पर चक्रपाणि)
क्रियागुणवत् समवायिकारणम् इति। (सु. सू.-40.3)
4. रस्यते आस्वाद्यते इति रसः।
रसाः स्वाद्वम्ललवणतिक्तोषणकषायकाः।
षड्द्रव्यमाश्रितास्ते च यथापूर्वं बलावहा।। (अ. हृ. सू. अ.-1)
5. सार्था गुर्वादयोः बुद्धिः प्रयत्नान्ता परादयः।
गुणाः प्रोक्ताः...।। (च. सं. सू.-1.49)

विश्वलक्षणा गुणाः। (नागार्जुन)

द्रव्यं गुणकर्माश्रयः गुणस्तु गुणकर्मानाश्रयः इति द्रव्यतो भेदः।

6. येन कुर्वन्ति तद्वीर्यम्। (च. सं. सू.-26.13)

वीर्यं तु क्रियते येन या क्रिया। (च. सं. सू.-26.65)

'कर्मलक्षणं वीर्यम्' (र. वै. सू. अ. 1.169)

गुर्वाद्याः वीर्यमुच्यन्ते शक्तिमन्तोऽन्यथा गुणाः।

परसामर्थ्यहीनत्वाद्गुण एवेतरे गुणाः।। (अ. सं. सू.-17/36-37)

7. अवस्थापाकापेक्षया विशिष्टः पाकः।

जाठरेणाग्निना योगाद्यदुदेति रसान्तरम्।

रसानां परिणामान्ते स विपाक इति स्मृतः।। (अ. हृ. सू.-9)

अमीमांस्यान्यचिन्त्यानि प्रसिद्धानि स्वभावतः। (सु. सू.-40.19)

8. रसादिसाम्ये यत्कर्म विशिष्टं तत्प्रभावजम्। (अ. हृ. सू.-26)

'क्रियतेऽनेनेति कर्म'

'यत्कुर्वन्ति तत् कर्म' । (च. सं. सू.-1)

प्रयत्नादि कर्म चेष्टितमुच्यते। (च. सं. सू.-1.49)

इहौषधकर्माणि ऊर्ध्वाधोभागोभयभागसंशोधनसंशमनसांग्राहिकाग्निदीपनपीडनलेखन-बृंहणरसायनवाजीकरणश्वयथुहरविलयनदहनदारणमादनप्राणघ्नविषप्रशमनानि।

(सु. सं. सू.-40.5)

9. संयोगे च विभागे च कारणं द्रव्यमाश्रितम्।

कर्त्तव्यस्य क्रिया कर्म कर्म नान्यदपेक्षते।। (च. सं. सू.-1.52)

2
DRAVYA

- Dravya Lakshana (Characteristics of Dravya)
- Panchabhoutikatwa
- Oushadhatwa
- Dravya Hetu/Yukti
  (Reasons for the superiority of Dravya)

Dravya Lakshana
(Characteristics of Dravya)

The category (Padartha) in which Karma and Guna reside and which is Samavayi karana is called Dravya[1]. Some interprete that the substance as the substratum in which both the Guna and Karma coexist with inherent relationship.

Prof. C. Dwarakanath while rendering English translation for Dravya paribhasha quotes—'Dravya is the substratum of Guna or quality, Karma or action and Samavayi karana or inherent cause'.

Panchabhoutikatwa

In the universe substances are composed of the five Bhutas i.e., Prithivi, Apa, Tejas, Vayu and Akasha. The elementary substances (Panchabhutas) with which every compound substance (Karya dravya) is constituted are known as Karana dravyas. The diversity of substances which arise out of the various modes of combination and permutation of these elementary substances are described as Karya dravyas. These compound substances exhibit different characteristics according to the preponderance of one or the other of the Bhutas over others in the collocation *(Vyapadeshastu bhuyashaha)*.

The various properties (qualities) ascribed to compound substances are stated to be held in a potential state in the elementary substances that compose them. These properties become actualised in the effect of Karya, which are described in terms of Rasa, Guna, Virya, Vipaka and Prabhava. It is a well known Ayurvedic concept that the properties which exist in the causative factors are present in the resultant factors and the modern science of physics which agrees with this concept also defines that the initial state of a system wholly determines its subsequent states.

Though every compound substance is constituted by all the five Bhutas, it is identified as—Parthiva, Apya, Taijasa, Vayavya and Nabhasa basing on the relative predominance of the particular Bhuta in its formation. To summarise, all the matter is constituted of five Mahabhutas and it is classified as animate (Chetana) and as inanimate (Achetana) substances.

Oushadhatwa

The basic factors for the formation of composition of substances (food/drug) as well as the human body are five Mahabhutas. By the use of or consumption of substances which are composed of the five Bhutas in varying properties and in different collocations, Vata, Pitta and Kapha of the body which are built up by the same kind of substances become vitiated, leading to the manifestation of different kinds of Vikaras (diseases). The phenomenon namely increase or decrease of Dosha, Dhatu and Malas either by diet or by drugs is explained with the concept of Samanya (generic concomitance) and Vishesha (variant factor). In the body, qualitities of Panchamahabhutas are augmented or increased by administering Dravyas possessing similar qualities and the same qualities result in diminution by the intake of Dravyas (Ahara/Oushadha) possessing opposite qualities[3]. Sushrutha explicitly states that the decrease, increase or equilibrium of the Doshas is due to Rasa, Guna and Vipaka of the Dravyas (Sus. 46). Charaka quotes that there is no substance in the world which is non-medicinal in nature.[4]

The diet is responsible for growth, strength, health, complexion and normal functioning of the senses. Irregularities of diet results in ill health. Thus the diet as well as drugs play a crucial role in preserving the health as well in curing the disease, i.e., Swasthyarakshana and Vyadhi-prashamana. For achieving the two goals—preservation of health (Swasthya-rakshana) and cure of the disease (Vikara-prashamana) the Dravya is administered in the form of Swarasa, Kalka, Kwatha, Phanta, Hima, Asava, Sneha etc. Charaka explains that there is nothing in the world which does not have therapeutic utility in appropriate conditions and situations. Chakrapani further clarifies that though every substance can be used as an therapeutic agent, it must be remembered that everything cannot be used for the treatment of every disease. A drug is useful in specific conditions and situations. So the selection of drugs is to be made in accordance with the propriety of its administration and therapeutic needs. Certain drugs which are unwholesome by nature like immature curd and poison can produce wholesome effect if used properly. Even straw and dust are useful for therapeutic purposes like fomentation etc.

Dravya Pradhnaya Hetu/Yukti

(Reasons for the Superiority of Dravya)[5]

1. **Vyavasthitattwa** (Stability):

Dravya is stable and the principles like Rasa, Guna, and Virya are unstable. Eg: Rasa present in unripe fruit may not present in ripe one.

2. **Nityatwa** (Constancy):

Dravya is a constant factor while its properties are inconstant. Eg: Variation in tastes in different preparations like Kalka, Kwatha.

3. **Swajatiya-avastha** (Unchangeability):

Dravya is unchangeable and maintain its own generic character. Eg: Parthiva dravya maintains its generic character and never changes into another Bhuta dravya.

4. **Panchendriya-grahana** (Sensory perceptibility):

Dravya is perceptible by all the five senses and not its properties like Rasa etc.

5. **Ashrayatwa** (Substratumness):

Dravya is the substratum for all the principles/properties.

6. **Arambha-samarthya** (Capacity of initiation):

Any usage is Dravya based but not Rasadi guna oriented. Eg: Pound Vidarigandhadi dravyas.

7. **Shastra-pramana** (Authenticity):

Authentic texts confirm that Dravya is the prime factor. Eg: In a recipe Dravya's name alone is mentioned like Matulunga, Agnimantha etc.

8. **Kramapekshitattwa** (Gradual dependency):

Rasadi gunas depend on Dravya in order of maturation. Eg: In unripe Dravya the properties are in immature state and in ripe drug the properties attain maturity.

9. Ekadesha-sadhyatwa (Part wise therapeutic action):

Curability of a disease by any one part of the drug. Eg: Latex of Snuhi.

●

References

1. यत्राश्रिताः कर्मगुणाः कारणं समवायि यत्।
   तद् द्रव्यं...।। (च. स. सू.-1.51)
   द्रव्यलक्षणन्तु क्रियागुणवत् समवायिकारणम्। (सु. सू.-40.3)
   द्रव्यमाश्रयलक्षणं पञ्चानाम्। (र. वै.-नागार्जुन)
   रसादीनां पञ्चानां भूतानां यदाश्रयभूतं तद् द्रव्यम्। (भा.)
2. सर्वं द्रव्यं पाञ्चभौतिकमस्मिन्नर्थे। (च. सू.-26.10)
   भूतेभ्यो हि परं यस्मान्नास्ति चिन्ता चिकित्सिते। (सु. शा.-1.17)
3. सर्वदा सर्वभावानां सामान्यं वृद्धिकारणम्।
   ह्रासहेतुर्विशेषश्च..।। (च. सू.-1.44)
4. अनेनोपदेशेन नानौषधिभूतं जगति किञ्चिद् द्रव्यमुपलभ्यते, तां तां युक्तिमर्थं च तं तमभिप्रेत्य। (च. सू.-26.12)
   धातुसाम्यक्रिया चोक्ता तन्त्रस्यास्य प्रयोजनम्। (च. सू.-1.53)
   अनेन निदर्शनेन नानौषधिभूतं जगति किञ्चिद् द्रव्यमस्ति। (सु. सू.-41.9)
5. पाको नास्ति विना वीर्य्याद्वीर्य्यं नास्ति विना रसात्।
   रसो नास्ति विना द्रव्याद् द्रव्यं श्रेष्ठतमं स्मृतम्।। (सु. सू.-40.18)
   वीर्य्यसंज्ञा गुणा येऽष्टौ तेऽपि द्रव्याश्रयाः स्मृताः।
   रसेषु न भवन्त्येते निर्गुणास्तु गुणाः स्मृताः।।
   द्रव्ये द्रव्याणि यस्माद्धि विपच्यन्ते न षड्रसाः।
   श्रेष्ठं द्रव्यमतो ज्ञेयं, शेषा भावास्तदाश्रयाः।। (सु. सू.-40.20-21)

●

3
DRAVYA VARGIKARANA

- Chetana and Achetana (Living & Nonliving)
- Karya-Karana (Effect-Cause)
- Utpatti (Evolution)
- Yoni (Source)
- Prayoga (Use)
- Rasa-skandha (Classification according to Rasa)
- Virya-bheda Vargikarana (Classification according to Virya)
- Dosha-karmanusara

Dwaividhyam (Quality of Dravya according to Dosha-karma)
  (a) Samoshodhana Dravya
  (b) Samshamana Dravya

- Oushadhi Vargikarana on the basis of Udbhava-KulaAkriti-Vayas
- Charaka-Sushruta and Vagbhatokta Dravya-vargikarana and Tulanatmaka jnana (Comparative knowledge of Dravya-vargikarana of Charaka-Sushruta and Vagbhata)
- Nighantu Vargikarana-paddhathi (Methods of classification of Dravya in Nighantus)

Dravya is classified into different groups according to their source, physical characters, pharmacological as well as pharmacotherapeutic actions.

Chetana-Achetana
(Living and Nonliving)

Dravya (matter) having sense organs is called 'Sendriya' (sentient) or 'Chetana', while the one devoid of them is called 'Achetana' or 'Nirindriya' (insentient)[1]. Although it is the soul and not the mind or body, which is sentient, still the sentient aspect of the soul manifests itself only when it is combined with mind and the body. This definition also applies to the vegetable kingdom, that is to say the vegetable kingdom is also sentient. Chakrapanidutta furnished certain examples to prove this:

1. Suryabhakta (Helianthus annus Linn.) moves according to the movement of the sun.

2. The Havali (Gicea acida)plant gets fruits just on hearing the sound of thunder.
3. Bijapuraka (Citrus medica) tree produces fruits only by the smell of fat of jackals.
4. Amra (Mangifera indica) trees when irrigated with the fat of fish, produces fruits in plenty.
5. Ashoka (Saraca indica) tree hit with the sole of the feet of a lady begets flowers.

Chakrapanidutta further quoted the references regarding the observations made by ancient Acharyas indicating that the members of vegetable kingdom have got life as well as consciousness full of happiness and miseries also.

In Manusmriti it is clearly indicated that plants possess 'Antahsanjna' (internal sense) and have the feelings of pleasure and displeasure.[2] The observations recorded in Vedas and Charaka Samhita (1000 BC) have been revalidated during 20th century by a well known biologist and physicist Dr. J.C. Bose. On May 10, 1901, the hall of the Royal society in London was packed with eminent scientists. They were watching Jagadish Chandra Bose conduct experiments to show that plants and metals have feelings. The plant with its roots, was carefully picked up and dipped up to its stem in a vessel containing bromide, a poison, Bose looked expectantly at the light spot on a screen meant to indicate the pulse of the plant. So, also did everyone else. The plant pulse beat, which the spot recorded as a steady to and fro movement like the pendulum of a clock, began to grow unsteady. Soon, the spot vibrated violently and then came to a sudden stop. It was almost like a poisoned rat breathing heavily and jerking its legs and tail in its struggle against death. The plant had died because of the poison. The experiment was greeted with thunderous applause. Bose arrived at the conclusion that plants and metals have life on the basis of the electric nature of living things. It was shown experimentally that, though plants do not have a brain, muscle, or heart, there are small cells in them, which behave in the same manner. The only difference between the response of a plant and of an animal is of time. A plant takes a longer time to respond. All these experiments carried out by modern scientists confirm that the conclusion drawn by seers of Ayurveda are the scientific truths and leave behind some questions regarding the instruments utilized by them to deduce such facts.

Karya–Karnana
(Effect–Cause)

Dravyas are divided into Karya and Karana (effect-cause) dravyas.

Dravyas (matter) in this universe have taken their origin from Panchamahabhuta (Prithvi, Apa, Vayu, Tejas, Akasha), Atma, Manas, Dik (direction) and Kala. These nine Dravyas are called the Karana dravya.

Drugs and other matter derived from these nine Karana dravya are called Karya dravyas as they perform Karya (effect).

Eg: Amalaki, Harithaki, Ghata etc.

Utpatti Bhedana
(Evolution)

Dravyas according to their Panchabhauthika constitution are classified into 5 types namely Parthiva, Apya, Taijasa, Vayavya, Akashiya. The basis for this classification is the predominance of particular Bhuta though every Dravya is made up of Panchabhutas.

Parthiva Dravya:

It consists of Gunas namely Guru (heavy), Sandra (dense), Manda (dull), Sthira (non-mobile), Sthoola (bulky) and tastes Madhura and Kashaya.

Apya Dravya:

It consists of Gunas namely Drava (liquid), Snigdha (oily), Sheeta (cool), Mridu (soft), Manda (dull), Pichchila (slimy), Guru (heavy) and tastes Madhura, Ishat kashaya, Amla and Lavana.

Taijasa Dravya:

It consists of Gunas namely Ushna (heat), Teekshna (sharp), Sukshma (penetrating), Laghu (light), Ruksha (harsh), Vishada (clear), Khara (rough) and tastes Katu, Ishadamla and Lavana.

Vayavya Dravya:

It consists of Gunas namely Laghu (light), Sheeta (cold), Ruksha (harsh), Khara (rough), Vishada (clear) and Sukshma (penetrating) and tastes Kashaya and Ishat tikta.

Akashiya Dravya:

It consists of Gunas namely Mridu (soft), Laghu (light), Shlakshna (smooth), Sukshma (penetrating), Vyavaya (instant spreading) Vishada (clear) and contains Avyakta rasa.

Yoni Bhedana

(Based on the Source)[3]

Dravyas are of 3 kinds viz. animal origin, vegetable origin and metals including minerals. Substances like honey, products of cow's milk, bile, fats, bone marrow, blood, flesh, faeces, urine, skin, semen, bone, ligament, horn, nail, hoof, hair, oxbile are some of the drugs of animal origin.

Jantava dravyas are further classified as follows:

A. Jarayuja: Animals giving birth to offspring (mammals). Eg: Human being, animals.

B. Andaja: Propagation of race takes place through eggs. Eg: Birds, snakes.

C. Swedaja: Propagation through sweat. Eg: Insects & micro organisms.

D. Udbhija: Which are entering into life by coming out of the earth. Eg: Frog.

Oudbhida dravyas are vegetable in origin. These are again divided into:

A. Vanaspati is the one having fruits only (without flowers). Eg: Vata, Udumbara etc.

B. Vaanaspati has flowers as well as fruits. Eg: Amra, Jambu etc.

C. Virudha – which are in the form of climbers and shrubs. Eg: Guduchi, Karavira.

D. Oshadhi are those which die out when their fruits mature. Eg: Shali, Godhuma.

Dravyas which are the transforming metals in earth crust are Parthiva. Eg: Saindhava lavana, Swarna etc.

Prayoga Bhedana

(Based on the Usage)

Based on the usage, the Dravyas are of 2 types:

1. Oushadha dravya
2. Ahara dravya

Oushada Dravya

It is of Virya pradhana and when taken in, it produces the effects of Virya viz., Sheeta and Ushna. Eg: Shunthi, Pippali.

Ahara Dravya

It is of Rasa pradhana and nourishes Rasadi dhatus and produces Sheeta and Ushnadi gunas.[4] Eg: Godhuma, Shalidhanya etc.

Rasa Skandha

(Classification According to Rasa)

According to Rasa, Dravyas are classified into six types i.e., Madhura-skandha, Amla-skandha, Lavana-skandha, Katu-skandha, Tiktha-skandha and Kashaya-skandha.

Virya Bheda vargikarana

(Classification According to Virya)

Chakrapani Dutt has classified dravya according to virya as follows Tikshnavirya Dravaya e.g. Sunthi. Madhyavirya Dravya e.g. Bihva. Mriduvirya Dravya e.g. Amalaki. Acharya Priyavat Sharma quotes Chandanadi taila and Agurvadi taila (Jwara-chikitsa—Charaka) as the examples for Virya bheda classification. A critical anaiysis of the Virya of drugs included in these formulations clearly indicate that both the tailas contain Ushna as well as Shita-virya drugs and basing on this it can be concluded that this reference can not be considered as the authentic reference in favour of drug classification according Virya.

Dosha Karmanusara

(According to Dosha-karma)

Dravya is of 3 types, namely, Shamana (Pacifying Doshas) Kopana (Deranging or Aggravating dhatus/doshas) and Swasthahitha (Maintaining homoeostasis).

Dravya which subdues the aggravated Doshas is known as Shamana dravya. Eg: Devadaru, Kushtha, Eranda, Dashamoola, Vidarigandhadi dravyas subside the aggravated Vata. Chandana, Ushira, Manjishtha, Shatavari, Sariba, Nygrodha, Utpala and Trinapanchamoola etc. act as Pitta-shamaka and Agaru, Karpura, Pippali, Vacha, Surasa, Brihati, Aragwadha, Valli & Kantaka panchamoola act as Kapha-shamaka dravya.

Dravya which aggravates Dosha is known as 'Kopana dravya'. Shuska Shaka (dried substances), Shuska Mamsa (dried meat), Nishpava, Jambu etc. aggravate Vata. Tilataila, Pinyaka, Sarshapa, Kuluttha, Matsya mamsa, Dadhi, Maricha etc. aggravate Pitta. Godhuma, Anupa mamsa, Navanna, Milk, Kilata aggravate Kapha.

The drugs which are helpful to maintain swasthyam (healthy state) are known as swasthahita dravya[6] eg., Rasayana & Vajeekarana dravya.

Rakta shali, Antariksha jala, Mudga, Saindhava lavana, Jivantishaka, Ghee of cow, Rohitha fish, Milk of cow, Tilataila, Draksha etc.

Dwaividhyam

(Quality of Dravya According to Dosha-Karma)

Samshodhana Dravya

Dravya which expunges the Doshas through Urdhwabhaga (mouth) or through Adhobhaga (anus) is called as Samshodhana dravya. Eg: Devadatilphala.[7]

Dravya which keeps Dosha in Samyavastha and which brings the Vishama dosha into Sama-doshavastha, is called Samana dravya'. Eg: Guduchi.

Udbhava Bhedana

(According to Udbhava)

Dravya is classified in to 4 types:

1. Sthalaja — which are propagated on land. Eg: Amalaki, Vibhitaka.
2. Jalaja (Acquatic) — which are propagated in water. Eg: Jalakumbhi, Kamala.
3. Vriksharuha (Epiphytic) — which grow on another tree and prepare their nourishment. Eg: Vanda.
4. Vrikshadana (Parasitic) — which grows on other trees and also depend on them for their nourishment. Eg: Akashavalli.

Kula Bhedana

This classification is based on different parts of the plant and mainly on reproductive organs. They are again divided into different divisions based on genus, species etc.

Akruti Bhedana

Dravyas (plants) are divided into 4 types based on their Akruti E.g. Vriksha (trees), Gulma (shurbs), Kshupa (herb), Lata (weak plants, climbers).

Ayu (Vayas) Bhedana

It is classified into 3 types, Ekavarshayu (annual), Dwivarshayu (biennials) and Bahuvarshayu (perennials):

Ekavarshayu — which lives for one year. Eg: Wheat.

Dwivarshayu — which lives for two years. Eg: Carrot.

Bahuvarshayu — which lives for more number of years. Eg: Ashwatha, Amra.

Charaka, Sushruta, Vagbhatokta Ganas

- In Charaka Samhita, Sutrasthana 1st chapter, classification of Dravya such as Jangama, Oudbhidha and Parthiva dravyas was described. And in same chapter (Sutrasthana) according to Doshaprabhava another classification of Dravya such as Dosha-prashamana, Dhatu-pradushana and Swasthahita was mentioned. It is generally observed that one Dravya may have various actions and similarly several Dravyas may possess similar actions. Basing on the similarity of actions Acharyas of Ayurveda attempted to classify drugs into groups. Charaka also illustrated another classification based on the part used such as Moolini, Phalini etc. In the 4th chapter of Sutrasthana Charaka has classified Dravyas into 50 Kashaya vargas according to their action (Karma). He again classified Ahara dravya into Shukadhanya, Shamidhanya, Gorasa varga etc. (in total 12 Vargas) in the 27th chapter of Sutrasthana. Agraioushadhis were described in the 25th chapter of sutrasthana.

- Sushruta classified Ahara dravya into Dravadravya and Annadravya. Dravadravya was again classified into 10 Vargas and Annadravya into 13 Vargas in the Sutrasthana 45-46 chapters. In Annadravya varga Sushruta described certain subvargas like Dhatu, Ratna, Lavana, Kshara, Pushpa, Kanda vargas independently. In Dravadravya he described new Vargas such as Sushruta Taila, Madhu, Mutravargas. Vidarigandhadi, Aragwadhadi etc in total 37 Vargas and 4 Vargas related to Samshodhana and 3 Samshamana vargas are described sushruta according to Dravya-karma in Sutrasthana 38, 39 chapters. Mishrika ganas like Triphala, Trikatu, Dashamoola etc. were also mentioned by him.

- Vagbhata in Ashtanga Sangraha described Dravadravya and Annadravya in 12 Vargas. Out of 50 Mahakashaya vargas which were described by Charaka only 45 Vargas were included in the 15th chapter of Sutrasthana and the 5 Vargas in the 6th chapter of Sutrasthana including Doshashamana vargas. He included in 14th chapter 25 Vargas described by Sushruta. Dhumopaga vargas, Trijataka, Chaturjataka, Panchavalkala, Madhyama Panchamoola were described independently by him.

Vagbhata, in Ashtanga Hridaya described 33 Ganas in the Shodhanadigana Sangrahadhyaya. Dravadravyas were described in 5 Vargas and Annadravyas in 7 Vargas. He mentioned Lavana, Kshara and Hingu in Annavarga.

Nighantu Vargikarana

Oushadha vargas were described under different classifications in Nighantus based on synonyms (Paryayanama), Bheda and Gunakarma etc. Dravyas were classified. As the number of medicinal plants have increased during Madhyama kala when compared to Samhita kala, for the purpose of detailed study Dravyas were divided into different Vargas. Dravyas having similar action were kept under one Varga and it was named after the important Dravya in that Varga. For example in Dhanwantari Nighantu, Guduchyadi varga, Shatapushpadi varga, Chandanadi varga, Karaviradi varga, Amradi varga, Suvarnadi varga and Misrikadi varga (7 Vargas) were described. Among those Vargas, Urdhwa, Adho-samshodhana dravyas are kept under Shatapushpadi varga, drugs which relieve different diseases are kept under Karaviradi varga etc. In Suvarnadi varga Taila, Kshira etc., Dravadravyas and Shakadhanya, Shamidhanya etc. Anna dravyas are also described. It clearly indicates that author of Dhanwantari Nighantu has not applied any specific criterion while grouping the drugs. In Kaiyadeva Nighantu, for fecilitating the study of synonyms of Dravyas, Nanartha varga was introduced in which different Dravyas having common synonyms were described.

In Bhavaprakasha Nighantu, Dravyas in which Phala and Kanda were in usage are kept under Haritakyadi varga, and aromatic (Sugandha dravya) drugs are described in Karpuradi varga, and the drugs having Valkala/Twak (bask) as useful part are kept under Vatadi vargas.

In addition to dravyas described by Ayurvedic classics the authors of Vrindamadhava, Chakradutta, Madanapala and Bhavaprakasha Nighantus, havet also included new Dravyas Eg: Parasika yavani, Dwipantara vacha etc. But a critical analysis indicates that Nighantus never adopted a specific criterian for classifying the drugs.

●

References

1. तत् (द्रव्यं) चेतनावदचेतनं च। (च. सू.-1)
   सेन्द्रियचेतनं द्रव्यं निरीन्द्रियमचेतनम्। (च. सू.-1)
   तमसा बहुरूपेण वेष्टिताः कर्महेतुना।
2. अन्तःसंज्ञा भवन्त्येते सुखदुःखसमन्विताः।। (मनुस्मृति)
3. तत्पुनस्त्रिविधं ज्ञेयं जाङ्गमौद्भिदपार्थिवम्। (च. सू.-1.69)
   उद्भिद्य पृथिवीं जायते इति औद्भिदं वृक्षादिः। (चक्रपाणिदत्त)
   मूलत्वक्सारनिर्यासनालस्वरसपल्लवाः।
   क्षारः क्षीरः फलं पुष्पं भस्मतैलानि कण्टकाः।।
   पत्राणि शुङ्गाः कन्दाँश्च प्ररोहाँश्चौद्भिदो गणः। (च. सू.-1.74-75)
   ....औद्भिदं तु चतुर्विधम्।
   वनस्पतिर्वीरुधश्च वानस्पत्यस्तथौषधिः।। (च. सू. अ.-1.72)
   अपुष्पाः फलवन्तो वनस्पतयः। (सु. सू.-1.29)
   पुष्पफलवन्तो वृक्षाः। (सु. सू.-1.29)
   प्रतानवत्यः स्तम्बिन्यश्च वीरुधः। (सु. सू.-1.29)
   'लतति वेष्टतेति लता प्रसरणाद्भूमिमारोहणाच्च वृक्षादीनाच्छादयति' (द्रव्यगुणसूत्रम्)
   ओषधयः फलपाकान्ताः। (च. सू.-1.72)
   फलपाकनिष्ठा ओषधयः। (सु. सू.-1.29)
   भूमेर्विकारः भौमं सुवर्णादिकम्। (योगेन्द्रनाथ)
4. (औषधाहारभेदेन) द्रव्यं तावद् द्विविधं वीर्यप्रधानमौषधद्रव्यं रसप्रधानमाहारद्रव्यञ्च। (च. सू.-2 चक्र.)
5. तत्राप्यौषधद्रव्यं त्रिविधं वीर्यभेदात् तीक्ष्णवीर्यं; यथा शुण्ठ्यादि, मध्यवीर्यं बिल्वाग्निमन्थादि, मृदुवीर्यञ्चामलकादि। (चक्रपाणिदत्त)
6. किञ्चिद्दोषप्रशमनं किञ्चिद्धातुप्रदूषणम्।
   स्वस्थवृत्तौ मतं किञ्चित् त्रिविधं द्रव्यमुच्यते।। (च. सू.-1.68)
   शमनं कोपनं स्वस्थहितं द्रव्यमिति त्रिधा।(अ. सं. सू.-1.37, अ. हृ. सू.-1.16)
7. शोधनं शमनञ्चेति समासादौषणं द्विधा। (अ. सं. ा.-1.48)
   स्थानाद्बहिर्नयेदूर्ध्वमधश्च मलसञ्चयम्।
   देहसंशोधनं तत्स्याद्देवदालीफलं यथा।। (शा. प्र. अ.-4)

●

4
GUNA VIJNANA

- Guna-nirukti (Etymology of Guna)
- Lakshana (Characteristics)
- Bhedha (Varieties)
- Guna-pradhanya Yukti (Reasons for the superiority of Guna)

Ayurvedic classics described twenty qualities/properties viz., Guru, Manda, Hima, Snigdha, Shlakshna, Sandra, Mridu, Sthria, Sukshma and Vishada and their opposite viz. Laghu, Tikshna, Ushna, Ruksha, Khara, Drava, Kathina, Sara, Sthula and Pichchhila. According to Charaka Mridu, Tikshna, Guru, Laghu, Snigdha, Ruksha, Ushna and Shita are relatively more important in view of their being essence of twenty. Prof. C. Dwarakanath interprets regarding the difference between Guna and Karma as follows:

"Eight Gunas become actualised and manifest themselves when the atoms of elementary substances are in action i.e., when they perform Karma, when the elementary substances are active in motion."[1] In another context Dwarakanath quotes Gunas or physical qualities/properties of substances are modes (or different manifestations) of Virya or energy. Gunadi Gunas as such can not initiate any action (Nischesta) unless they attain Virya form (State of potentiation).

Nirukti
(Etymology of Gunas)

The quality through which the whole universe is attracted towards the Dravya is 'Guna'.

Lakshana
(Characterstic)

Guna is that which is located in Dravya inherently is the causative factor for production of similar Gunas in the body and devoid of any action.[1]

Bheda
(Varieties)

I. Samanya (or) Shariraka gunas

These are 2 types:

1. Gurvadi (Physico pharmacological) gunas[2]

1. Guru x Laghu	6. Sandra x Drava
2. Manda x Tikshna	7. Mridu x Khatina
3. Shita x Ushna	8. Sthira x Sara
4. Snigdha x Ruksha	9. Sukshma x Sthoola
5. Slakshna x Khara	10. Vishada x Pichchila

2. Paradi (Para pharmacological) gunas[3]

1. Para	6. Vibhaga
2. Apara	7. Pruthaktwa
3. Yukti	8. Parimana
4. Sankhya	9. Samskara
5. Samyoga	10. Abhyasa

II. Vaiseshika (Specific) **guna**

1. Shabda	4. Rasa
2. Sparsha	5. Gandha
3. Rupa	

III. Adhyatmika (Psychological) **guna**[4]

1. Iccha (desire)	4. Duhkha (misery)
2. Dwesha (aversion)	5. Prayatna (effort)
3. Sukha (pleasure)	6. Buddhi (intellect)

Yogindranath Sen incorporated Manoguna in Adhyatmika gunas and mentioned number of Gunas as 42.

Gurvadi Gunas & Their Action

1. **Guru** (Heavy)

Which produces bulkiness (Brimhana) to the body is Guru guna. It is having dominance of Prithivi and Jala bhuta and acts as Vatahara, Kaphakara, Tarpana, Brimhana, Chirapaki.[5]

Eg: Masha, Ikshu.

2. **Laghu** (Light)

Which imparts lightness (Laghava) to body is Laghu guna.[6] It is having dominance of Vayu, Akasha, Agni bhuta and acts as Kaphahara, Vatakara, Langhana, Vranaropana, Sheeghrapaki.

Eg: Mudga.

3. **Manda** (Dull or slowly acting)

Which passifies (Shamana) is Manda guna.[7] It is having Prithivi and Jala bhutad dominance and acts as Kapha-vardhaka, Pitta-shamaka, Chirakari.

Eg: Amalaki, Ativisha.

4. **Tikshana** (Sharp/Active)

Which cleans (Shodhana) is Tikshana guna.[8] It is of Agnibhuta dominance and acts as Kapha-vatahara, Daha, Sravana, Lekhana.

Eg: Danti, Maricha.

5. **Hima/Shita** (Cooling)

Which condenses (Sthambhana) is Shita guna.[7-9] Hemadri quoted it as Hima. It is of Jala mahabhuta dominance. It acts as Pittahara, Sleshmakara, Stambhana, Murcha-Daha-Trishna-Sweda nashaka. It is considered as Karmanumeya and Sparshanendriya-grahya guna.

Eg: Chandana, Ushira.

6. **Ushna** (Heating)

Which induces perspiration (Swedana) is Ushna guna.[10] It is of Agnibhuta dominance and acts as Vata-sleshmahara, Pittakara, Pachana, Murchcha, Daha, Trishna, Sweda-karaka. It is also considered as Karnanumeya and Sparshanendriya-grahya guna.

Eg: Maricha, Chitraka.

7. **Snigdha** (Oily/Soothing)

Which produces moisture (Kledana) is Snighda guna.[11] It is a guna of Jala mahabhuta dominance. It acts as Vatahara, Sleshma-vardhaka, Balya, Vrishya (aphrodisiac), Varnya and produces Mridutwa in the body.

Eg: Taila, Ghrita, Shigru etc.

8. **Ruksha** (Harsh/Drying)

Which dries (Shoshana) is Ruksha guna.[12] It is of Prithivi, Vayu, Agni mahabhuta dominance. It acts as Vata-vardhaka, Kapha-shamaka, Stambhana, Avrishya and produces Rukshatwa/Kathinya to the body and also destroys Bala and Varna of the body.

Eg: Yava, Musta.

9. **Slakshna** (Smooth)

Which stimulates growth (Ropana) is Slakshna.[13] It is of Agni-bhuta dominance and acts as Kaphakara, Jeevaniya, Balya and Sandhanakara.

Eg: Abhraka, Haridra.

10. **Khara, Parusha** (Rough/Harsh/Coarse)

Which slenders, attenuates (Lekhana) is Khara.[14] Sushruta mentioned it as Karkasha guna. It is of Vayu bhuta dominance.

Eg: Vacha, Shilajatu.

11. **Sandra** (Thick/dense)

Which nourishes (Prasadana) is Sandra guna.[15] It is of Prithivi-bhuta dominance and acts as Rakta and Chakshu prasadana. It causes Sthulatva and Stroto-avarodha.

Eg: Kakoli, Kshriakakoli.

12. **Drava** (Liquid)

Which dissolves or mixes (Vilodana) is Drava guna.[16] It is of Jala bhuta dominance. It causes Ardratva in the body.

Eg: Jala (water).

13. **Mridu** (Soft)

Which relaxes (Slathana) is Mridu guna.[17] It is of Akasha and Jala bhuta dominance. It relieves Daha, Paka and Srava.

Eg: Yashtimadhu.

14. **Kathina** (Hard/Acting strongly)

Which fastens, hardens, solidifies (Dridhikarana) is Kathinya[18]. It is dominant of Prithivi bhuta.

Eg: Ashwagandha, Shatavari.

15. **Sthira** (Non-mobile)

Which supports (Dharana) is Sthira.[19] It is dominant of Prithivi bhuta. It is Kapha-vardhaka, and acts as Mutra and Purisha-sthambhaka.

Eg: Asthi, Sukti, Bala, Atibala etc.

16. **Sara/Chala** (Mobile)

Which produces motion or action or stimulation (Prerana) is

Sara or Chala.[20] Vagbhata quoted Chala guna opposite to Sthira guna instead of Sara guna. Hemadri mentioned the term Chala for Sara guna. It is of Jala bhuta dominance. It acts as Vata and Mala pravartaka and Anulomana.

Eg: Haritaki, Trivrit.

17. **Sukshma** (Penetrating/Thinning)

Which penetrates (Vivarana) is Sukshma guna.[21] It is of Agni, Vayu and Akasha bhuta dominance. It is having capacity to penetrate into thinner and smaller channels of the body and causes their dilatation.

Eg: Eranda taila, Lavana.

18. **Sthoola** (Bulky/Fattening)

Which covers (or) protects (Samvarana) is Sthula guna.[22] It is of Prithivi bhuta dominance. It causes Sthulatwa (obese) and Srotorodha (obstruction of channels).

Eg: Dadhi, Pinyaka.

19. **Vishada** (Transparent/Clear)

Which clears (Kshalana) is Vishada guna.[23] It is of Prithivi, Vayu, Agni and Akasha bhuta dominance and acts as Kaphakara, Jeevaniya, Balya and Sandhanakara.

Eg: Jivanti.

20. **Pichchhila** (Slimy/Gelatinous)

Which forms coating (Lepana) is Pichchila guna.[24] It is mentioned as an important property of Mamsa dhatu in Samhitas. It is of Jala bhuta dominance and acts as Kaphakara, Jeevaniya, Balya and Sandhanakara.

Eg: Asthisamharaka.

Sushruta has mentioned some gunas normaly Vyavaya, Vikasi (discussed under karma chapter) Sugandha, Durgandha, Asukari and Sushka (Bhavamishra).[25]

Paradigunas and Their Action

1. **Paratwa** (superiority)

Importance attached to a particular substance among the group is called Paratwa.

Eg: Vidanga is superior among Krimighna drugs.

2. **Aparatwa** (Inferiority)

Inferiority attributed to substance which are not fit for selection is known as Aparatwa.

Superiority and inferiority in relation to place, time, age, measurement, Vipaka, Virya, Rasa may be illustrated as follows:

1. Jangala desha is superior to Anupa desha.
2. The measurement of the body deliberated in Sharira sthana of classics are superior to other measurements.
3. Vipaka, Virya and Rasa which are Hita (wholesome) are superior to Ahita (unwholesome).

3. **Yukti** (Propriety)

Yukti refers to the logic selection of the drug in the treatment. Chakrapani comments that Yukti implies selection of proper therapy with due regard to the nature of Doshas vitiated. The inappropriate selection of therapy is considered to be useless.[26]

4. **Sankhya** (Number)

It is useful for enumeration of Doshas, Dravyas etc.[27]

5. **Samyoga** (Combination)

Mixing or combination of two things is called as Samyoga.[28]

Eg: Fighting between two sheeps, Dhatri and Nisha for Prameha.

6. **Vibhaga** (Division)

Dissociation or distinction made between two things is called Vibhaga.[29]

Eg: Bhallataka in Sushkharshas and Kutaja in Raktarshas.

Grahya and Agrahya lakshanas of Haritaki.

7. **Prithaktwa** (Separation)

Concept of division or differentiation to identify the substance from one another is called as Prithaktwa.

Eg: Meru and Himalayas are separate entities. Sahaja and kritrima kasturi.

Palankasha means Gokshura in Mutraroga chikitsa and Guggulu in Medoroga chikitsa.

8. **Parimana** (Measurement)

That quality which is useful for measuring the substances or objects is known as Parimana.[30]

Eg: Anjali, Anguli etc. Triphala (one haitaki, 2 vibhitaka and 4 Amdaki).

9. Samskara (Transformation)

Factor which is responsible for bring out a change is known as Samskara.[31]

Eg. Shalidhanya is made into Laja.

10. Abhyasa (Repetition)

Continuous use of the same substance is called Abhyasa.[32]

Eg: Regular intake of rice etc.

Gunopalabdhi (Assessment of Gunas)

Guna of the substance (diet/drug) can be identified by inference after the observation of actions on the body. The most potent Gunas (Virya) can also be assessed by Nipata as well as Adhivasa.

Guna Pradhana Yukti

(Reasons for the Superiority of Guna)

1. Rasavhibhava:

Gunas supercede Rasas in their action.

Eg: Though Patola is of Tiktha rasa, due to Ushna guna it is acting as Vatahara.

2. Vipaka-karanatwa:

Vipaka is controlled by Gunas. Shita, Snigdha, Gugu, Pichchila gunas are contributing for the genesis of Guru vipaka (Karana) and Laghu, Ruksha, Vishada, Teekshana gunas are (Karana) contributing for the genesis of Laghu vipaka. The ability to produce action of Rasa is bestowed with Vipaka. Vipaka is controlled by Guna.

3. Bahulyata:

Gunas are more in number.

4. Bahudhopayogita:

Usage is in many forms like that of Abhyanga, Parisheka, Avagaha etc. But Rasa is used through mouth only.

5. Aneka karmatwata:

Gunas present in Rasas perform many actions.

6. Mahavishyatwata:

Guna is of many varieties.

7. Upadesha:

Guna is declared to be superior to the rest of Gunas by authentic texts.

Eg: Guru, Snighdha, Ushna gunas acts as Vataghna.

8. Apadesha:

It is used during comparison (Upamana).

Eg: The individual is of Tikshna swabhava.

9. Anumana:

Through inference Guna can be known.[33]

Eg: If the Dravya is of Shita guna it acts as Pittahara.

●

References

1. समवायी तु निश्चेष्टः कारणं गुणः। (च. सू.-1.15)
अथ द्रव्याश्रिता ज्ञेया निर्गुणा निष्क्रिया गुणाः।। (कारिकावली गुणग्रन्थ)
2. सार्था गुर्वादयो बुद्धिः प्रयत्नान्ता परादयः।
गुणाः प्रोक्ता..........।। (च. सू.-1.49)
गुर्वादयस्तु गुरुलघुशीतोष्णस्निग्धरूक्षमन्दतीक्ष्णस्थिरसरमृदुकठिनविशदपिच्छिलश्लक्ष्ण-खरस्थूलसूक्ष्मसान्द्रद्रवाः विंशतिः। (चक्रपाणि)
गुरुमन्दहिमस्निग्धश्लक्ष्णसान्द्रमृदुस्थिराः ।
गुणाः ससूक्ष्मविशदा विंशतिः सविपर्ययाः।। (अ. हृ. सू.-1.18)
3. अर्था शब्दादयो ज्ञेया गोचरा विषया गुणाः। (च. शा.-1.31)
परापरत्वे युक्तिश्च सङ्ख्या संयोग एव च।
विभागश्च पृथक्त्वञ्च परिमाणमथापि च।।
संस्कारोऽभ्यास इत्येते गुणा ज्ञेयाः परादयः।
4. इच्छा द्वेषः सुखं दुःखं प्रयत्नश्चेतना धृतिः।
बुद्धिः स्मृतिरहङ्कारो लिङ्गानि परमात्मनः।। (च. शा.-1.72)
5. यस्य द्रव्यस्य बृंहणे कर्मणि शक्तिः स गुरुः। (हेमाद्रि)
सृष्टविण्मूत्रो विशदो गुरुः। गौरवं पार्थिवमाप्यञ्च। (र. वै.-3.116)
6. लङ्घने लघुः। (हेमाद्रि)
लघुस्तद्विपरीतः स्याल्लेखनो रोपणस्तथा। (सु. सू.-46.526)
7. यस्य शमने शक्तिः स मन्दः। (हेमाद्रि)

8. यस्य शोधने शक्तिः स तीक्ष्णः। (हेमाद्रि)
दाहपाककरस्तीक्ष्णः स्रावणो। (सु. सू.-46.518)
तीक्ष्णं पित्तकरं प्रायो लेखनं कफवातहृत्। (भा. प्र., पू. खं.)
9. स्तम्भने हिमः। (हेमाद्रि)
स्तम्भनं स्वेदापनयनम्। (अ. हृ. सू.-9.19)
जलं स्तम्भनीयानाम्। (च. सू.-25.40)
10. स्वेदने उष्णः। (हेमाद्रि)
उष्णस्तद्विपरीतः स्यात् पाचनश्च विशेषतः। (सु. सू.-46.515)
11. यस्य क्लेदने शक्तिः स स्निग्धः। (हेमाद्रि)
स्नेह-मार्दवकृत् स्निग्धो बलवर्णकरस्तथा। (सु. सू.-46.523)
स्निग्धं वातहरं श्लेष्मकारि वृष्यं बलावहम्। (भा. प्र., पू. ख.)
12. यस्य शोषणे शक्तिः स रूक्षः। (हेमाद्रि)
रूक्षस्तद्विपरीतः स्याद्विशेषात् स्तम्भनः खरः। (सु. सू.-46.523)
13. यस्य रोपणे शक्तिः स श्लक्ष्णः। (हेमाद्रि)
श्लक्ष्णः स्नेहं विनाऽपि स्यात् कठिनोऽपि हि चिक्कणः। (भा. प्र., पू. खं.)
14. यस्य लेखने शक्तिः स खरः। (हेमाद्रि)
15. यस्य प्रसादने शक्तिः स सान्द्रः। (हेमाद्रि)
सान्द्रः स्थूलः स्याद् बन्धकारकः। (सु. सू.-46.527)
16. यस्य विलोडने शक्तिः स द्रवः। (हेमाद्रि)
द्रवत्वं स्यन्दनकर्मकारणम्। (भा. प्र., पू. खं.)
द्रवः प्रक्लेदकरो व्यापी। (भा. प्र., पू. खं.)
द्रवः प्रक्लेदनः। (सु. सू.-46.527)
17. यस्य श्लथने शक्तिः स मृदुः। (हेमाद्रि)
18. यस्य दृढ़ीकरणे शक्तिः स कठिनः। (हेमाद्रि)
19. यस्य धारणे शक्तिः स स्थिरः। (हेमाद्रि)
स्थिरो वातमलस्तम्भी सरस्तेषां। (भा. प्र., पू. खं.)
20. यस्य प्रेरणे शक्तिः स सरः। (द्र. वि.), प्रेरणे चलः (हेमाद्रि)
सरस्तेषां प्रवर्त्तकः। (भा. प्र. पू. ख.)
सरोऽनुलोमनो प्रोक्तः। (सु. सू.-46.529)
अनुलोमनो वातमलप्रवर्त्तनः। (डल्हण)
21. यस्य विवरणे शक्तिः स सूक्ष्मः। (हेमाद्रि)
सूक्ष्मस्तु सौक्ष्म्यात् सूक्ष्मेषु स्रोतःस्वनुसरः स्मृतः। (सु. सू.-46.531)
देहस्य सूक्ष्मच्छिद्रेषु विशेद्यत् सूक्ष्ममुच्यते। (भा. प्र., पू. खं.)
22. यस्य संवरणे शक्तिः स स्थूलः। (हेमाद्रि)
स्थूलः स्थौल्यकरो देहे स्रोतसामवरोधकृत्। (भा. प्र., पू. खं.)

23. यस्य क्षालने शक्तिः स विशदः। (हेमाद्रि)
विशदो विपरीतोऽस्मात् क्लेदाचूषणरोपणः। (सू. सू.-46.524)
क्लेदच्छेदकरः ख्यातो विशदो व्रणरोपणः। (भा. प्र., पू. खं.)
24. यस्य लेपने कर्मणि शक्तिः स पिच्छिलः। (हेमाद्रि)
पिच्छिलो जीवनो बल्यः सन्धानः श्लेष्मलो गुरुः। (सु. सू.-46.524)
25. 'व्यवायी चाखिलं देहं व्याप्य पाकाय कल्पते।' (सु. सू.-46.529)
पूर्वं व्याप्याखिलं कायं ततः पाकं च गच्छति।
व्यवायी तद्यथा भङ्गा फेनञ्चाहि समुद्भवम्।। (शार्ङ्गधर)
'विकासी विकसन्नेवं धातुबन्धान् विमोक्षयेत्।' (सु. सू.-46.530)
सन्धिबन्धाँश्च शिथिलान् करोति हि विकासि तत्।
विश्लिष्यौजश्च धातुभ्यो यथा क्रमुककोद्रकः।। (शार्ङ्गधर)
आशुकारी तथाऽऽशुत्वाद्धावत्यम्भसि तैलवत्। (सु. सू.-46.530)
आशुराशुकरो देहे धावत्यम्भसि तैलवत्। (भा. प्र., पू. खं.)
द्रवः क्लेदकरो व्यापी शुष्कस्तद्विपरीतकः। (भा. प्र., पू. खं.)
26. युक्तिश्च योजना या तु युज्यते। (च.सू.-26.31, च. वि.-1; चक्रपाणिदत्त)
या युज्यते तादृशी दोष-देश-काल-मात्राद्यपेक्षिणी योजना युक्तिः। (च. वि.-1)
दोषाद्यपेक्षया भेषजस्य समीचीनकल्पना। (च. वि.-1; चक्रपाणिदत्त)
बुद्धिः पश्यति या भावान् बहुकारणयोगजान्।
युक्तिस्त्रिकाला सा ज्ञेया त्रिवर्गः साध्यते यया।।
न नामज्ञानमात्रेण रूपज्ञानेन वा पुनः।
ओषधीनां परां प्राप्तिं कश्चिद्वेदितुमर्हति।
योगविन्नामरूपज्ञस्तासां तत्त्वविदुच्यते।। (च. सू.-1.122-123)
मात्राकालाश्रया युक्तिः सिद्धिर्युक्तौ प्रतिष्ठिता।
तिष्ठत्युपरि युक्तिज्ञो द्रव्यज्ञानवतां सदा।। (च. सू.-2.16)
27. ....संख्या स्याद्गणितम्। (च. सू.-26.32)
गणितं व्यवहारहेतुरेक-द्वि-त्र्यादिसङ्ख्यया।
सङ्ख्या विकल्पप्राधान्यबलकालविशेषतः।
सा भिद्यते यथाऽत्रैव वक्षन्तेऽष्टौ ज्वरा इति।। (च. नि.-1.12)
28. योग सह संयोग उच्यते। द्रव्याणाम्। (च. सू.-26.32)
संयोगः पुनर्द्वयोर्बहूनां वा द्रव्याणां संहतीभावः। (च. वि.-1.21.3)
29. विभागस्तु विभक्तिः स्याद्वियोगो भागशो ग्रहः। (च. सू.-26.33)
30. परिमाणं पुनर्मानम्। (च. सू.-26.34)
31. संस्कारः करणं मतम्। (च. सू.-26.34)
करणं हि स्वाभाविकानां द्रव्याणामभिसंस्कारः।
संस्कारो हि गुणान्तराधानमुच्यते। (च. वि.-1.21.2)

32. भावाभ्यसनमभ्यासः शीलनं सततक्रिया। (च. सू.-26.34)
33. कर्मभिस्त्वनुमीयन्ते नानाद्रव्याश्रया गुणाः। (सु. सू.-46.514)
गुणा य उक्ता द्रव्येषु शरीरेष्वपि ते तथा।
स्थानवृद्धिक्षयास्तस्माद् देहिनां द्रव्यहेतुकाः।। (सु. सू.-41.12)

5
Rasa Vijnana

- Nirukti (Etimology)
- Artha (Meaning)
- Lakshana (Characteristics)
- Sankhaya-nirdharana (Number of Rasas)
- Panchabhautikatwa
- Nivritti-vishesha-karma (Evolution of Rasas – Special order)
- Rasa–Anurasa (Difference of Rasa–Anurasa)
- Rasa-vaishishtya – Bhautika sanghatana
- Ritu-prabhava (Effect of seasons & determination of Bhautika evolution)
- Rasa – Dosha-karma
- Bhautika nishpatti-nirdharana
- Rasopalabdhi
- Rasa Rupantara (Transformation of Rasa)
- Vargikarana
- Shadrasa lakshana — Guna–Karma (Characteristics, functions & properties of Rasas)
- Rasa-Guna vyavastha (Arrangement of Guans of Rasa as best–medium–worst)
- Aushadha–Ahara prayogakrama (Order in the usage of Rasa in the context of Aushadha-ahara)

Nirukti
(Etymology)

Rasa or taste is something experienced by an individual while consuming a Dravya.

Artha
(Meaning)

Rasa is special sense known through the 'Rasanendriya' (tongue or taste bud). The word 'Rasa' is also referred in Ayurvedic literature for Parada (Mercury), Sharira Rasa Dhatu, and Swarasa (juice) of the herb.[1]

Lakshana
(Characteristics)

Taste perception is the characteristic feature of Rasa. It is basically provided by two Mahabhutas i.e., Jala & Prithivi.

Sankhya Nirdharana
(Number of Rasas)

A seminar was organised by Punarvasu Atreya regarding the determination of number of Rasas. After considering the various views expressed by different Rishis, it was concluded by Atreya that the Rasas are six only i.e. Madhura, Amla, Lavana, Katu, Tikta and Kashaya.

No.of Rasa	*Types*	*Proposed by*
1.	Apya (water)	Bhadrakapya
2.	Bhedaniya (weight reducing) Upashamaniya (weight increasing)	Shakunteya Brahmana
3.	Bhedaniya, Upashamaniya, Sadharana	Moudgalya
4.	Swaduhita (liked & good) Swadahita (liked & not good) Aswaduhita (disliked & good) Aswadahita (disliked & not good)	Hiranyaksha Koushika
5.	Bhauma, Apya, Agneya, Vayavya, Akasheeya	Kumarasira Bharadwaja
6.	Guru, Laghu, Sheeta, Ushna, Snigdha, Ruksha	Vayorvid
7.	Madhura, Amla, Lavana, Katu, Tikta, Kashaya, Kshara	Vaidehanimi
8.	Madhura, Amla, Lavana, Katu, Tikta, Kashaya, Kshara, Avyakta (tasteless)	Badisha Dharmargava
9.	Aparisankhya (Indefinite)	Kankayana
10.	Madhura, Amla, Lavana, Katu, Tikta, Kashaya	Punarvasu Atreya

Punarvasu Atreya concluded the above seminar by stating that the Rasas are only six in number and furnished solutions to the above different queries as below.[2]

There are only six types of tastes viz. Madura (sweet), Amla (sour), Lavana (saline), Katu (pungent), Tikta (bitter) and Kashaya (astringent). The source material for the manifestation of all these tastes is Jala mahabhuta, nourishment and emaciation are their actions, combination of these two leads to the manifestation of tastes having a general action; palatability or otherwise is the subjective reaction (Bhakti); wholesomeness or unwholesomeness constitutes the specific action; manifestations of (Vikara) the five Mahabhutas are the substrata and they are conditioned by nature, modification, combination, location and time; the attributes of the material substrates are heaviness, lightness, cold, heat, unctuousness, dryness etc., because of its corrosive nature (Ksaranat) it is known as Ksara or alkali; it is not a taste by itself; this is manifested by the combination of many tastes and it possesses itself many tastes dominated by pungent and saline ones; it is the object of many senses and it involves a special method of preparation. Imperceptibility of taste is effected only in Jala mahabhuta or in the after taste or where the quantity of material having a specific taste is not added or added in inadequate quantity.

It is not correct to say that the tastes are innumerable, simply because of the innumerability of the specific material substrate for each one of these elements (substrata, quality, action and variation in taste) depend on certain concomitant variations. However in spite of such innumerable variation the taste as such remains the same. Different tastes may manifest themselves in many different forms, depending on the various permutations and combinations but this does not amount to any variation in the original qualities and as such the question of innumerability of tastes does not arise. That is why the wise do not advocate any action in combined tastes.

Panchabhautikatwa[3]

Rasas	*Charaka*	*Sushruta*	*Vagbhata*	*Nagarjuna*
Madhura	AP+Prithivi	AP+Prithivi	AP+Prithivi	AP+Prithivi
Amla	Prithivi+Agni	Prithivi+Agni Jala+Agni*	Prithivi+Agni	AP+Agni
Lavana	AP+Agni	AP+Agni Prithivi+Agni*	AP+Agni	AP+Agni
Katu	Agni+Vayu	Agni+Vayu	Agni+Vayu	Agni+Vayu
Tikta	Vayu+Akasha	Vayu+Akasha	Vayu+Akasha	Vayu+Akasha
Kashaya	Vayu+Prithivi	Vayu+Prithivi	Vayu+Prithivi	Vayu+Prithivi

* According to Dalhana.

Nivritti Visesha Karma
(Evolution of Rasas)

The moon is the presiding diety of water. The water in the atmosphere (before it falls on the grounds) is by nature cold and light, and its Rasa is not manifested at this state. The moment it starts falling from atmosphere and after it falls on the ground, it gets impregnated with the qualities of the five Mahabhutas and it nourishes the individuals belonging to the vegetable and animal kingdom. At this state, the six tastes manifest themselves in these individuals.

Rasa-Anurasa
(Difference of Rasa-Anurasa)

The gustatory effect of the initial as well as final contact of a dry as well as wet substance with the tongue is known as Rasa or taste. When such an effect is not distinctly perceptible but is inferred only by its actions, it is known as Anurasa (after taste). It is included in one of the six tastes and there is no separate seventh taste.[4]

The above concept is interpreted differently by some commentators. The Rasa of a substance is only the taste which is perceptible in the dry state of the substance. Conversely the taste which is perceptible in wet state of a substance but which does not follow in the dry state is its Anurasa. For example, while wet (green and ripe) Pippali produces sweet taste, in its dry state it produces pungent taste. So the Rasa of Pippali is pungent and its Anurasa is sweet.

Rasa	*Anurasa*
1. Found in dry state	Wet state
2. Expressed in the beginning	In the end
3. Experienced immediately	Lately
4. Predominant state	Secondary or subsidiary state

Rasa Vaishishtya-Bhautika Sanghathana

Basing on the actions of Rasas, the Bhautika sanghathana is as follows:

1. Ushnatwa and Abhishyandatwa of Lavana rasa will provide us a clue that it contains Agni and Jala bhutas.

2. Urdhwabhaghahara (or) Vamana dravyas are having pre-

dominance of Agni and Vayu bhutas. Adhobhaghahara (or) Virechana dravyas are having Jala and Prithivi bhuta predominance.

Ritu Prabhava

(Effect of Seasons & Determination of Bhautika Evolution)

Ritu	*Formed Rasa*	*Bhuta dominance*
Shishira	Tikta	Vayu + Akasha
Vasanta	Kashaya	Vayu + Prithivi
Grishma	Katu	Vayu + Agni
Varsha	Amla	Prithivi + Agni
Sharat	Lavana	Jala + Agni
Hemanta	Madhura	Prithivi + Jala

Rasa-Dosha-Karma

(Actions of Rasas on Tridosha)[5]

Anti-vata	*Anti-pitta*	*Anti-kapha*
Swadu	Kashaya	Tikta
Amla	Tikta	Katu
Lavana	Madhura	Kashaya

Promoting vata	*Promoting pitta*	*Promoting kapha*
Tikta	Amla	Madhura
Katu	Lavana	Amla
Kashaya	Katu	Lavana

Bhauthika Nishpatti Nirdharana

Rasa	*Action*	*Bhautika nishpatti*
1. Swadu	Kaphavardhaka, Antipitta, Antivatika	Jala, Prithivi
2. Amla	Kaphavardhaka, Pittavardhaka, Antivatika	Prithivi, Agni
3. Lavana	Pittavardhaka, Kaphavardhaka, Antivatika	Jala, Agni
4. Katu	Vatavardhaka, Pittavardhaka, Antikapha	Vayu, Agni
5. Tikta	Vatavardhaka, Antipitta, Antikapha	Vayu, Akasha
6. Kashaya	Vatavardhaka, Antipitta, Antikapha	Vayu, Prithivi

Rasopalabdhi[6]

Charaka says *'Rasonipate dravyanam'* i.e., taste is identified after the contact of Dravya with tongue.

According to Bhadanta Nagarjuna, that the taste can be perceived by means of 3 methods. They are—

1. Pratyaksha - through direct means
2. Anumana - through inference
3. Aptopadesha - instructions of elders

Process involved in Rasopalabdhi is:

Food or drug brought into contact

↓

With tongue (or) taste buds

↓

Food mixes with Bodhaka kapha i.e, saliva

↓

Prapaka (chemical change)

↓

Stimulation of gustatory centres

↓

Taste perception

Rasa Rupantara

(Transformation of Rasa)

According to Bhadanta Nagarjuna, the factors responsible for changes in Rasa of a Dravya are as follows:

1. Sthana

Storage of the Dravya for sometime changes its Rasa.

Eg: If cooked rice which is of Madhura Rasa is mixed with water and stored for some days it transforms into Dhanyamla which is of Amla rasa. The word 'Sthana' is also related to the vessel (Container).

Eg: If milk is stored in Amla rasa vessel, its Madhura rasa changes to Amla rasa.

2. Samyoga

Rasa may be changed due to mixing.

Eg: When tamarind which is of Amla rasa is mixed with lime, it becomes Madhura rasa.

3. Agni

Rasas of the Dravyas are altered on cooking.

Eg: When tamarind is cooked (or) cooked and dried it becomes sweetish.

4. Atapa

Exposure to sunlight changes the Rasa.

Eg: When Tumbura phala which is of Kashaya rasa is dried in sunlight, it becomes Madhura.

5. Bhavana

Soaking the Dravya may change its Rasa.

Eg: Tila which are of Kashaya, Tikta, Madhura rasas when soaked in Yashtimadhu kashaya, change their taste into Madhura.

6. Desha

Rasa may also change based on Desha-vishesha.

Eg: Amalaki phala in some places is sweetish in taste.

7. Kala

By leaving it for sometime Dravya may change its taste.

Eg: Kadali phala which is of Kashaya rasa changes its taste to Madhura rasa due to Kala prabhava.

8. Parinama

By change in their form.

Eg: Kshira which is of Madhura rasa and changes into Amla rasayuktha Dadhi (curd).

9. Upasarga

Rasa changes when infected by insects etc.

Eg: Ikshu (sugar cane) when infected by insects changes its taste to Tikta (or) Amla rasa.

10. Vikriya

By using peculiar procedures Rasa alters.

Eg: When a Talaphala is cooked on fire and rubbed on earth changes its taste to Tikta rasa.

Vargikarana

Depending on Effect of Tridoshas

Dosha Prakopa			*Dosha Shamaka*		
Vata	*Pitta*	*Kapha*	*Vata*	*Pitta*	*Kapha*
Katu	Katu	Madhura	Madhura	Kashaya	Katu
Tikta	Amla	Amla	Amla	Tikta	Tikta
Kashaya	Lavana	Lavana	Lavana	Madhura	Kashaya

Depending on Behaviour of Ushna & Sheeta Characters

Sheeta	*Ushna*
Madhura	Katu
Tikta	Amla
Kashaya	Lavana

Depending on the Digestive Process

Vidahi	*Avidahi*
Katu	Madhura
Amla	Tikta
Lavana	Kashaya

Shadrasa Lakshana : Guna-Karma

(Characteristics, Functions and Properties of Rasas)

Lakshana

1. Madhura rasa :
   1. Coating with sweet taste
   2. Feeling of Pleasure
   3. Strength to body
2. Amla rasa :
   1. Clearance of oral cavity
   2. Tingling sensation of teeth
   3. Blinking of eyes
3. Lavana rasa :
   1. Dryness
   2. Burning sensation of buccal cavity and throat
4. Katu rasa :
   1. Stimulation of tip of tongue
   2. Burning sensation over the tongue
   3. Increases secretions from eyes, nose and oral cavity
5. Tikta rasa :
   1. Disallow the other taste perception
   2. Reduces desire to eat
6. Kashaya rasa :
   1. Feeling of stiffness of tongue
   2. Dry and stiffness in throat
   3. Catching pain in heart

Gunas (Properties)

There cannot be an attribute within another attribute. So, Rasa itself being an attribute of drugs, diets etc. there cannot really be any attribute assigned to Rasa as such. The attributes so mentioned in fact relate to those of drugs, diets etc. which constitute the sub-strata for Rasa (tastes).[7]

Rasa		Guna
1. Madhura	:	Snigdha, Sheeta, Guru
2. Amla	:	Snigdha, Ushna, Laghu
3. Lavana	:	Snigdha, Usha, Guru
4. Katu	:	Ruksha, Ushna, Laghu
5. Tikta	:	Ruksha, Sheeta, Laghu
6. Kashaya	:	Ruksha, Sheeta, Guru

Karma
(Functions)

Madhura Rasa

Drugs and diets having sweet taste are wholesome to the body and as such they add to the growth of Rasa (body fluid) blood, muscle, fat, bone, marrow, Ojas, semen and longevity. They are soothing to the six sense organs. They promote strength and complexion, alleviate Pitta, Vata and effects of poison.

They relieve thirst and burning sensation, promote healthy skin, hair, voice, and strength. They are soothing, invigorating and nourishing. They bring about stability and heal up emaciation and consumption. They are soothing to the nose, mouth, throat, lips and tongue and relieve convulsions. They are much liked by the bees and ants. They are unctuous, cold and heavy.

Amla Rasa

Drugs and diets having sour taste add to the deliciousness of food, stimulate appetite, nourish and energise the body, enlightens the mind, strengthen the sense organs, promote strength, alleviate Vata, nourish the heart, cause salivation, help in swallowing, moistening and digestion of food. They are refreshing, light, hot and unctuous.

Lavana Rasa

Drugs and diets having saline taste help in carmination, production of stickiness, digestion, osnosia, excision and incision. They are sharp, mobile, Vikashi (clear or antispasmodic) and laxative, Avakasakara (deobstruent). They alleviate Vata, cures stiffness, obstruction and accumulation. They nullify the effect of all other tastes, cause salivation, liquefy Kapha, clear the channels of circulation, bring about tenderness of all the bodily organs, and cause deliciousness of food. They are essential ingredients of food. They are neither very heavy, unctuous nor hot.

Katu Rasa

Drugs and diets having pungent taste keep the mouth clean, promote digestion, help in absorption of food, cause secretion through nose, lacrimation, help in the elimination of waste products which are sticky in nature and produce oleation and fomentation therapies, cause deliciousness in food, cure itching, ally excessive growth of ulcers, kill germs, corrode the muscle tissues, break blood clots and other obstructions, clarify the passages and alleviate Kapha. They are light, hot and unctuous.

Tikta Rasa

Drugs and diets having bitter taste are by themselves not delicious but when added with other things, they promote deliciousness. They are antitoxic and germicidal. They cure fainting, burning sensation, itching, obstinate skin diseases including leprosy, thirst and fever. They promote firmness of the skin and muscles. They promote carmination and digestion, purify milk, cause drying and help in the depletion of moisture, fat, muscle fat, bonemarrow, lymph, pus, sweat, urine, stool, Pitta and Kapha. They are unctuous, cold and light.

Kashaya Rasa

Drug and diets having astringent taste are sedative and constipative. They produce pressure on the affected part and cause granulation, absorption and stiffness. They alleviate Kapha and Raktapitta (a disease characterized by bleeding from various parts of the body). They absorb the body fluid and are dry, cold and heavy.

Side Effects on Excessive Usage of Rasas

Madhura Rasa

Excessive intake of Madhura Dravya causes vitiation of Kapha resulting in obesity, tenderness, laziness, hypersomnia, heaviness, loss of appetite, loss of the power of digestion, abnormal growth of muscles in the mouth and throat, dysuria, cough, coryza, Alasaka (intestinal torpor), fever preceded with cold, Anaha (constipation) sweetness in mouth, vomiting, loss of sensation and voice, scrofula, cervical lymphadenitis, elephantiasis, Galasopha (pharyngitis), adhesion in the bladder, vessels, throat and eye diseases like Abhishyanda (conjunctivitis).

Amla Rasa

Excessive usage of Amla rasa causes thirst, morbid sensitiveness of teeth, closure of eyes, horripilation, liquefication of Kapha, aggravation of Pitta, vitiation of Rakta, decomposition of muscle, flabiness of body, oedema in patients suffering from emaciation, consumption, cachexia, and weakness.

Due to heating property they cause suppuration of wounds caused by ulceration, trauma, contagious bites, burn, fracture, swelling, dislocation, poisonous urine, contact with poisonous animals (viz. snakes like Karanda), bruise, excision, incision, separation, perforation and crushing. It also causes burning sensation in throat, chest and cardiac region.

Lavana Rasa

Excessive usage of lavana rasa causes vitiation of Pitta, aggravation of Rakta, thirst, fainting, heating sensation, erosion, depletion of muscle tissue, sloughing in the parts of the body afflicted with obstinate skin diseases including leprosy, aggravation of poisonous symptoms, bursting of inflamed parts, dislodgement of teeth, reduction of manhood, obstruction of the function of senses and production of premature wrinkling, graying and baldness.

It also causes diseases like Raktapitta (a condition characterized by bleeding from different parts of the body), Amlapitta (acid dyspepsia), Visarpa (an acute spreading disease of the skin), Vatarakta (gout), Vicharcika (a type of skin eruption), alopecia etc.

Katu Rasa

Excessive usese of katu Rasa destroys manhood by virtue of its Vipaka. It affects potency by its taste and causes unconsciousness, wearingness, asthma, emaciation, fainting, choking, giddiness, burning sensation in throat, production of great heat and thirst, and diminution of strength.

Because of dominance of Vayu and Agni mahabhutas it also causes giddiness, burning sensation, tremor, piercing and stabbing pain in legs, hands, back etc.

Tikta Rasa

Tikta rasa if used in excess, by virue of its unctuousness, roughness and non sliminess, depletes the plasma, blood, muscle, fat, bone marrow and semen. It produces roughness in the circulatory channels, reduces strength, causes emaciation, weariness, unconsciousness, giddiness, dryness of mouth and produces other diseases due to the vitiation of Vata.

Kashaya Rasa

Kashaya Rasa if used in excess, causes dryness of mouth, affliction of the heart, distention of abdomen, obstruction of speech, construction of circulating channels, black complexion and destruction of man-hood. It gets digested slowly and obstruct the passage of flatus, urine, stool and semen, causes emaciation, weariness, thirst, stiffness and by virtue of its roughness and dryness. It produces diseases like hemiplegia, spasm, convulsions, facial paralysis etc. due to the vitiation of Vata.

Rasa-Guna Vyavastha

(Table Showing the Degree of Activity of Rasas in Relation to Guna)

Guna	*Uttama*	*Madhyama*	*Avara*
Ruksha	Kashaya	Katu	Tikta
Snigdha	Madhura	Amla	Lavana
Ushna	Lavana	Amla	Katu
Sheeta	Kashaya	Madhura	Tikta
Guru	Madhura	Kashaya	Lavana
Laghu	Tikta	Katu	Amla

Aushada-Ahara Prayoga Karma

(Order in the Usage of Rasa in the Context of Aushadha & Ahara)

According to Kashyapa, the utilisation of Rasas in various disorders should be in the order as follows:[8]

Kapha disorders	*Pitta disorders*	*Vata disorders*
Katu	Tikta	Lavana
Tikta	Madhura	Amla
Kashaya	Kashaya	Madhura

While consuming food the following Rasa pattern is suggested by Sushruta.

First stage	:	Madhura
Middle stage	:	Amla, Lavana
Last stage	:	Tikta, Katu, Kashaya

According to Bhavamishra

Madhura rasa shall be taken both at the first and also at the end of principal meal.

Salt and ginger if taken before meal act as an appetizer and clean the tongue and prepares it ready to relish the taste of different diets.

Rasa Pradhanyahetu

1. Agama

According to Shastra (Agama), Rasa is the most important factor among all principles.

Eg: Food is dependent on Rasa and life is dependent on food.

2. Upadesha

Rasas have been advocated in the treatment of Doshas.

Eg: Madhura, Amla, Lavana alleviate Vata.

3. Anumana

Through inference, the therapeutic action of Rasas is assessed.

Eg: The drugs that are Madhura may increase Kapha.

4. Rishi-vachana

Vedas are the words of Rishis and they employ the usage related to Rasas in the performance of Yajna.

Eg: Some Madhura Dravya should be brought for Yajna.

Research on Rasa

Prof. P.V. Sharma has attempted to evolve a methodology for the objective determination of Rasa and the summary is given below. (Ref. Nagarjuna, May, 1970)

Charaka has said that the Rasa of a drug may be known by contact with the gustatory organ; but this method involved so many difficulties:

1. The observation is purely subjective and liable to vary from individual to individual.

2. Perception may vary due to any abnormality or disease in the organ.
3. As solubility of the substance is an essential factor for perception of taste, Rasa of an insoluble drug may not be known.
4. Some substances may not be put on the tongue due to ethical or psychological reasons such as urine, faeces etc.
5. Poisonous substances, if put on tongue, may prove fatal and as such an unknown drug may not be advised to be put on tongue.

On account of these and other similar difficulties the subjective test will not hold good in all circumstances and will not achieve the desired standard. Hence some objective method has to be evolved to know the Rasa of an unknown drug.

Dravya having 'Madhura' rasa take part mainly in the formation of tissues and producing energy in the body; which according to modern physiology is the function of protein, fat and carbohydrate. As vegetable fats are less used in medicine tests for protein and carbohydrate were done for determination of Madhura rasa in this study. Drugs having 'Amla' rasa (sour) are acidic in nature which can be seen by the test with the litmus paper. So Dravyas having acidic reaction were labelled as having Amla rasas. 'Lavana' dravyas are of saltish taste and should contain sodium chloride. So Dravyas containing sodium chloride were classified as Lavana dravya. 'Katu' dravyas mainly contain essential oil and phenol; 'Tikta' dravyas mainly contain alkaloid and glycoside. So for these Rasas test for these constituents were done and Dravyas containing essential oil and phenol were labelled as 'Katu' dravyas whereas those containing alkaloid and glycoside were labelled as 'Tikta' dravyas. 'Kashaya' dravyas are astringent in nature due to its tannin content. So Dravyas containing tannin in their chemical analysis were labelled as 'Kashaya' dravyas. Besides this coumarin and sterol were also tested in the 'Katu' and 'Tikta' dravyas.

In this study Madhura rasa was found in all Dravyas of the Mishra vargas. In 30% of the Dravyas of Mishra varga Madhura rasa not mentioned in any of Nighantu. Protein and carbohydrate being the essential constituent of the plant kingdom are usually present to some extent in all Dravyas. Dravyas containing a higher percentage of carbohydrate and protein besides sweetish taste may be classified as having Madhura rasa while other as having Madhura Anurasas. In the same way 60% Dravyas contained Lavana rasa which was not confirmed by any of the Nighantus, as both the percentage of Nacl and saltish tests should be deciding factor in a Dravya to label as Lavana otherwise only presence of Nacl in traces carries no sense. About other Rasas all Nighantus differ to a great extent. Even then the observations of the present study are mostly in conformity with most of the Nighantus regarding major Rasas. In this way, the remaining Rasas observed in this study may be taken as Anurasa. Analysis of the Dravyas by this method may help in deciding the Rasas as well as Anurasa and also bring some new informations regarding the drug.

Quantitative determination of Rasa

Prof. C. Dwarakanath suggested one method namely 'Taste Threshold Test' for the quantitative determination of the Rasa. In this experiment the test drug of 10gm. weight is dissolved in a litre of water. Every cubic centimetre of such a solution contains 0.01 gm of the drug. Measure of 10CC of such solution is taken and by adding 90CC of distilled water 100CC of the solution is prepared. Each cubic centimetre of this solution will contain 0.1gm of the drug. Following this method, drug solutions of varying strengths can be made up and the threshold of taste can be evaluated.

•

References

1. (क) रसनेन्द्रियग्राह्यवस्तुनि रसः।
'रसनेन्द्रियग्राह्योऽर्थः स रसः' या 'रसनेन्द्रियग्राह्यवस्तुनि' या 'रस्यत आस्वाद्यत इति रसः।' रसनार्थो रसः। (च. सू.-1.64)
(ख) रसति भक्षयति सर्वान् लोहानिति रसः।
(ग) रसति अहरहर्गच्छतीति रसः।
(घ) रसति शरीरे आशु प्रसरति इति रसः।
2. षडेव रसा इत्युवाच भगवानात्रेयः पुनर्वसुः—मधुराम्ललवणकटुतिक्तकषायाः।
(च. सू.-26.9)
3. भूम्यम्बुगुणबाहुल्यान्मधुरः।
भूम्यग्निगुणबाहुल्यादम्लः।

तोयाग्निगुणबाहुल्याल्लवणः।
वाय्वग्निगुणबाहुल्यात् कटुकः।
वाय्वाकाशगुणबाहुल्यात् तिक्तः।
पृथिव्यनिलगुणबाहुल्यात् कषायः। (सु. सू.-42.4)

4. व्यक्तः शुष्कस्य चादौ च रसो द्रव्यस्य लक्ष्यते।
विपर्ययेणाऽनुरसो रसो नास्ति सप्तमः।। (च. सू.-26.28)
तत्र व्यक्तो रसः। अनुरसस्तु रसेनाभिभूतत्वादव्यक्तो व्यक्तो वा किञ्चिदन्ते।
(अ. सं. सू.-17.4)
....तत्र व्यक्तो रसः स्मृतः।
अव्यक्तोऽनुरसः किञ्चिदन्ते व्यक्तोऽपि चेष्यते।। (अ. हृ. सू.-9.3)

5. कट्वम्ललवणाः पित्तं स्वाद्वम्ललवणाः कफम्।
कटुतिक्तकषायाश्च कोपयन्ति समीरणम्।। (च. सू.-1.67)

6. प्रत्यक्षतोऽनुमानादुपदेशतश्च रसानामुपलब्धिः। (र. वै. अ.-3.108)
रसो निपाते द्रव्याणाम्। (च.सू. 26)

7. गुर्वादयो गुणा द्रव्ये पृथिव्यादौ रसाश्रये।
रसेषु व्यपदिश्यन्ते साहचर्योपचारतः।। (अ. हृ. सू.-9.4)

8. पूर्वं मधुरमश्नीयान्मध्येऽम्ललवणौ रसौ।
पश्चाच्छेषान् रसान् वैद्यो भोजने..............।। (सु. सू.-46.466)
भोजनाग्रे सदा पथ्यं लवणार्द्रकभक्षणम्।
अग्निसन्दीपनं रुच्यं जिह्वाकण्ठविशोधनम्।।
लवणाम्लकटूष्णानि विदाहीन्यत्ति यानि तु।
तद्दोषं हर्तुमाहारं मधुरेण समापयेत्।। (भा. प्र. नि.)

6
VIPAKA

- Nirukti (Etimological derivation)
- Lakshana (Characteristics)
- Vipaka nirdharana siddhanta (Concepts of determination of Vipaka)
- Vipaka : guna-karma (Properties & functions)
- Vipaka taratamyata (Strength of Vipaka)
- Vipaka upalabdhi (Perception of Vipaka)
- Rasa-vipaka bheda (Difference between Rasa-vipaka)
- Vipaka pradhanya hetu (Reasons for the superiority of Vipaka)

Nirukti
(Etymology)

'Vipaka' means Vishesha (or) Vishishta paka (specific digestion).

Lakshana of Dravya Rasa[1]
(Characteristics)

Vagbhata exclusively defined 'Vipaka' as the factor which is the final outcome of the biotransformation of Rasa through the action of Jatharagni.[2]

The term Paka generally means to 'prepare', 'to render fit', 'to cook', 'to digest' etc. The term Vipaka means Vishesha or Vishishta paka. In the context of Ayurveda the term Paka comprehends various chemical reactions to which food and drugs are subjected to in the 'Ama-pakvashaya' during the process of digestion and absorption, and in the tissues (Dhatus) all over the body in the course of metabolism in which various kinds of powerful chemical substances such as enzymes, oxygen, hormones, etc. take part. In Avastha-paka (gastro intestinal digestion) no chemical change takes place and the digestion at this stage is merely a physical change. On the other hand the Nishta-paka (highly complex chemical reactions implied in the tissue metabolism) which starts at the end of Avastha-paka (gastrointestinal digestion) generates radical changes in the substances involving change in their tastes also.

Vipaka Nirdharana Siddhantha
(Concepts of Determination of Vipaka)

Charaka described regarding the assessment of Vipaka without giving the definition. Sushruta quoted that the good or bad effects of ingested drugs depend on Vipaka (final transformation).[2A] Sushruta concludes that Vipaka synthesises the final effect of the drug. Paka other than Avastha-paka is considered as Vipaka by Shivadas Sen.

Difference between Avasthapaka & Nishtapaka

Avastha-paka	*Nishta-paka*
1. Madhura, Amla, Katu vipakas	1. Rasa Mala separation
2. Increase of Kapha and Pitta	2. Increase of Mala forms of Kapha, Pitta

Sankhya
(Number of Vipakas)

1. Shavidha Vipaka-vada
   a. Yatharasa Vipaka-vada
   b. Aniyata Vipaka-vada
2. Panchavidha Vipaka-vada
3. Trividha Vipaka-vada
4. Dwividha Vipaka-vada

Shadvidha Vipaka-vada

Some commentators are of the view that Vipakas are according to the Rasas. They quoted that, 'From the seeds of Shali, Yava, Mudga etc. the same plants take their origin, and in the same way, Rasas like Madhura, Amla etc. do not leave their properties and go into Vipakas like Madhrua vipaka, Amla vipaka etc. This is also known as Yatharasa vipaka-vada.

Vipaka is according to the dominant Rasa involved at that time. This is known as Aniyata vipaka-vada. Vrihi dhanya is of Madhura rasa but it transforms into Amla vipaka. Though Pippali is of Katu rasa it transforms into Madhura vipaka. Amalaki which is of Amla rasa is having Madhura vipaka. By this it is proved that Vipaka is not according to Rasa as commented in Yatharasa vipaka-vada. This concept was not accepted by most of the commentators.

Panchavidha Vipaka-vada

According to Sushruta, Ahara which is of Panchabhautika constitution will be having Parthiva, Apya, Taijasa, Vayavya, Nabhasa vipakas. This Panchavidha vipaka-vada is considered as another type of Dwividha (Guru, Laghu) vipaka-vada.[3]

Trividha Vipaka-vada

According to Charaka, Vagbhata, Parashara and other Acharyas, Vipaka is of 3 types—Madhura, Amla and Katu. Madhura and Lavana rasa give rise to Madhura vipaka, Amla rasa gives rise to Amla vipaka and Katu, Tikta and Kashaya rasas go in to Katu vipaka. But according to Parashara—Madhura, Lavana, Tikta, Kashaya rasas transform into Madhura vipaka, Amla rasa gives rise to Amla vipaka, Katu rasa gives rise to Katu vipaka.[4]

Some Acharyas are of view that the Trividha vipaka-vada is based on Tridosha-siddhanta as follows—[5]

Madhura vipaka	-	Kapha vardhaka
Amla vipaka	-	Pitta vardhaka
Katu vipaka	-	Vata vardhaka

Dwividha Vipaka-vada

According to Sushruta & Nagarjuna, Vipaka is of 2 types—namely Guru and Laghu i.e., Prithivi and Jala bhuta predominance in Guru and Agni, Vayu, Akasha bhuta predominance in Laghu.[5A] As this is based on Gunas and Bhutas it is known as Guna vipaka-vada or Bhuta vipaka-vada. According to Sushruta Guru vipaka is Madhura vipaka and Laghu vipaka is Katu vipaka. Nagarjuna condemning the Trividha vipaka-vada proposed that vipaka is of Chira-kalika and Achira-kalika based on Dravyapaka.

Sushruta condemning the Trividha vipaka-vada illustrated that the Prakruta rasa of Pitta is Katu and in Vidagdhavastha it is Amla. So, Amla vipaka is not accepted. Amlatwa is Avasthika but not Prakruta. But Vipaka nirnaya (determination) must be done based on Prakruta rasa. If Vipaka nirnaya is done based on Vikruta rupa, Lavana vipaka must also be accepted because in Vidagdha avastha Kapha gets the taste Lavana.

To summarise:

Madhura rasa	-	Madhura vipaka
Amla rasa	-	Amla vipaka
Lavana rasa	-	Madhura vipaka
		Lavana vipaka

Rasa	*Charaka*	*Sushruta* and the views of others quoted by him*	*Ashtanga Sangraha*	*Ashtanga Hridaya*	*Parashara quoted by Sangraha*	*Ayurveda Sutra of Yoganand a nath*
Madhura (sweet)	Madhura	Madhura	Madhura	Madhura	Madhura	–
Amla (sour)	Amla	Amla	Amla	Amla	Amla	–
Lavana (saltish)	Madhura	Lavana	Madhura	Madhura	Madhura	–
Katu (acid or pungent)	Katu	Katu	Katu	Katu	Katu	Lavana
Tikta (bitter)	Katu	Tikta	Katu	Katu	Madhura	Madhura
Kashaya (astringent)	Katu	Kashaya	Katu	Katu	Madhura	Amla

*Sushruta considered Guru and Laghu vipakas only which are otherwise called as Madhura and Katu vipakas. He has explained Vipaka basing on Pancha-mahabhutas but not according to Rasas of the Dravya.

Katu rasa	-	Katu vipaka Lavana Vipaka
Titka rasa	-	Katu vipaka Tikta vipaka Madhura vipaka
Kashaya rasa	-	Katu vipaka Kashaya vipaka Madhura vipaka Amla vipaka

Note : A critical review of different concepts of Vipaka, indicate that it is more appropriate to name the Vipaka basiug on Guna in view of the actions attributed to Vipaka based on Guna like Guru-Laghu, Snigdha-Ruksha, Ushna and sheeta.

Vipaka : Guna-Karma[6]

(Properties and Functions)

Types of Vipaka	*Properties*	*Effect on Doshas*	*Effect on Dhatus*	*Effect on Malas*
Madhura	Snigdha, Guru	Kapha vardhaka	Shukrala	Increases quantity of stool and urine (Srushta vinmutra)
Amla	Snigdha, Laghu	Pitta vardhaka	Shukrahara	Srushta vinmutra
Katu	Ruksha, Laghu	Vata vardhaka	Sukrahara	Decreases quantity of stool and urine (baddha vinmutra)
Guru	Guru	Kapha vardhaka, Vata-pittahara	—	Srushta vinmutra
Laghu	Laghu	Vata-pitta Vardhaka, Kaphahara	—	Baddha vinmutra

Srushta vinmutra = free evacuation of stool and urine.

Baddha vinmutra = difficulty in evacuation of stool and urine.

According to Nagarjuna, the effect of Vipaka is not Niyata (Uniform). Honey which is having Laghu vipaka acts as Shleshma shamaka, and water which is having Laghu vipaka acts as Shleshma vardhaka.

Vipaka Taratamyata

(Strength of Vipaka)

According to the Guna vishishtata of Dravyas, Vipaka is of Alpa, Madhya, Uttama strengths. According to Kaviraja Gananath Sen—

Vipaka	*Uttama*	*Madhyama*	*Avara*
Madhura	Madhura	Amla	Lavana
Katu	Kashaya	Katu	Tikta

Vipaka Upalabdhi

(Preception of Vipaka)

By observing the final action, Vipaka can be inferred. 'Karmanishta' is the completion or conclusion of actions.[7] Chakrapani interprets it as 'Kriya-parisamapti'. The term 'Kriya' refers to action; 'Pari' means the conclusion or completion. In other words, Vipaka refers to the completion of actions in their entirety.

Eg: Srushta Vinmutra — Madhura vipaka and Amla vipaka.

Baddha Vinmutra — Katu vipaka.

Rasa-Vipaka Bheda

(Difference between Rasa and Vipaka)

Rasa	*Vipaka*
1. Taste Sensation	1. State of metabolic transformation
2. Immediate response	2. Delayed response
3. Effect localised and extended to the level of digestion	3. Systemic effect after metabolism
4. Immediate psychological response	4. Delayed response of well being or otherwise
5. Perceivable	5. Inferrable

Vipaka Pradhnaya-hetu

(Reasons for Superiority of Vipaka)

1. '*Samyakmithya vipakatwam*'—All the ingested Dravyas after undergoing final transformation produce either good or bad effects.
2. The vitiations and palliation of Doshas depend on Vipaka.
3. The formation of Dhatus also depends on Vipaka.
4. Samyak vipaka engenders Gunas and Mithya vipaka causes vitiation of all the Doshas.
5. Even wholesome diet may become etiological factor if it undergoes Mithyapaka.
6. Authentic texts declare that Vipaka is most important among all the principles.[8]

After discussing about the relative importance of various principles namely Rasa, Virya and Vipaka, Sushruta concluded that Vipaka can not exist without Virya; Virya is not possible without Rasa and existence of Rasa without Dravya is not possible and hence 'Dravya' is most important among all the principles of drug-action.

He further quites that the origin of Dravyas and Rasas is simultaneous and interdependent, just as the body and soul is simultaneous and interdependent. Even eight Gunas which have been named as Viryas belong to Dravya but not to Rasa because the Gunas themselves are without any quality.

The Dravyas alone can be metabolised in the body and not the six tastes themselves, hence Dravyas should be regarded as the most important, the rest (Rasadi gunas) are dependent upon the drugs.

●

References

1. जाठरेणाग्निना योगाद्यदुदेति रसान्तरम्।
रसानां परिणामान्ते स विपाक इति स्मृतः।। (अ. हृ. सू.-9.20)
रसानां जरणनिष्ठाकाले यद् रसविशेषः उत्पद्यते स विपाकः। (अरुणदत्त)
विपाक इति पाकः पचनं द्रव्याणां स्वरूपरसयोः परावृत्तिः। सा च स्वरूपान्तरत्वेन रसान्तरत्वेन परिणतिः, तस्या विशेषो विपाकः। (गंगाधर)
अवस्थापाकापेक्षया विशिष्टः पाकः विपाकः। (शिवदास)
परिणामलक्षणो विपाकः।
2. ....सम्यङ्मिथ्याविपक्वानि गुणं दोषं वा जनयति।
3. पञ्चभूतात्मके देहे ह्याहारः पाञ्चभौतिकः।
विपक्वः पञ्चधा सम्यग्गुणान् स्वानभिवर्धयेत्।। (सु. सू.-46.526)
4. पाकास्त्रयो रसानामम्लोऽम्लं पच्यते, कटुः कटुकम्। चत्वारोऽन्ये मधुरम्।
(पराशर; अ. सं. सू.-17.19)
5. कटु-तिक्त-कषायाणां विपाकः प्रायशः कटुः।
अम्लोऽम्लं पच्यते स्वादुर्मधुरं लवणस्तथा।। (च. सू.-26.58)
त्रिधा विपाको द्रव्यस्य स्वाद्वम्ल कटुकात्मकः। (अ. हृ. सू.-1.17)
स्वादुः पटुश्च मधुरमम्लोऽम्लं पच्यते रसः।
तिक्तोषणकषायाणां विपाकः प्रायशः कटुः।। (अ. हृ. सू.-9.21)
द्रव्येषु पच्यमानेषु येष्वम्बुपृथिवीगुणाः।
निवर्तन्तेऽधिकास्तत्र पाको मधुर उच्यते।।
तेजोऽनिलाकाशगुणाः पच्यमानेषु येषु तु।
निवर्तन्तेऽधिकास्तत्र पाकः कटुक उच्यते।। (सु. सू.-40.14-15)
गुणकारणत्वाद् गुणद्वैविध्याच्च। (र. वै.-1.51)
द्वौ द्वैविध्यदर्शनात् परिणामस्य। (र. वै.-1.50)
यथा खदिरसारादीनि चिरादग्निसंयोगे परिणामं गच्छन्ति, पललादीनि अचिरादिति।
(भा. उ.)

6. शुक्रहा बद्धविण्मूत्रो विपाको वातलः कटुः। (च. सू.-26.61)
पित्तकृत् सृष्टविण्मूत्रः पाकोऽम्लः शुक्रनाशनः। (च. सू.-26.62)
मधुरः सृष्टविण्मूत्रो विपाकः कफशुक्रलः। (च. सू.-26.61)
मधुरो लवणाम्लौ च स्निग्धभावात्त्रयो रसाः।
वातमूत्रपुरीषाणां प्रायो मोक्षे सुखा मताः।।
कटुतिक्तकषायास्तु रूक्षभावात्त्रयो रसाः।
दुःखाय मोक्षे दृश्यन्ते वातविण्मूत्ररेतसाम्।। (च. सू.-26.59-60)

7. विपाकः कर्मनिष्ठया। (च. सू.-26.66)
विपाकं द्रव्याणां कर्मणः परिनिष्ठया। (अ. सं. सू.-17.31)

8. आगमे हि द्विविध एव पाको—मधुरः कटुकश्च। (सु. सू.-40.13)
तयोर्मधुराख्यो गुरुः कटुकाख्यो लघुरिति। (सु. सू.-40.13)

7
VIRYA

- Etymology of the word Virya
- Lakshana of Virya (Characteristics of Virya) & Swarupa-nirdharana (Determination of character of Virya)
- Analysis of Virya Concept
- Sankhya (Number of Virya)
- Panchabhoutikatwa of Virya
- Functions of Virya
- Determination of Virya (Virya-upalabdhi)
- Virya-nirdharana Samanya Siddhantha & Apavada (Generalrules with exceptions about Virya)
- Reasons to consider Virya as the important factor among the principles of drug-action (Virya-pradhanya-hetu)
- Research on Virya

In the context of drug-action, the word Virya, as envisaged in the Ayurvedic classics by the ancient Acharyas, connotes different meanings in different contexts and ultimately projects into the potential factor of any drug by virtue of which it performs certain actions in the body. This comprehensive term is employed to explain lesser or greater potential factors in the drug in relation to different processes and procedures to achieve a desired effect in the body.

The Ayurvedic principles of drug action have been described in the form of Rasa, Guna, Virya, Vipaka and Prabhava. If these are the principles through which the drug operates, the word 'Virya', then, should also be used for actions due to Rasa, Vipaka, Guna and Prabhava. As Prabhava could not be rationally and practically proved, it was put into the category of empirical treatment and as the other four could be rationally and practically demonstrated they were put into another group. Right in the beginning Virya was divided into two groups—Chintya virya and Achintya virya. Chintya virya indicating Virya in general and Achintya virya indicating Prabhava.

Etymology of the Word Virya

According to the various Sanskrit dictionaries and Koshas, it is apparent that the word Virya is derived from the root Veera or Vira meaning 'Vikranti' or specific power to express vigour etc.[1]

The word Virya is used simply for physical capacity of a human being and references are available from Manusmruti, Vedas, and Bhagavata Purana in the support of this idea.

According to Vedic literature and the commentary of Sayana thereon, 'Virya' means, the special capacity (Samarthya) not only necessary for physical and mental activity but also that which is necessary for worldly capacity to possess different kinds of wealth, like Pashu, Putra, Dhana etc. has been meant by it. The 'Sabdakalpadruma' has quoted in support of it.

Amarakosha, Nayananda and Ramanada—all these authorities have described the meaning of Virya as 'Utsaha'. The ordinary Utsaha is not known as 'Virya' but such over whelming exertion requires extraordinary vitality and for such purpose the required amount of vitality is produced by 'Virya'.

In the ancient Sanskrit literature the meaning of word Virya is ascribed to Shukra dhatu as well as for male genital organ.

In the Ayurvedic literature the Virya is used for the Shakti or energy through which drug can act in the body. Intactness of Virya in different pharmaceutical preparations was described by Narayandas in his 'Paribhasha' as follows — In Kalka and Kashaya the Virya remains intact upto one Yama (3 hours), in Churna for 3 Paksha (45 days), Ghrita and Modakas along with Guda for six months, Guggulu preparation for 3 months, Siddha rasa and Bhasma for 3 years, and medicated oils for a considerable long time, the Virya respectively remains intact.

Lakshana evam Swarupa-nirdharana

(Characteristics and Determination of Character of Virya)

According to Charaka, the power which performs work or action is Virya. He said that there is no action without Virya. All actions take place only because of Virya.[2]

The term Virya means power, potency and efficacy. It also conveys the meaning manliness and valour. Prof. Dwarkanath opines—

the term Virya conveys the idea of energy. The energy of a body is its capacity for doing work and the measure of energy is work. Energy may be potential or kinetic. Described in terms of Virya, the former (potential energy) is Sheeta and the latter (kinetic energy) is Ushna. The chemical energy locked up in the food substances/ drugs represents Sheeta virya. Substances (food or drug) from which energy is readily released in Paka karma (Vipaka) under the influence or the action of Kayagni (or bio-chemical reactions) involving oxidation, which in part manifests as heat, are Ushna in Virya.

Discussing the number of Viryas, Charaka has quoted the contemporary views which indicate Ashtavidha and Dwividha virya concepts and at the same time he did not mention his own opinion. Unlike Charaka, Sushruta firmly opines that Virya are two only i.e., Ushna & Sheeta. He also quotes the contemporary view of Ashtavidha virya-vada.

Vagbhata truly followed Charaka and quoted the contemporary views of Ashtavidha virya and Dwividha virya-vada. A critical appraisal of Brihatrayee indicates that Sushruta alone accepted the Dwividha virya concepts while Charaka simply made a mention about these concepts without quoting his agreement to them. Vagbhata after quoting the concept of Ashta viryas and Charaka's definition of Virya substantiated Guna virya-vada i.e., Ashtavidha virya and Dwividha virya.

Table—The reasons for considering 8 Gunas as Viryas[2A]

Reason	*Explanation*
1. Samagra guna sarata	8 Gunas remain constant and can't be changed during Kayagni paka
2. Shaktyutkarshata	Are extremely potent in their actions
3. Vyavahara mukhyatwa	Accorded priority of consideration
4. Bahulyata	Much abundant in Dravya

Analysis of Virya Concept

Charaka defines the term 'Virya' as the power that performs work. He further observes that all actions take place only because of Virya and there is no action which is not due to Virya. Chakrapani Datta while emphasizing the view that Gunas are only modes of Shakti observes that the term Virya is meant for Rasa, Guna, Vipaka or Prabhava of a Dravya. Dalhana also opines Virya as Shakti whether it is of two or eight kinds. Shivadasa Sen observes that Virya is a special power. Acharya Yadavji interprets Virya as active principle of the drug. Prof. P.V.Sharma differing with Yadavji's concept argues that active principle is also a Dravya and Virya being a Guna cannot be equated with active principle. Prof. C. Dwarakanath equating Virya with energy interprets Ushna and Shita viryas as kinetic and potential energies.

Sankhya
(Number of Virya)

Different concepts of Virya were described in different texts. Mainly 3 concepts were mentioned namely—

1. Guna viryavada
    (a) Shakti viryavada
    (b) Paribhashika viryavada consisting of Dwividha and Ashtavidha viryavada
2. Karma viryavada
3. Dravya viryavada

Let us consider these concepts one by one with their implications.

1. Guna Viryavada

(a) Shakti Viryavada

Charaka system has delineated Virya as Shakti and defined it in its own verses as *'Ena kurvanti tat viryam'*. Chakrapani Datta has implied the term Virya in general for Rasa, Guna, Vipaka & Prabhava. So this Vada was named as Shakti viryavada or general Virya concept or Bahuvidha viryavada.

(b) Paribhashika Viryavada

Sushruta has denoted the Virya as the generator of any drug action. Maharshi Sushruta put forth the Dwividha viryavada i.e Ushna & Sheeta viryas which represent Agni (heat) and Soma (cold) of the universe.[3] He has also quoted contemporary Ashtavidha viryavada which considers 8 Gunas out of 20 Gunas as Virya. But Vishada, Pichchhila were mentioned in the place of Guru and Laghu. The eight Gunas are — Sneha, Ruksha, Vishada, Pichchhila, Sheeta, Ushna, Mrudu and Tikshna. He has also stated the Dwividha viryavada known as Ushna and Sheeta.[4]

Dalhana commenting on Sushruta's verses stated Achintya and Chintya viryas. The former was denoted as Prabhava.

Vagbhata followed the Charaka school of thought and also Sushruta's observations. But regarding Ashtavidha viryas Guru and Laghu were mentioned instead of Vishada and Pichchhila.

Hemadri has made a reference to the view that 'Viryas are many' and observed that 'though Virya has been described of two types, it can still be as many as there are actions to be performed'. In this view, all actions, regardless of Gunas, are due to Virya and, therefore, there can be as many Viryas as there are actions. The other significant clarification offered by Hemadri which have direct bearing on the subject now under study is 'that which evokes taste perception is Rasa and all the rest are Gunas'. Particular or distinct Vishishta rasa or taste that occur as the result of Kayagnipaka is Vipaka and produced Guna at this stage is Virya.

Arunadatta has stated that Gunas are only Viryas but not Rasas as the latter cannot withstand the influence of Kayagnipaka and undergo changes.

2. Karma Viryavada

Bhadanta Nagarjuna has envisaged the Karma viryavada by furnishing a definition for Virya as *'Karmalakshanam viryam'*. Guna viryavada was subjected to severe criticism by Acharya Nagarjuna. He has described certain Viryas such as Chardaniya virya, Anulomana virya etc. Nimi has mentioned 15 types of Viryas such as Urdhwabhagahara virya, Adhobhagahara virya etc.

3. Dravya Viryavada

Shivadas Sen has observed that—Virya is a special power. The uniqueness of Virya has been stressed by him as he observes—Shakti is Virya. It alone is capable of performing powerful actions. These actions do not suffer from any limitations due to non-attachment of Viryas to Rasas. Virya is intimately correlated to Gunas viz., Ushna, Shita etc. Since Virya inheres inseparably in Dravays, it is considered to be complementary to Rasas. Shivadas Sen propounded a different type of definition of Virya as follows—It is not the quality of the substance, but it is the fraction of substance itself, capable of performing a special action, and also derived from the very important part of the Panchabhautic structure of the Dravya itself. He has also mentioned Krttrima and Sahaja viryas. Acharya Yadavji supporting the concept of active principle as Virya indirectly prefers Dravya viryavada.

To sum up and summarize, the fundamental principle of drug action 'Virya' has been dealt with in different aspects such as Shakti, Utkrishta gunas and Karmas.

Table—Classification of Viryas

Dalhana & Shivadas Sen's	*Guna viryavada*				*Hemadri*	*Nimi's (15)*
	Shakti Viryavada	*Paribhashika viryavada*				
		Charaka	*Sushruta*	*Vagbhata*		
1.		Mridu	Mridu	Mridu		Adhoba-
(i) Chintya	Bahuvidha	Tikshna	Tikshna	Tikshna		gahara
(ii) Achintya		Guru	Pichchila	Guru	Bahu	Urdhwa-
(Dalhana)	(Chakra-	Laghu	Vishada	Laghu	virya-	bhaga-
	pani postu-	Snigdha	Snigdha	Snigdha	vada	hara
	lates this	Ruksha	Ruksha	Ruksha		Ubha-
2.	theory)	Ushna	Ushna	Ushna		yatobha-
(i) Sahaja		Sheeta	Sheeta	Sheeta		gahara
(ii) Krittima						Samgra-
(Shivadas						hika
Sen)						Samsha-
						mana
						Deepana
						Jeeva-
						niya
						Prana-
						ghna
						Madana
						shitika-
						rana
						Shotha-
						kara
						Shotha-
						ghna
						Pachana
						Dharana
						Ropana

Panchabhoutikatwa of Virya

Ahara (dietic) and Oushada (medicinal) substances are constituted by Pancha mahabhutas. Acharyas have enumerated the various Panchabhautic combinations for the formation of principles of drug action.

Sushruta mentioned about the composition of Panchabutas of different Virya as follows—

1. Tikshana and Ushna - Agni bhuta
2. Guru and Sheeta - Jala bhuta
3. Snigdha - Jala bhuta
4. Mridu - Jala & Akasha bhutas
5. Ruksha - Vayu bhuta
6. Laghu - Agni, Akasha & Vayu bhutas

Functions of Virya[5]

Table—Various effects and functions of eight Viryas

Virya	*Effect on doshas*	*Systemic effects*
1. Ushna	Vatahara, Kaphahara, and Pittavardhaka	Deepana, Pachana, Daha-janana, Murchchhana, Swedana, Vamana, Virechana, Vilayana, Bhrama, Trishna-janana, Ashupaka, Avrishya
2. Sheeta	Pittahara, Vata-kapha-vardhaka	Prahladana, Vishyandana, Sthirikarana, Prasadana, Kledana, Jivaniya, Sthambhana, Rakta-prasadana, Balya
3. Snigdha	Vatahara, Kaphavardhaka	Snehana, Brimhana, Santarpana, Vajikarana, Vayah-sthapana
4. Ruksha	Vatavardhaka, Kapha-pittahara	Sangrahana, Peedana, Virukshana, Ropana
5. Guru	Kaphavardhaka Vatahara	Upalepana, Brimhana, Balya
6. Laghu	Kaphahara Vatavardhaka	Lekhana, Langhana, Dhatu-kshaya
7. Mridu	Pittahara	Rakta-prasadana, Mamsa-prasadana
8. Tikshna	Kaphahara	Sangrahi, Achushana, Avadarana, Sravana
9. Vishada	Kaphahara	Kleda-chushana, Virukshana, Uparohana
10. Pichchhila	Kaphavardhaka	Upalepana, Purana, Brimhana, Vajikarana

Determination of Virya
(Virya Upalabdhi)

The criteria of identification or determination of the principles of drug action namely Rasa, Vipaka and Virya are furnished by Agnivesha.

'Rasa (taste) of the Dravyas (drug/diet) can be ascertained immediately after their contact with the tongue (Nipata), their Vipaka by the final action (Nishta karma) and Virya during their association with the body (Adhivasa) or immediately after their contact with the body (Nipata)'.[6]

Rasa or taste is known by direct perception and Vipaka can only be inferred from its action on Dosha, Dhatu, Mala, Agni and Srotas. As regards Virya, it may sometimes be inferred from its action, e.g. Sheeta virya of Saindhava lavana or Usna virya of Anupa mamsa (meat of marshy animals) canbe inferred from their action on the body. In certain Dravyas the Virya (potency) can also be known by direct perception e.g. knowledge of the Tikshna virya of Rajika is based on olfactory perception.

Pichchhila (slimness), Vishada (non-slimness), Snigdha (unctuousness) and Ruksha (ununctuousness) can be known by direct visual perception. Tikshna virya of Maricha can be determined immediately after its contact with the tongue (Nipata). Virya can also be ascertained while it is in the process of digestion and metabolism (Adhivasa). Chakrapani interprets Adhivasa as Shareera-nivasa and spectrum of action of Virya lies between Nipata (Rasa) and Karmanishtha (Vipaka).

Sushruta quotes the following criteria for identification of different Viryas.

Mrudu, Sheeta	- Sparsha grahya
Pichchhila, Vishada	- Chakshu + Sparsha grahaya
Snigdha, Ruksha, Tikshna	- Mukhaduhkhotpadana

Determination of Virya/Guna by Nishtha karma, Nipata & Adhivasa

While discussing the pharmaco-dynamics of drugs it is clearly mentioned by Charaka that the factor responsible for the manifestation of action/effect is known as Virya *(Ena kurvanti tat viryam)*. Sushruta also expresses the same concept mentioning that the principle by which drug acts is Virya (Su. 41). Drugs act by virtue of their own nature (Dravya prabhava) or by virtue of qualities (Guna prabhava) or both. Either Dravya prabhava or Guna prabhava responsible for drug action can be called as Virya. The term 'Guna' includes Rasa, Guna, Virya, Vipaka and Prabhava. Basing on this statement of Charaka, one can classify the concept of Virya as Dravya viryavada and Guna viryavada. Dravya prabhava means the nature of Dravya but it should not be interpreted as Prabhava which is included under Pancha Rasadi gunas i.e. Rasa, Guna, Virya, Vipaka and Prabhava.

A careful and critical appraisal of the actions attributed to Rasa and Vipaka indicates that all the their actions are explained in terms of their Gunas.

So it may be interpreted that any action is preferred by the most potent Guna (Utkrushta Sampanna guna) which otherwise renamed as Virya. Hence the determination of Guna is done by—

Nipata	- Contact at the tongue level (the term Rasa is employed for Guna) or contact with the body.
Nishta karma	- Final action (the term Vipaka is given).
Adhivasa	- Stay in the body (the term Virya is given).

The ingested drug starts its action immediately (initial-action of Guna/Virya) and commences its journey to reach Adhishtana (site of action) which is the seat of final action (Vipaka). The different phases which contribute for final action takes place between Nipata and Nishthapaka stage. Chakrapani in his Bhanumati vyakhya on Sushruta Samhita quotes that—Rasa starts its action immediately after the administration of the drug; Virya exercises its action during Parinamavastha (during metabolic process) and Vipaka acts at the end of Parinama (metabolism). Transforming Gunas (Virya) of the Dravya which are in the transit (Guna/Virya) also contribute certain actions before their final synthesis to perform Nishtha karma. According to Hemadri the principle that evokes taste perception is Rasa and all the rest are Gunas. Vishishta rasa (particular or distinct taste) which occurs as the result of Kayagnipaka is Vipaka. The Guna which generates at the end of Paka is Virya. It can be interpreted in a different way i.e. Rasanagrahya guna is Rasa, Vishishta guna transformed during Kayagnipaka is Vipaka and finally synthesised Guna at the end of the Vipaka is Virya. Basing on this it can be concluded the Gunas/Virya of a Dravya can be ascertained by Nipata, Adhivasa and Nishtha karma.

To sum up the primary physical qualities such as Guru, Laghu, Ushna, Sheeta etc. are coinherent in the Bhutas i.e. Prithivi, Ap,

Tejas, Vayu & Akasha on which the constitution of Rasas depend. In other words, the characteristic taste (Rasa) of substances are correlated to the Gunas (primary physical qualities) of the Bhutas which collocate in their formation.

The criterion for the assessment of Rasa viz. Nipata should be considered as the index of Guna/quality of the drug. The primary physical qualities of the substances are subjected to physico-chemical reactions or Pakas for further synthesis and potentiation of them. The potentiated/charged Gunas conferred with Virya status exercise (Nishta karma) their final action to produce therapeutic effect (Phala). Barring Rasa, the remaining principles of drug action are assessed by inference. In case of substances having 'Avyakta rasa' (unknown taste) the interrelated principles of drug action can be assessed by Anumana-Pramana (inference) only. Hence the objective assessment of Rasapanchaka is not absolutely possible but by precise evaluation of the pharmacological action (Karma), the principles of drug action can be inferred in a most rational way.

Virya-Nirdharana : Samanya Siddhantha & Apavada
(General Rules with Exceptions about Virya):

The general rule is that a substance which is Madhura in Rasa (sweet in taste) and Madhura in Vipaka is Sheeta in Virya. The substance which is Amla in Rasa and Vipaka is Ushna in Virya. Similarly that which is Katu in Rasa and Vipaka is Ushna in Virya. In this category usually by assessing Rasa of a Dravya one can conclude the Virya of that particular Dravya. It is also observed that in exceptional cases Virya may not be in accordance with Rasa. In the following tables the general rule and the exceptions to the general concept with examples are furnished.[7]

Table—Samanya Siddhanta of Virya

Rasa Samanya Siddhanta	*Virya and Vipaka*
Madhura Rasa	Sheeta virya, Madhura vipaka
Amla Rasa	Ushna virya, Amla vipaka
Katu Rasa	Ushna virya, Katu vipaka.

Table—Charaka quoted following exceptions to Samanya Siddhanta

Dravya	*Rasa*	*Virya*
1. Anupa Mamsa	Madhura	Ushna
2. Amalaki	Amla	Sheeta
3. Saindhava Lavana	Lavana	Anushna
4. Guduchi	Tikta	Ushna
5. Maha Panchamula	Kashaya, Tikta	Ushna

From the above tables it is clear that the Dravyas which follow the general rule is identified as Samana pratyarabdha dravyas and the substances which differ with this rule are categorized as Vichitra pratyarabdha dravyas.

Virya Pradhanya Hetu

(Reasons to Consider Virya as the Important Factor among the Principles of Drug Action)

Among the Rasapanchaka, Virya is considered as the most important factor in the process of drug action. Reasons substantiating the importance of Virya furnished by Sushruta are given below:

1. Aushadha-karma Karaka

The actions of drugs brought about on account of their potency. The actions namely Shodhana, Shamana, Grahi, Agni-deepana, Peedana, Lekhana, Brimhana, Rasayana, Vajeekarana, Swayathukara, Vilayana, Dahana, Dharana, Pranaghna, Visha-prashamana etc. are produced by Virya only. Virya is of two types i.e. Ushna and Sheeta in accordance with the nature of universe which is formed of Agni (heat) and Soma (cold). Some consider Virya to be of eight types i.e. Sheeta-Ushna, Snigdha-Ruksha, Vishada-Pichchhila and Mridu-Tikshna.

2. Rasabhibhava[8]

Vriya suppresses the action of Rasa and performs its own function owing to its overpowering property. Examples are:

a. Brihat Panchamoola though Tikta rasa alleviate Vata due to their Ushna virya.
b. Kulutha (Kashaya rasa) and Palandu (Katu rasa) also alleviate Vata due to their Snigdha virya.
c. Ikshu through Madhura rasa increases Vata due to Sheeta virya.
d. Ardra Pippali (Katu rasa) alleviates Pitta due to its Mridu and Sheeta virya.

e. Amalaki (Amla rasa) and Saindhava lavana (Lavana rasa) alleviate Pitta due to their Mridu and Sheeta Virya.
f. Kakamachi (Tikta rasa) and Matsya (Madhura) increase Pitta due to their Ushna virya.
g. Mulaka (Katu) increases Kapha due to its Snigdha virya.
h. Kapittha (Amla rasa) and Madhu (Madhura) alleviate Kapha due to their Ruksha virya.

If Vata alleviating Rasas (Madhura-Amla-Lavana) possess Ruksha-Laghu-Sheeta gunas they do not pacify Vata.

If Pitta alleviating Rasas (Kashaya-Tikta-Madhura) possess Tikshna-Ushna-Laghu gunas, they do not pacify Pitta.

If the Kapha alleviating Rasas (Katu-Tikta-Kashaya) possesses Snigdha-Guru-Sheeta gunas they are not capable of pacifying Kapha. Hence it can be concluded that Virya is the most important principle among the principles of drug action.

3. Agama

Acharyas (Aptas) consider Virya is the most superior principle of drug action (Rasa-vaishesha).

Research on Virya

1. Action of Ushna & Sheeta Virya Drugs on Skeletal Muscle

Total 24 drugs of 12 each belonging to Ushna and Sheeta viryas have been selected at random. Their aqueous extracts (10% water infusion) were tested for their activity against contractions of frog skeletal muscle (frog rectus abdominis) by using Burn model (1954).

Two similar dose response curves with acetylecholine were taken (1r, 2r doses) before and after injecting 1 ml 10% solution of the trial drug.

However, statistical analysis showed insignificant inhibition of both the Viryas. Therefore the skeletal muscle experiment does not reveal any specificity about the nature of Ushna and Sheeta virya drugs (Nishteswar K. et. al).

2. Effect of Ushna & Sheeta Virya Drugs on Frog Heart Muscle

The aqueous extracts of 16 Ushna and 16 Sheeta vriya drugs were screened on 32 healthy frog hearts. Conventional method for this experiment was followed as suggested by Burn (1952). The effect of Ushna and Sheeta virya drugs in different doses (0.2ml and 0.4ml) was assessed on the basis of heart rate (chronotropic activity) and amplitude (inotropic) activity of isolated frog heart during and after perfusion.

Sheeta virya group has shown significant decrease of amplitude ($P<0.05$) at the dose of 0.4ml while Ushna virya drugs have shown significant depressant action at 0.2ml and 0.4ml doses ($P<0.01$).

It is evident that more depressant effect on amplitude was exercised by Ushna virya group in comparison to Sheeta virya group. Both Sheeta and Ushna virya drugs have shown insignificant decrease of heart rate.

Hence the action of Ushna and Sheeta virya drugs cannot be associated with positive and negative chronotropic and ionotropic effect since both the groups have not shown a specific action on frog heart rate and amplitude (Nishteswar K. et.al.).

3. Effect of Sheeta and Ushna Virya Drugs on B.M.R.

Two Sheeta virya drugs namely Yashtimadhu and Shatavari and two Ushna vriya drugs namely Chitraka and Jatiphala have been taken for this study. In healthy volunteers initially B.M.R. was recorded with Mc Kission metaboler. Then the drug was administrated three times for only one day (Chitraka and Jatiphala 2 gm each and Yashtimadhu and Shatavari 5 gm each).

A significant increase ($P<0.05$) has been observed with Yashti, while increase in B.M.R. with Shatavari is not very significant.

The action of Ushna virya drugs is quite opposite i.e., they bring about a decrease in B.M.R. after administration. Both Chitraka and Jatiphala have shown a very significant action ($P<0.05$).

Therefore Sheeta and Ushna viryas, which represent the Saumyatwa and Agneyatwa of a drug or food, may be responsible for synthesizing or metabolizing the Dhatus due to their Santarpaka or Apatarpaka actions. (Nishteswar K. et.al.)

4. Study of Virya vis-à-vis 'pH' Value of Drugs

Total 25 Ushna and 25 Sheeta virya drugs have been screened for 'pH' value in cold water and hot water with 'pH' meter. 10 gms of each drug was soaked in 100 ml of distilled water and kept for one hour. After one hour the 'pH' of the sample was tested. Then the sample was kept on water bath for 30 minutes and again 'pH' was recorded.

In the end all the screened drugs have shown acidic reaction. It is evident from the present study that Ushna and Sheeta virya drugs does not exhibit specific difference in 'pH' values (Nishteswar K. and Dhyani S.C.)

The above experiments carriedout for evaluating Virya have not communicated the specific nature of Virya. Invitro studies designed with frog's heart and skeletal muscle can be categorized as Nipata study of Virya which also did not give any lead. Effects of Virya on B.M.R in human volunteers which falls under Adhivasa category have shown significant response. In view of the Agni and Soma concepts which is interpreted as acidic and alkaline nature of substance, pH value was assessed and this experiment also failed to show any specificity regarding Virya. Animal studies provide analogies and serve as useful models only to evaluate different actions (Karma) but not the principles of drug action. It is rightly said that a cat or a rat cannot act as an ideal model for man. Clinical pharmacology (Dravyaguna) which involves the study of various aspects of drug action and metabolism in humans, both in health and in disease and which is also a part of medicine (Kaya-chikitsa) should be preferred for evaluating Ayurvedic principles of drug action. While evaluating these principles one should follow unbiased and uncompromising adherence to the Shastric descriptions.

•

References

1. येन कुर्वन्ति तद्वीर्यम्। (च. सू.-26.13; सु. सू.-41.5)
वीर्यं तु क्रियते येन या क्रिया। (च. सू.-26.65)
कर्मलक्षणं वीर्यम्। (र. वै. सू.-1.169)
वीर्यं द्रव्यस्य तज्ज्ञेयं यद्योगात्क्रियते क्रिया। (अ. सं. सू.-17.12)
2. समग्रगुणसारेषु शक्त्युत्कर्षविवर्तिषु।
व्यवहाराय मुख्यत्वाद्बह्वग्रग्रहणादपि।। (अ. हृ. सू.-9.15)

3. नानात्मकमपि द्रव्यमग्नीसोमौ महाबलौ।
व्यक्ताव्यक्तं जगदिव नातिक्रमति जातुचित्।।

(अ. हृ. सू.-9.17, अ. सं. सू.-17.15)

4. गुर्वाद्या वीर्यमुच्यन्ते शक्तिमन्तोऽन्यथा गुणाः। (अ. सं. सू.-17.36)
मृदु-तीक्ष्ण-गुरु-लघु-स्निग्ध-रूक्षोष्ण-शीतलम्।
वीर्यमष्टविधं केचित् केचिद् द्विविधमास्थिताः।।
शीतोष्णमिति...। (च. सू.-26.64-65)
वीर्यं पुनर्वदन्त्येके गुरु स्निग्धं हिमं मृदु।
लघुरूक्षोष्णं तीक्ष्णं च तदेवं मतमष्टधा।। (अ. हृ. सू-9.12)

5. तत्रोष्णं भ्रम-तृड्-ग्लानि-स्वेद-दाहाशुपाकिताः। शमं च वातकफयोः करोति.....।

(अ. हृ. सू.-9.18)

ह्लादनं जीवनं स्तम्भं प्रसादं रक्तपित्तयोः। (अ. हृ. सू.-9.19)

6. वीर्यं यावदधिवासान्निपाताच्चोपलभ्यते। (च. सू.-26.66)
यावदधिवासादिति यावच्छशरीरनिवासात्। निपाताच्चेति शरीरसंयोगमात्रात्। किञ्चिद् वीर्यमधिवासादुपलभ्यते; यथा—आनूपमांसादेरुष्णत्वं किञ्चिच्च निपातादेव लभ्यते; यथा—मरिचादीनां तीक्ष्णत्वादि, किञ्चिच्च निपाताधिवासाभ्यां; यथा—मरिचादीनामेव। शीतोष्णा स्पर्शग्राह्याः, पिच्छिलविशदौ चक्षुःस्पर्शाभ्यां, स्निग्धरूक्षौ चक्षुषा, तीक्ष्णो मुखे दुःखोत्पादनात्। (सु. सू.-41.15)

7. शीतवीर्येण यद्द्रव्यं मधुरं रसपाकयोः।
तयोरम्लं यदुष्णं च द्रव्यं कटुकं तयोः।।
तेषां रसोपदेशेन निर्देश्यो गुणसंग्रहः।
वीर्यतोऽविपरीतानां पाकतश्चोपदेक्ष्यते।। (च. सू.-26.45-46)
यथा पयो यथा सर्पिर्यथा च चव्यचित्रकौ ।
तस्माद् रसोपदेशेन न सर्वं द्रव्यमादिशेत्।
दृष्टं तुल्यरसेऽप्येवं द्रव्ये द्रव्ये गुणान्तरम्।। (च. सू.-26.52)

8. मधुरं किञ्चिदुष्णं स्यात् कषायं तिक्तमेव च यथा महत् पञ्चमूलं यथाऽब्जानूपमामिषम् लवणं सैन्धवं नोष्णमम्लमामलकं तथा अर्कागुरुगुडूचीनां तिक्तानामुष्णमुच्यते ।

(सु.सू.-40.5)

●

8
PRABHAVA

- Nirukti (Etymological derivations of Prabhava)
- Lakshana (Characteristics)
- Karma (Actions)
- Pradhanyata-nirupana (Superiority of Prabhava)
- Dravya Pratyayarabdhata

Nirukti

The principle by which the substance possesses the capacity to engender specific action is called Prabhava.

Lakshana
(Characteristics)

The property of a substance which produces specific actions different from and contrary to those ascribed to Rasa, Guna, Virya and Vipaka is known as Prabhava.[1]

Eg: Danti and Chitraka.

Both Danti and Chitraka are pungent in tastes as well as in Vipaka and they are hot in potency (Ushna virya). But in spite of this similarity, Danti acts as a purgative while Chitraka does not. The purgative effect of Danti therefore can be explained only by taking recourse to its Prabhava—the cause for specific action. The antitoxic property of toxins, actions leading to the upwards and or downward elimination of Doshas and various effects of precious stones (Ratna) when worn over the body etc. are due to their specific action which are beyond all plausible explanations.

Drugs with similar chemical structure will have similar actions. But it is not possible to predict the activity of drug entirely on the basis of chemical structure. Drugs with similar structures are having entirely different actions.

Eg: Antazoline & Tolazoline appear chemically similar but former is an antihistamine and the latter is an adrenergic blocking agent. In the same way many dissimilar chemical agents are having same action. Eg: Phenobarbitone, Chloralhydrate and Paraldehyde are all depressants of central nervous system.

Karma of Prabhava

(Actions of Prabhava)

According to Ahcarya P.V. Sharma, classification of Prabhava-janya karma is—

1. Aushadhiya karma (Pharmacological action)
   Eg: Danti, Trivrit etc.
2. Agadiya karma (Toxicological action)
   Eg: Anti-toxicity of Shirisha.
3. Rakshoghna karma (Bacteriological action)
   Eg: Guggulu, Jatamamsi.
4. Manasa karma (Psychological action)
   Eg: Mantras, worship, wearing stones etc.
5. Bhautika karma (Physical action)
   Eg: Extraction of foreign body with magnet.

Pradhanyata Nirupana

(Superiority of Prabhava)

According to Nagarjuna, following six reasons establish superiority of Prabhava:

1. Achintya : Its action is inexplicable
2. Daiva pratighatata : Bacteriological action
3. Visha pratighatata : Antitoxic activity
4. Karma vaishishtya : Because of its specific action
5. Adbhuta karma : Mantras, worship, wearing stones etc. come under wonderful actions
6. Agama : Shastra's explained it as an important principle

Sushruta advocates that the drugs whose mode of action is indisputable and inexplicable and which are well-known by their usage should be used by the intelligent physicion (only) on the basis of authoritative scriptures (agama). The drugs, properties and actions of which are evident need not be tested for their mode of action by the wise physician. The drugs of Ambasthadi gana will never cause purgation, no matter even if thousands of reasons are advanced for it, hence the wise should have faith in the authoritative scriptures and not in any logic.[2]

Acharya P.V. Sharma opines that Virya acts as dosha pratyanika (anti-dosha) while Prabhava acts as Vyadhi-pratyanika (anti-disease). Hence Virya is said as explainable while Prabhava is inexplicable because of its adherence to natural composition.

Dravya Pratyarabdhata

Basing on physical composition, Dravyas are of two types:

1. Samana pratyayarabdha dravyas
2. Vichitra pratyayarabdha dravyas

Samana Pratyayarabdhata

Ordinarily the Bhutas or elemental substances which contribute to the constitution of Rasa, Virya, Vipaka etc. also contribute to the composition of substances which are the substrate of them. These substances are usually classified under the category of Samana pratyayarabdhata. The qualities and actions of such substances are determined and actualised according to their secondary qualities such as the Rasa, Virya and the rest. Examples of this category of substances are as follows.

The drugs and diets which are Madhura in Rasa and Vipaka and of Sheeta virya, those with Amla rasa or Katu rasa and Vipaka are of Ushna virya. In the case of such of the drugs and diets where Virya and Vipaka are in conformity with Rasa, their properties are explained in terms of Rasa only. Such drugs are called Samana pratyayarabdha dravya. As for example the properties of Ksheera and Ghrita both of which are Madhura in Rasa and Vipaka and Sheeta in Virya can be ascertained in terms of their tastes only. This principle does not apply in the cases of such of the drugs and diets which are not in conformity with Rasa and these drugs are called Vichitra pratyayarabdha dravya. The word Vichitra pratyayarabdha is coined by Vagbhata for the original concept rendered by Charaka.

Substances which possess Madhura rasa and Guru guna are by nature anti-Vatika, Sheeta virya and Madhura vipaka. Accordingly, it is but natural for Godhuma which possesses these qualities to be anti-Vatika; milk is Sheeta virya and the flesh of the swine is Madhura vipaka. These three examples illustrate here the substances classified under the category Samana pratyayarabdha which act by virtue of their Rasa, Guna, Virya and Vipaka.

Vichitra Pratyayarbdhata

In the substances belonging to this category, the collocations of the molecules responsible for the determination of their characteristics i.e., Rasa, Guna, Vipaka and Virya are of an different order from those of the Bhutas or elemental substances which collocate to constitute these molecules. It is because of this structural peculiarity that the effects produced by these substances are at variance with those ascribed to the different secondary qualities mentioned above.

A substance possessing Madhura rasa and Guru guna increases Vata because of its Katu vipaka.

Some drugs having sweet taste are of Ushna virya. Eg: The meat of aquatic and marshy animals.

Some drugs having astringent and bitter tastes are also of Ushna virya. Eg: Drugs belonging to Mahat Panchamula group.

Arka, Agaru and Guduchi having bitter taste, are all Ushna virya in nature. Saindhava lavana which is possessing Sheeta virya and Amalaki which is Amla in Rasa are not Ushna in nature.

Some scholars interprete that Charaka discussed the concept of Vikruti-vishama-samvaya which is similar to Vichitra pratyayarabdhata discribed by Vagbhata. In fact the concept of dissimilar Virya (not according to Rasa) discussed by Charaka in Sutrasthana (a. 26) was followed by Vagbhata and was discussed under the heading of Vichitra pratyayarabdhata.

Vikriti Vishama Samaveta Samavaya

Rasas and Dravyas in the form of drugs, alleviate diseases, and they are also responsible for the vitiation of Doshas.

There are two types of combination of Rasas and Doshas.

(a) Similar to the nature of the constituent factors (Prakrityanu guna)—this combination is called Prakriti sama samavaya.

(b) Dissimilar to the nature of the constituent factors (Prakrityananu guna)—this combination is named as Vikriti vishama samavaya.

Tanduliyaka having Madhura rasa is devoid of Snigdha and Vrishya properties (actions of Madhura rasa). Tila according to its Rasa (Katu-Tikta-Madhura) should alleviate Pitta and Kapha but it aggravates Pitta and Kapha. Varataka (Katu-Tikta rasa) acts as Vatahara instead of Vatakara. The concept Vikriti-vishama samaveta savmavaya explains the action of Rasas on bodily Doshas in the form of aggravation or palliation whereas the concept of Vichitra Pratyayarabdhata discusses the interrelationship between Rasa and other Gunas like Virya and Vipaka.

Chakrapani Dutta further clarifies about Vikriti vishama samavayatwa with a lucid explanation stating that the drug possessing Virya and Vipaka in accordance with its Rasa exercises its action through Rasa (Prakriti sama samavayatwa). Basing on the Chakrapani's interpretation it may be concluded that Vichitra pratyayarabdha dravya's action can be explained in a most rational way with its Virya and Vipaka and Vikriti vishama samavayi dravyas action is attributed to its Prabhava which is empirical in nature.

•

References

1. रसवीर्यविपाकानां सामान्यं यत्र लक्ष्यते।
विशेषः कर्मणां चैव प्रभावस्तस्य स स्मृतः।। (च. सू.-26.67)
रसादिसाम्यं यत् कर्म विशिष्टं तत् प्रभावजम्। (अ. हृ. सू.-9.27)
रसेन वीर्येण गुणैश्च कर्म द्रव्यं विपाकेन च यद्विदध्यात्।
सद्योऽन्यथा तत्कुरुते प्रभावाद्धेतोरतस्तत्र न गोचरोऽस्ति।। (अ. सं. सू.-17)
2. अमीमांस्यान्यचिन्त्यानि प्रसिद्धानि स्वभावतः।
आगमेनोपयोज्यानि भेषजानि विचक्षणैः।। (सु. सू.-40.22)
प्रत्यक्षलक्षणफलाः प्रसिद्धाश्च स्वभावतः।
नौषधीर्हेतुभिर्विद्वान् परीक्षेत कथञ्चन।।
सहस्रेणापि हेतूनां नाम्बष्ठादिविरेचयेत्।
तस्मात्तिष्ठेत मतिमान्नागमे न तु हेतुषु।। (सु. सू.-40.23-24)

•

9

Dravyagata Padarthas & Paresparika Sambandha

- Rasadi Guna Paraspara Sambandha (Mutual relationship between Rasidugunas)

A substance which is Madhura (sweet) in Rasa and Vipaka, is Sheeta in Virya. That which is Amla in Rasa and Vipaka is Ushna in Virya. Similarly, that which is Katu in Rasa and Vipaka is Ushna in Virya.[1]

The action of some substances are due to their Rasa only; the action of some substances are due to their Vipaka only; the action of some substances are due to their other qualities (Gunas) in them; the action of some substances are due to their Virya only and some substances act by Prabhava only.[2]

Substances in which mutually conflicting and incompatible qualities co-exist, in such cases, the numerically homologous among them combine to counteract the action or powers of the less active qualities.

Where Rasa, Guna, Virya, Vipaka and Prabhava of a substance are of equal power and strength, in such cases, the Vipaka may supercede the actions ascribed to Rasa; Virya may supercede the actions of both Rasa and Vipakas and Prabhava may overcome all of them.[3]

Vipaka is not possible without Virya, Virya is not possible without Rasa and the Rasa is not possible without Dravya, hence Dravyas is considered to be supreme among all the principles.

Rasadi Gunas : Paraspara Sambandha

The natural relationship among the Rasadi guna:

Rasa	*Guna*	*Virya*	*Vipaka*
1. Madhura	Snigdha, Sheeta, Guru	Sheeta	Madhura
2. Amla	Snigdha, Ushna, Laghu	Ushna	Amla
3. Lavana	Snigdha, Ushna, Guru	Ushna	Madhura

Rasa	*Guna*	*Virya*	*Vipaka*
4. Katu	Ruksha, Ushna, Laghu	Ushna	Katu
5.Tikta	Ruksha, Sheeta, Laghu	Sheeta	Katu
6.Kashaya	Ruksha, Sheeta, Guru	Sheeta	Katu

The above table, showing inter-relationship is nothing but the reflection of the concept of Samana pratyayarabdhata.

In a drug,
Vipaka > Rasa, Virya > Rasa-Vipaka
Prabhava > Rasa-Vipaka-Virya (Charaka)

Example:

(1) Honey — Madhura rasa-Katu vipaka. Because of Katu vipaka its suppresses Kapha (Vipaka dominates).

(2) Anupa mamsa — Madhura rasa-Madhura vipaka Ushna virya and acts as Pittakara (Virya dominates).

(3) Sura — Amla rasa-Amla vipaka-Ushna virya Because of Prabhava—Stanyajanana (Prabhava dominates)

Where there is association of dissimilar qualities, the more potent quality will supercede the quality of lower potency and exhibit its own effects or qualities.[4]

The drug action of any Dravya will depend upon either Rasa (or) Virya (or) Vipaka (or) Prabhava.

●

References

1. शीतं वीर्येण यद् द्रव्यं मधुरं रसपाकयोः।
तयोरम्लं यदुष्णञ्च यद् द्रव्यं कटुकं तयोः।।
तेषां रसोपदेशेन निर्देश्यो गुणसंग्रहः।। (च. सू. 26.45-46)

2. किञ्चिद्रसेन कुरुते कर्म वीर्येण चापरम्।
द्रव्यं गुणेन पाकेन प्रभावेण च किञ्चन। (च. सू.-26.71-72)
तद्द्रव्यात्मना किञ्चित्किञ्चद्वीर्येण सेवितम्।
किञ्चिद्रसविपाकाभ्यां दोषं हन्ति करोति वा।। (सु. सू.-40/17)

3. रसं विपाकस्तौ वीर्यं प्रभावस्तानपोहति।।
बलसाम्ये रसादीनामिति नैसर्गिकं बलम्। (च. सू. 26.72-73)

4. यद्यद्द्रव्ये रसादीनां बलवत्वने वर्तते ।
अभिभूयेतरांस्तत्तत् कारणत्वं प्रपद्यते ।
विरूद्धगुणसंयोगे भूयसाल्पं हि जीयते । (अं.स.सू. 27)

10
KARMA

- Nirukti (Etymology)
- Lakshana (Characteristics)
- Swarupabheda (Nature)
- Vargikarana (Classification)
- Prachina–Arvachina Karma-siddhanta (Drug action from ancient & modern perspective)
- Parikshana-vidhi (Drug testing)
- Detailed description of certain actions with examples:
  Deepana, Pachana, Samshodhana, Samshamana, Anulomana, Bhedana, Rechana, Lekhana, Grahi, Sthambhana, Madakari, Pramadi, Vyavayi, Vikashi
- Modern Pharmacological Action

Nirukti
(Etymology)

Factor responsible for action of drug is known as Karma.

Lakshana
(Characteristics)

Karma present in Dravya (matter) is the cause of combination and separation. Karma is the action relating to something to be achieved. It does not require any other factor for its action. Commenting on this, Chakrapani quotes that by definition, Karma implies only the action relating to something to be achieved (like the action of drugs) and not something like Vamana karma or Adrishta karma.[1]

Swarupa Bheda
(Nature)

Action or activity is the characteristic feature of Karma. It is the cause and Karma is effect.

According to Chakrapani, Vamana, Virechana, Deepana, Sangrahaka etc. are considered as Karma. Chetana, Prayatna etc. are considered as Karma by Charaka. Sushruta considered Vamana,

Virechana, Deepana, Sangrahaka etc. as Karmas. In Vaisheshika Darshana, Utkshepana, Apakshepana, Akunchana, Prasarana etc. are considered as Karmas.[2]

Vargikarana
(Classification)

The administered drug acts on various bodily components namely on Dosha, Dhatu, Mala, Agni and Srotas. The classification based on them is as follows. Basing on the Adhishtana (site of action), the classification of Karma is as follows:

I. Based on Dosha

1. Vata prakopaka
2. Vata shamaka
3. Pitta prakopaka
4. Pitta shamaka
5. Kapha prakopaka
6. Kapha shamaka

II. Action on Dhatu and Upadhatu

1. Jeevaniya
2. Balya
3. Brimhana
4. Snehana
5. Medo vardhaka
6. Medo kshapana
7. Rakta prasadana
8. Raktotkleshana
9. Shukra nashana
10. Shukrala
11. Shukra shodhana
12. Stanya janana
13. Stanya shodhana
14. Artava janana
15. Artava nashana etc.

III. Action on Mala

1. Mutra virechaniya
2. Mura sangrahaniya
3. Mutra virajaniya
4. Ashmari bhedana
5. Bhedaniya
6. Purisha sangrahaniya
7. Purisha virajaniya
8. Sweda sangrahaka
9. Swedopaga etc.

IV. Action on Srotas

1. Pranavaha srotas
   a. Hridya
   b. Ahridya
2. Udakavaha srotas
   a. Trishna nigrahana
   b. Trishnakara
3. Annavaha srotas
   a. Deepana
   b. Pachana
   c. Rochana
   h. Chardi nigrahana
   i. Rechana
   j. Virechanopaga

d. Vidahi
e. Vishtambhi
f. Vamanopaga
g. Vamaka
k. Grahi
l. Stambhana
m. Triptighna
n. Krimighna etc.

Bhedas (Classification)

Karma

- 1. Samsodhana
  2. Samshamana
- 1. Sthanika
  2. Sarvadaihika
  3. Visishta
- 1. Antahparimarjuna
  2. Bahirparimarjana

Prachina-Arvachina Karma-Siddhantha
(Drug Action from Ancient & Modern Perspective)

Drug may act by:

1. Dravya prabhava
2. Guna prabhava
3. Dravya-guna prabhava[3]

Drug action discussed by Charaka is as follows:

Karma	: The factor which does the act.
Virya	: Factor responsible for the manifestation of the effect is known as Virya.
Adhikarana	: Site of action (where Dravya acts)
Kala	: Time taken for drug action (when they act is the time)
Upaya	: Methods adopted for achieving action (how they act is Upaya). It is interpreted as mode of action by some.
Phala	: Therapeutic effect of the drug (what they accomplish is the achievement).

Chakrapani Dutta has taken Nasya karma as example and explained it as follows:

Drayva	: Apamarga/any Sirovirechana dravya
Karma	: Nasya karma
Virya	: Ushna
Adhikarana	: Siras
Kala	: Heaviness in head (diseased state), Vasanta ritu (period of Nasya karma),
Upaya	: Method of performing Nasya karma

Phala : Relief from headache and feeling of heaviness in the head

According to Modern Pharmacology

A drug may act by virtue of its physical properties, chemical properties or metabolic activity. Physical action of a drug is defined as the one which entirely due to the physical properties of a drug. Certain drugs act by the physical properties like osmosis (osmotic diuretics and purgatives), adsorption (kaolin in the treatment of diarrhoea), lubrication (liquid paraffin), surface tension (entrimide for cleaning the skin), radio activity (131 I in hyperthyroidism), radio opacity (barium sulphate as barium meal), electrical charge (anti coagulant effect of heparin by virtue of its negative charge) etc.

Chemical action is the one where drug action can be represented as a chemical reaction. Neutralization of gastric acid by sodium carbonate, administration of hydrochloric acid in the treatment of hypochlorhydria and the elimination of metals like copper and lead with the help of chelating agents are a few examples of chemical action.

Metabolic activity is the one in which a drug acts by altering the functions of cell membrane or may act on the intercellular structures and various enzyme systems.

Drug may produce specific actions by—

1. Stimulation

Increase in the activity of specialised cells is called stimulation.

Eg: Stimulation of respiration by leptazol.

2. Depression

Decrease in the specialised function of a cell is called depression.

Eg: Depression of central nervous system by barbiturates.

3. Irritation

It indicates that a drug produces effects on growth, nutrition and morphology of living tissue. It is not restricted to specialised cells, but can occur in all the body tissues. Precipitation of proteins by astringent effect, tissue damage due to deeper penetration by corrosive effect, dehydration, damage to cell wall and inhibition of cellular enzymes are some of the examples of irritation.

4. Replacement

When the production of endogenous substances is reduced certain drugs may be used.

Eg: Insulin in diabetes mellitus, thyroxin in myxoedema etc.

5. Anti-infective activity

Drugs having specific action on causative organisms in terms of prevention, arrest, and eradication are used in therapeutics.

Eg: Antibiotics & anti-microbial drugs.

6. Modification of immune status

Certain agents (corticosteroids), vaccines and sera act by altering the immune status.

Receptor theory of drug action

This is a recent theory in the modern pharmacology and according to it the site (either on the cell membrane or inside the cell) at which a drug molecule attaches itself to produce action is called a receptor. A drug combines with a receptor (Samyoga) to form a drug receptor complex and that brings about the final action. The drugs which produce effect combine with the receptors and this combination is rapidly broken (Vibhaga) to facilitate further combination to take place. When a drug occupies a receptor and remains there further action through that receptor is blocked.

Parikshana-vidhi
(Drug Testing)

According to Ayurveda, Parikshana is done by Pratyaksha, Anumana and Aptopadesha. Rasa and Virya present in Dravya are tested by tongue through Pratyaksha pramana. Virya and Vipaka are tested for their action through Anumana pramana. Karma phala is tested on the body by Pratyaksha pramana and then Dravyagata karma is tested by Anuaman pramana. Sharira-krishatwa (leanness of body) is tested by Pratyaksha pramana and the Lekhana karma of the Dravya can be inferred by this.[4]

Snigdha and Ruksha gunas are having actions like Shrishta vinmutra and Baddha vinmutra respectively which are inferred by perceiving the effect.

If Sahadevi root is tied to the head, it suppresses Vishama jwara. This is illustrated in Shastra and it is considered as Aptopadesha.

According to Modern pharmacology, animal experiments are carried out to evaluate drug action. References regarding detecting the toxic substances in the food, by using animals like monkey and birds are available in Sushruta Samhita.

Experimental Evaluation of Anti-inflammatory Actions

The anti inflammatory action can be evaluated against the experimentally produced oedema and chronic inflammation. Irradiation of the shaven back skin of a guinea pig with ultraviolet light causes erythema. Odema can be produced by local injection of substances like formaldehyde, histamine and carrageenin. An irritant like croton oil diluted with cotton seed oil or air is injected subcutaneously in the rat, usually on the back. After drug treatment the animal is killed, the pouch (which forms after injection) is dissected, its exudate contents measured and compared with that control animals. Polyarthritis induced in rats by injection of dead tubercule bacilli suspended in liquid paraffin is the method frequently used for evaluating the anti-inflammatory activity.

Detailed Descriptions of Certain Actions with Examples

1. Dipana

The drug which does not digest Ama but only stimulates Antaragni (or) Jatharagni is known as Dipaniya. Eg: Misi.[5]

Arundadatta mentioned that Dipaniya drug sometimes may also act as Amapachaka. Some commentators illustrated that it is due to Prabhava. According to Sushruta, Deepaniya dravya is of Agnibhuta predominance and according to some, it is of Prithivi and Vayubhuta predominance. Charaka mentioned Pippali, Pippalimula, Chavya, Chitraka, Shunthi, Amlavetasa, Maricha, Ajamoda, Bhallataka and Hingu under Dipaniya Dasaimani gana.

2. Pachana

The drug which digests Ama but does not directly stimulates the Agni is Pachaniya. Eg: Nagakeshara.[6]

Arunadatta quoted that which increases the Pachana shakti of Agni is known as Pachana. He mentioned it as Shamana bheda and Charaka mentioned it as Langhana bheda. Charaka mentioned Dipana, Pachana and Dipana-Pachana drugs under Dipaniya Dasaiemani. But Sharngadhara mentioned them separately and given Chitraka as an example for Dipana-Pachana.

Sushruta mentioned Pippalyadi and Dasamula gana as Ama-pachaka, Vachadi and Haridradi gana as Dosha-pachaka, Mustadi gana as Pachaka.

Jarana and Jaraniya are words used for Pachana. Pachana dravya according to Arunadutta is of Agni bhuta pradhana and according to Chakrapan it is of Vayu and Agni bhuta predominance.

3. Samshodhana

The drug which sends up or pushes down the excretory products of digestion after dislodging them from their respective regions is called Samshodhana. Eg: Devadali.[7]

Though by the term Samshodhana, Vamana, Virechana, Asthapana, Siro-virechana, Rakta-mokshana etc. should be mentioned, here by the term Deha-samshodhana only Vamana and Virechana must be accepted. Ubhayatobhagahara dravyas are considered to be of Prithivi, Jala, Agni and Vayubhuta predominance.

4. Samshamana

A drug which neither expunges the Doshas nor disturbs the equilibrium of Doshas but passifies the aggravated Doshas is called Samshamana. Eg: Guduchi.[8]

Samshamana dravya is of Akasha bhuta predominance according to Sushruta and Vayu, Jala, Prithivi bhuta predominance according to Nagarjuna.

According to Sushruta and Vagbhata, Samshamana dravya is of 3 types namely, Vata samshamana, Pitta samshamana and Kapha samshamana.

5. Anulomana

The drug which carries out the Paka of Malas and facilitates their easy elimination through anus by breaking the contact (Bandh) is called Anulomana. Eg: Harithaki.[9]

According to Dalhana, the expulsion of Vata and Mala through Adhomarga (anus) is known as Anulomana.

6. Bhedana

The drug which pushes the Malas downwards after breaking down the scybal (hardened faecal mass) irrespective of their state i.e., clinging or not clinging to the walls is called Bhedana. Eg: Katuki.[10]

Charaka mentioned Suvaha, Arka, Urubaka, Agnimukha under Bhedana Dasaemani.

7. Sramsana

The drug which takes no part in digestion but which drives downwards the products that remain impacted in the intestines is called Sramsana. Eg: Kritamala. (Aragwadha) According to Yogendranath Sen, Sramsana is nothing but Virechana.[11]

8. Rechana

The drug which liquifies the Malas irrespective of their Paka and expunges them is called as Rechana. It is of Jala mahabhuta predominance. Expulsion of Doshas through Adhobhaga (anus) is known as Virechana. Eg: Trivrit.[12]

According to Charaka, Dravyas having Ushna, Tikshna, Sukshma, Vyavayi and Vikashi gunas by the nature of their potency (Virya) reach the heart, by Sukshma and Vyavayi gunas they reach Sthula and Sukshma srotas, spread all over the body and by Agneya guna, the Dosha sanghata are melted (Vileena) and by Teekshna guna melted Doshas undergo Bhedana. The Mala thus reach Amashaya and due to the Adhobhaga prabhava, and also due to Prithivi, Jala mahabhuta predominance, the Doshas are expelled out through Adhomarga. According to Charaka, Virechana is of 3 types namely:

1. Sukha virechana. Eg: Trivrit
2. Teekshna virechana. Eg: Snuhi ksheera
3. Mridu virechana. Eg: Aragwadha.

9. Lekhana

The drug which dries and scrapes either Dhatu (Pitta, Kapha & Sapta dhatus) or Mala (vitiated Doshas and Purishadi malas) is called Lekhana. Eg: Vacha, Yava, honey.[13]

According to Shalya Tantra, Chedana of the excessive growth over Vrana by using Kshara and Shastras is called Chedana. According to Dalhana, the Shoshana of Kapha and Medas is called Lekhana. Gangadhara Sen opined that the mechanism which causes Vidarana of skin by Gharshana is Lekhana.[14]

Sushruta mentioned Salasaradi gana is having action of Kaphamedo-visoshana. Charaka mentioned Musta, Kushta, Haridra, Vacha, Chitraka etc. under Lekhaniya Dasaemani.

10. Grahi

The drug which being both Deepaniya (appetizer) and Pachaniya (digestant), helps in the absorption of Drava (moisture) on account of its Ushna guna/virya is called as Grahi. Eg: Shunthi, Jeeraka.[15]

Grahi dravya is of Vayubhuta-pradhana (Sushruta) or of Prithivi, Vayubhuta predominance (Nagarjuna).

Sushruta mentioned Vayubhutadhikyata as a cause for Drava shoshana and according to Sharngadhara the cause for this action is Ushna virya.

According to Adhamalla, it is of 2 types mainly—

1. Pakwa sangrahaka
2. Ama sangrahaka

and the Dravya which digests the Ama present in Grahani and absorbs the Drava by causing Agni-deepti is known as Ushna sangrahaka and in Atisara, the method of Sthambhana of Pakwamala is known as Sheeta sangrahaka. Sheeta sangrahaka is of Vata guna predominance.

Sushruta mentioned Nyagrodhadi gana as Sangrahi, Rodhradi gana as Stambhaka and Priyangwadi, Ambhashtadi ganas as Pakwatisara-nashaka.

11. Sthambhana

The drug which possesses Ruksha guna, Sheeta virya, Kashaya rasa and Laghu vipaka (Katu vipaka) increases Vata and causes stasis of Malas (or arrests the secretions) is known as Sthambhaniya. Eg: Kutaja, Shyonaka.[16] Sushruta mentioned that Rodhradigana is having the action of Sthambhana.

Grahi	*Stambhaka*
1. Katu rasa	1. Kashaya rasa
2. Ushna virya	2. Sheeta virya
3. Agni-deepti, Amapachaka	3. Agni-sadaka
4. Vata shamaka	4. Vata-vardhaka

12. Madakari

The drug which is Tamas in nature, destroys the Buddhi (faculty of intelligene) is called Madakari. Eg: Madya.[17]

According to Sushruta, Madya, having qualities quite opposite to Ojas mingles (combines) with Jatharagni and reaches Hridaya. From there it reaches Indriya and Manas by passing thorugh Dhamanis in upward direction and causes Mada. Madakari dravya's mode of action can also be interpreted as described by Sushruta.

13. Pramathi

The drug which by virtue of its inherent Virya (strength/power) removes the Dosha-sanchaya (accumulated Doshas/Malas) from Srotas (body channels) is called Pramathi. Eg: Maricha, Vacha.[18]

14. Vyavayi

Drug which spreads first through out the body and then undergoes Paka is called Vyavayi. Eg: Bhanga, Ahiphena.[19]

According to Dalhana it spreads all over the body in Apakwa stage and undergoes Paka later just like toxic substances.

15. Vikashi

The drug which separates or dissociates Ojus from Dhatus and causes laxation of Sandhi (ligaments etc.) is called as Vikashi. Eg: Kramuka, Kodrava.[20]

Dalhanacharya discussing about the differences between Vyavayi and Vikashi gunas mentioned that Vikashi dravya spreads all over the body without undergoing Paka (digested) and causes Dhatu-shaithilya.

Adhamalla mentioned that Vyavayi is having Sara guna vishesha and Vikashi is having Tikshna guna vishesha. He further opines that vikashi dravya decreases the Doshabala.

Charaka while mentioning the Gunas of Madya, quotes that Vyavayi and Vikashi gunas of the Madya destroys the Sthira and Shlakshna gunas of Ojas respectively. By this it is clear that both Vyavayi and Vikashi gunas act as Oja-nashaka (destroys the immunity).

Some of the important Karmas though not mentioned in CCIM syllabus are given below:

16. Abhisyandi

The drug by its Picchila and Guru gunas obstructs Rasavaha

srotas and imparts the feeling of heaviness and it is called Abhisyandi. Eg: Curd.[21]

According to Dalhana the Dravya which causes Kledana to the Dosha, Dhatu, Mala and Srotas (channels) is called Abhishyandi.

According to Chakrapani the Dravya which destroys the Dosha-sanghata is Abhishyandi.

17. Yogavahi

The drug which absorbs the Gunas of the associated drugs (synergistic in nature) while undergoing Paka is called as Yogavahi. Eg: Madhu, Jala, Taila, Ghrita and Parada.[22]

18. Rasayana

The drug which destroys old age problems and diseases is called as Rasayana. Eg: Guduchi, Rudanti, Guggulu, Haritaki.[23]

The person who consumes the Rasayana drugs attains longevity, memory, maintains intellect, freedom from diseases, maintains youth, excellence of lusture, complexion and voice, excellent potentiality of the body and the sense organs, Vak-siddhi (i.e, what he says comes true), respect and brilliance.

According to Bhavamishara Rasayana dravya is Vayahsthapaka, Chakshushya, Vrishya and Brimhana. Jeevaniya, Vayahsthapana and Balya karma are considered as different types of Rasayana.

19. Vajikarana

The drug which causes Harsha (sexual arousal) towards women is called as Vajikarana. Eg: Nagabala, Kapikachchu beeja.[24]

Adhamalla, the commentator of Sharngadhara Samhita interprets that Vajikarana dravya imparts Harshatwa (sexual arousal) to both the sexes. Basing on this interpretation it can be concluded that Vajikarana drug is useful to treat impotence (males) and frigidity (females). Vajeekrana drugs are also useful to treat infertility of both the sexes.

In Ayurveda Vrishya is of 3 types:

1. Shukra-vriddhikara. Eg: Masha.
2. Shukra-srutikara. Eg: Sankalpa.
3. Shukra-vriddhi-srutikara. Eg: Milk.

20. Shukrala

The drug which increases seminal secretions/production is called Shukrala. Eg: Ashwagandha, Musali, Shatavari.[25]

Shukrajanana — Jeevaka, Rishabhaka etc.

According to Sharngadhara it is of 4 types.

1. Shukrajanaka and Shukra pravartaka } Eg: Kshira, Masha, Bhallataka
2. Sukra rechana - Eg: Brihathi Phala
3. Sukra sthambhaka - Eg: Jatiphala
4. Sukra shoshaka - Eg: Haritaki or Katinga

21. Sukshma

The drug which has access to all the minute parts of the body is called as Sukshma.[26]

Eg: Saindhava, Madhu, Eranda taila.

23. Vidahi

The drug which causes thirst, acid eructations (Amlodgara) and heart burn (Hridaya daha) and lately digests is called as Vidahi.

Eg: Kulattha.

24. Chedana

The drug which forcibly uproots the accumulated Doshas (including Krimis) is called as Chedana. E.g. Maricha, Shilajita, Kshara.[27]

●

References

1. एकद्रव्यमगुणं संयोगविभागेष्वनपेक्षकारणमिति कर्मलक्षणम्।(र. वै. सू.-1.1.17)
   यत् कुर्वन्ति तत् कर्म। (च. सू.-26.13)
   कर्म पञ्चविधमुक्तं वमनादि। (च. सू.-26.10)
2. इहौषधकर्माण्यूर्ध्वाधोभागोभयसंशोधनसंशमनसंग्राहकाग्निदीपनपीडनलेखनबृंहण-रसायनवाजीकरणश्वयथुकरविलयनदहनमादनप्राणघ्नविषप्रशमनानि वीर्य्यप्राधान्याद्भवन्ति। (सु. सू.-40.5)
3. न तु केवलं गुणप्रभावादेव द्रव्याणि कार्मुकाणि भवन्ति, द्रव्याणि हि द्रव्यप्रभावाद् गुणप्रभावात् द्रव्यगुणप्रभावाच्च (कार्मुकाणि भवन्ति)। (च. सू.-26.13)

4. तद्द्रव्यमात्मना किञ्चित् किञ्चिद्वीर्येण सेवितम्।
किञ्चिद्रसविपाकाभ्यां दोषं हन्ति करोति वा।। (सु. सू.-40.17)
कर्मभिस्त्वनुमीयन्ते नानाद्रव्याश्रया गुणाः।
गुणा या उक्ता द्रव्येषु शरीरेऽपि ते तथा।
स्थानवृद्धिक्षयौ तस्माद् द्रव्यहेतुकाः।।
सामान्यं एकत्वकृद्विशेषस्तु पृथक्त्वकृत्। (च. सू.-1.45)
सर्वदा सर्वभावानां सामान्यं वृद्धिकारणम्।
ह्रासहेतुर्विशेषश्च..। (च. सू.-1.44)

5. पचेन्नामं वह्निकृच्च दीपनं तद्यथा मिशिः। (शा. पू. खं.-4.1)
दीपनीयं वह्नेरुद्दीपनाय हितम्। (गंगाधर)
दीपनमन्तरग्नेः संधुक्षणं तस्मै हितम्। (योगीन्द्रनाथ सेन)
दीपनमग्निगुणभूयिष्ठं (तत्समानत्वात्)। (सु. सू.-41.10)

6. पचत्यामं न वह्निं च कुर्याद् यत्तद्धि पाचनम्।
नागकेशवरद्...।। (शा. पू. खं.-4.1)
जरणीयं पाचनम्। (योगीन्द्रनाथ)
पाचनं पाचयेद्दोषान् सामान् शमनमेव तु। (अ. हृ. सू.-14.7)

7. स्थानाद्बहिर्नयेदूर्ध्वमधो वा मलसञ्चयम्।
देहसंशोधनं तत् स्याद्देवदालीफलं यथा।। (शा. पू. खं.-4.8-9)
तत् पार्थिवाप्य-तैजस-वायव्यम्। (र. वै.-4.6)

8. न शोधयति यद्दोषान् समान्नोदीरयत्यपि। (अ. हृ. सू.-14)
समीकरोति विषमाञ्छमनं तद्यथाऽमृता।। (शा. पू. ख.-4.2-3)
आकाशगुणभूयिष्टं संशमनम्। (सु. सू.-41.10)

9. कृत्वा पाकं मलानां यद्भित्वा बन्धमधो नयेत्।
तच्चानुलोमनं ज्ञेयं यथा प्रोक्ता हरीतकी।। (शा. पू. खं.-4.3-4)
अनुलोमनो वातमलप्रवर्तनः। (डल्हण)
सरोऽनुलोमनः प्रोक्तः। (सु. सू.-46.529)

10. मलादिकमबद्धं यद्बद्धं वा पिण्डितं मलैः।
भित्वाधः पातयति तद्भेदनं कटुकी यथा।। (शा. पू. खं.-4.5-6)

11. पक्तव्यं यदपक्त्वैव श्लिष्टं कोष्ठे मलादिकम्।
नयत्यध स्रंसनं तद्यथा स्यात् कृतमालकम्।। (शा. पू. खं.-4.4-5)

12. विपक्वं यदपक्वं वा मलादि द्रवतां नयेत्।
रेचयत्यपि तज्ज्ञेयं रेचनं त्रिवृता यथा।। (शा. पू. खं.-4.6-7)

13. धातून् मलान् वा देहस्य विशोष्योल्लेखयेच्च यत्।
लेखनं तद्यथा क्षौद्रं नीरमुष्णं वचा यवाः। (शा. पू. ख.-4.10-11)
लेखनमनिलानलगुणभूयिष्ठम्।

14. शल्यतन्त्रे कठिनोत्पन्नमांसानां व्रणानां शस्त्रेण क्षौमादिभिर्वा घर्षणं लेखनमित्युच्यते।
(यादव जी; सु. चि.-1.38)
लेखनं ईषच्चर्मविदरणं घर्षणेन, तस्मै हितं लेखनीयम्। (गंगाधर)
लेखनः कठिनोत्सन्नमांसानां व्रणानाम्। (हाराणचन्द्र)
लेखनं पत्तलीकरणम्। (डल्हण)
लेखनः कफमेदसोः। (डल्हण)
15. पुरीषस्यातिसरतः संग्रहणं संग्रहः, तत्र हितं पुरीषसंग्रहणीयम्। (योगीन्द्रनाथ)
पुरीषसंग्रहणंपुरीषस्य स्तम्भनं, तस्मै हितम्। (गंगाधर)
दीपनं पाचनं यत् स्यादुष्णत्वाद् द्रवशोषकम्।
ग्राहि तच्च यथा शुण्ठी जीरकं गजपिप्पली।। (शा. पू. खं.-4.11-12)
16. स्तम्भनं स्तम्भयति यद् गतिमन्तं चलं ध्रुवम्। (च. सू.-22.11)
रौक्ष्यात् शैत्यात् कषायत्वात् लघुपाकाच्च यद्भवेत्।
वातकृत् स्तम्भनं तत् स्याद्यथा वत्सकटुण्टुकौ।। (शा. पू. खं.-4.12-13)
17. बुद्धिं लुम्पति यद् द्रव्यं मदकारि तदुच्यते।
तमोगुणप्रधानं च यथा मद्यसुरादिकम्।। (शा. पू. खं.-4.21-22)
18. निजवीर्येण यद् द्रव्यं स्रोतेभ्यो दोषसञ्चयम्।
निरस्यति प्रमाथी स्यात् तद्यथा मरिचं वचा।। (शा. पू. खं.-4.23-24)
19. व्यवायी चाखिलं देहं व्याप्य पाकाय कल्पते।
पूर्वं व्याप्याखिलं कायं ततः पाकं च गच्छति। (सुश्रुत)
व्यवायि तद्यथा भङ्गा फेनं चाहिसमुद्भवम्।। (शा. पू. खं.-4.19-20)
20. विकासी विकसन्नेवं धातुबन्धान् विमोक्षयेत्। (सु. सू.-46.530)
सन्धिबन्धांस्तु शिथिलान् यत्करोति विकासि तत्।
विश्लेष्यौजश्च धातुभ्यो यथा क्रमुककोद्रवः।। (शा. पू. खं.-4.20-21)
21. पैच्छिल्याद्गौरवाद् द्रव्यं रुद्ध्वा रसवहाः सिराः।
धत्ते यद्गौरवं तत् स्यादभिष्यन्दि यथा दधि।। (शा. पू. ख.-4.24)
22. गृह्णाति योगवाहि द्रव्यं संसर्गवस्तुगुणान्। (भावप्रकाश)
एतदेव हि योगवाहित्वं यत्स्वगुणपरित्यागेनांशेन सादृश्यात्परस्य शक्तिपूरणम्।
(इन्दु)
23. रसायनं च तज्ज्ञेयं यज्जराव्याधिनाशनम् ।
यथाऽमृता रुदन्ती च गुग्गुलुश्च हरीतकी । (शार्ङ्गधर)
24. येन नारीषु सामर्थ्यं वाजिवल्लभते नरः।
व्रजेच्चाभ्यधिकं येन वाजीकरणमेव तत्।। (च. चि.-2.4.51)
यस्माद् द्रव्याद्भवेत् स्त्रीषु हर्षो वाजीकरं च तत्।
यथा नागबलाद्याः स्युर्बीजं च कपिकच्छुजम्।। (शा. पू. खं.-4.14-15)
क्षीणानाञ्चाल्पवीर्याणां बृंहणं बलवर्धनम्।

तर्पणं समधातूनां वाजीकरणमुच्यते।। (वैद्यकसंग्रह-2)
शुक्रस्रुतिकरं किञ्चित् किञ्चिच्छुक्रंविवर्धनम्।
स्रुतिवृद्धिकरं किञ्चित् त्रिविधं वृष्यमुच्यते।। (द्रव्यगुणविज्ञानम्)
दुग्धं माषाश्च भल्लातकफलमज्जामलानि च।
प्रवर्त्तकानि कथ्यन्ते जनकानि च रेतसः।। (शा. पू. ख.-4.16)

25. यस्माच्छुक्रस्य वृद्धिः स्याच्छुक्रलं हि तदुच्यते।
यथाश्वगन्धा मुशली शर्करा च शतावरी।। (शा. पू. खं.-4.15-16)

26. देहस्य सूक्ष्मच्छिद्रेषु विशेद्यत् सूक्ष्ममुच्यते। (शा. पू. खं.-4.18)

27. श्लिष्टान् कफादिकान् दोषानुन्मूलयति यद् बलात्।।
छेदनं तद्यथा क्षारा मरिचानि शिलाजतु। (शा. पूर्व.-4.9)

11
MODERN PHARMACOLOGICAL ACTIONS

I. Central Nervous System

Anaesthetics: The term anaesthesia means loss of sensation and the drug which induces this is called anaesthetic.

Eg: Ether, Chloroform, Nitrous oxide, Theopental sodium.

Hypnotic: The drug which produces sleep resembling natural sleep is called as the hypnotic.

Eg: Barbiturates.

Sedative: A drug which reduces excitement is called sedative and is commonly used as an anxiolytic.

Eg: Benzodiazepines.

Hypnotics and sedatives both induce depression of the central nervous system, the difference being mainly quantitative.

Anti convulsant: Drug, which is used to abolish convulsions is called anti-convulsant.

Eg: Carbamazepine, Phenytoxin.

Analagesic: Analgesics are drugs which relieve pain without causing loss of consciousness.

Eg: Morphine (Narcotic analgesic), Salicylates (Non-opioid analgesic)

Antipyretic: Antipyretics are the drugs which reduce elevated body temperature.

Eg: Paracetemol.

Anti-inflammatory: A drug which reduces inflammation is called anti-inflammatory drug.

Eg: Oxyphenbutazone, Diclofenac, Indomethacin, Piroxicam, Ibuprofen, Nimesulide.

Analeptics: Analeptics are the drugs which cause central nervous system stimulation and in larger doses they cause generalised convulsions.

Eg: Nuxvomica, Caffeine.

Tranquillizer: A drug which have the ability to calm without causing hypnosis or anaesthesia.

Eg: Reserpine, Alprazolam.

Psychotropics: Drug which selectively modify the behaviour pattern are known as psychotropic (or) psychoactive drugs.

Anxiolytics: The drugs which reduce anxiety are called anxiolytics. These drugs are sometimes called as 'minor tranquillizers'.

Eg: Meprobamate, Benzodiazepines.

Anxiolytics have a calming effect in anxiety states associated with neurotic personality.

Anti-depressants: The drugs which relieve depression are called anti-depressants. They are also called as mood elevators (or) psychic energiser (or) psycho-analeptics.

Eg: Lithium carbonate, Amitriptyline, Imipramine, MAO inhibitors.

Caffeine and Amphetamine stimulate the central nervous system and can act as 'psychic energizers' and they are not true antidepressants.

Psychotmimetic (Hallucinogens): The drugs which are capable of producing psychosis—'a state characterised by maladoptive behaviour in which an individual reacts inappropriately to his environment'. These drugs are also known as psychotomimetic or hallucinogens.

Eg: Lysergic acid diethylamide (LSD).

Anorectic: The drug which acts as appetite suppressant is called anorectic action. These drugs are used in the treatment of obesity.

Eg: Fenfluramine.

Antihistaminic drug: The drugs which block the actions of histamine on receptors are known as antihistamines. They are of two types i.e.,

1. H_1 receptor antagonistics and

2. H_2 receptor antagonistics

Eg: H_1 receptor antihistaminic agents are CPM (Chlorphenimanine maleate).

II. Drugs Actions Related to Respiratory Disorders

Antitussives: Drugs which are used in symptomatic treatment of cough are called antitussives.

Expectorants: Expectorants are the drugs which increase the production of demulcent respiratory tract fluid that covers and protects the irritated mucosa. These drugs liquify the viscid fluids facilitating their easy expulsion. They can stimulate the output of respiratory tract fluid either directly or reflexly.

Eg: Volatile oils like Eucalyptus, Lemon, Ammonium salts, Potassium salts, Vasicine, Ipecacuanha.

Mucolytic Agents: These drugs make the sputum thin and less viscid, so that it can be easily expectorated.

Eg: Bromhexine.

Bronchodilator: The drug which dilates the bronchioles and relieve breathlessness is called bronchodilator.

Eg: Adrenaline, Ephedrine, Salbutamol.

III. Cardio-vascular Drugs

Vasodilator: Drug which dilates the blood vessels is called as vasodilator and the drugs are useful in the management of congestive heart failure and ischaemic heart diseases.

Antifibrillatory: The drug which prevents the development of atrial (or) ventricular fibrillation.

Antihypertensive: The drugs which reduces the elevated blood pressure is called as an anti hypertensive agent.

Eg: Reserpine.

Anticoagulant: The drug used for preventing clotting of blood inside the intact vasculature.

Eg: Heparine.

Haematinic: A drug which increases the haemoglobin and relieves anaemia is called haematinic.

Eg: Iron.

IV. Renal Function

Diuretics: Drugs which increase the rate of urine formation are called diuretics.

Eg: Frusemide.

Antidiuretics: Drugs which decrease the rate of urine formation are called antidiuretics.

Eg: ADH.

V. Drugs used in Disorders of Gastro Intestinal Tract

Appetizers: Drugs which increase the appetite are appetizers. Eg: Chirata.

Digestants: The digestants are the drugs which aid the digestion in gastrointestinal tract.

Eg: Pepsin, Renin, pancreatin.

Carminatives: The drugs used to expel gas from the stomach or intestines in the treatment of flatulence and of colics.

Eg: Dimethy Polysiloxane.

Appetite Supressants: Drugs which suppress the appetite are appetite suppressants (or) anorexiants.

Emetics: The drugs that produce vomiting are termed as emetics.

1. Centrally acting by stimulation of CTZ.
   Eg: Apomarphine, Morphine and Hydergine.
2. Peripherally acting.
   Eg: Mustard, Antimony and Potassium tartrate (tartar emetic) and hypertonic sodium chloride.
3. Both peripherally and centrally acting.
   Eg: Ipecacuanha.

Laxatives: Drugs which are used to promote defaecation are called laxatives.

1. Stimulant or irritant laxatives.
   Eg: Anthraquinone group.
2. Osmotic Laxative.
   Eg: Milk of magnesia, Magnesium oxide.
3. Bulk laxatives.
   Eg: Methyl cellulose, Agar agar.

4. Emollient laxative.

   Eg: Liquid paraffin, Dioctyl sodium, Sulfo succinate.

Antacids: Gastric antacids are the substances which, on ingestion, react with gastric acid and lower the acidity of gastric contents.

1. Nonsystemic antacid—

   Eg: Aluminium hydroxide gel.

2. Systemic antacid—

   Eg: Sodium bicarbonate.

Immuno Suppressants: Drugs which are used to suppress the immunity are called immuno suppressants.

Eg: Anti Lymphocytic Serum (ALS), Cyclophosphamide, Cyclosporine.

Immuno Stimulants: A variety of agents to enhance immunological and non-specific host defences and thus to modify the defences are immunostimulants. Immuno-modulaters are useful to enhance immunity and play a vital note in immuno deficiency disorders like AIDS.

Eg: BCG, Amantadine, Tilorane.

Anti-oxidants: Drugs which are used to prevent the toxic effects of free radicals are known as anti-oxidants. Eg. Vit. C, Vit. E

●

12
Audbhidadi Gana

Akriti (Shape), Guna (Properties), Karma (Actions), Jati (Class), Karya, Prasiddhi, Sadharmya (Similarities) of following Ganas—

- Dashamula - Vividha Panchamula - Panchavalkala
- Panchapallava –Triphala - Trikatu - Trimada
- Chaturushana – Panchakola - Sadushana
- Chaturbeeja – Jeevaniya gana - Ashtavarga
- Trijataka – Chaturjataka - Panchatikta
- Panchamla – Maha Panchavisha - Upavisha
  Jangama dravya (Drugs of animal origin)
- Kshirashtaka – Mutrashtaka - Pitta Panchaka
  Bhauma ganas (Drugs of mineral origin)
- Lavana panchaka – Ksharadwaya - Ksharashtaka

Charaka has mentioned the Dasaemani dravyas in Sutrasthana (4th chapter). Sushruta (38th chapter of Sutrasthana) has described Ganas including Dashamula, Triphala etc. In Dhanwantari Nighantu, Mishraka ganas were described. Acharya Priyavrata Sharma classified Audbidhadi ganas basing on different concepts of similarities (Sadharmyata) under heading of Mishra Vargikarana.

1. Akritigata sadharmyata

Moola	-	Brihat Panchamula
Kanda	-	Panchasurana
Pallava	-	Panchapallava etc.

2. Guna sadharmyata

Rupa	-	Sukla varga, Rakta varga
Shabda	-	Kakarashtaka
Rasa	-	Trikatu
Gandha	-	Sarvagandha
Sankhya	-	Ashtavarga
Sparsha	-	Mahasneha etc.

3. Karma sadharmyata - Mahavisha, Upavisha

4. Jati sadharmyata - Tri-sharkara
5. Karya sadharmyata - Kshara yoni, Sneha yoni
6. Prasiddha sadharmyata - Pancha-sara, Pancha-ghrita

Audbhidadi Ganas

Brihat Panchamula

Bilva, Agnimantha, Shyonaka, Patala, Gambhari.

Properties: Tikta, Kashaya, Madhura rasa, Ushna virya, Katu vipaka, Deepana, Pachana, Kapha-vatahara.

Indications: Shwasa, Kasa.

Laghu Panchamula

Shalaparni, Prishniparni, Brihati, Kantakari, Gokshura.

Properties: Kashaya, Tikta, Madhura rasa, Anushna, Balya, Brimhana, Vata-pittahara.

Indications: Jwara, Shwasa, Ashmari.

Dalhana suggests Eranda in the place of Gokshura.

Dashamula

Both Brihat and Laghu Panchamula are together called as Dashamula.

Properties: Tridoshahara.

Indications: Shwasa, Kasa, Shiroruja, Shotha, Jwara, Tandra, Anaha, Parshwapida.[1]

Kantaka Panchamula

Karamarda, Gokshura, Saireyaka, Shatavari, Himsra (Gridhranakhi).

Valli Panchamula

Vidari, Sariba, Guduchi, Haridra, (according to some Manjishta) Ajashringi (Karkatashringi-Dalhana).

Properties: Kantaka and Valli Panchamula are Kapha-shamaka.

Indications: Raktapitta, Shotha, Prameha, Shukra-dosha.

Trina Panchamula

Kusha, Kasha, Nala, Darbha, Ikshu.

Properties & Indications: In Mutra-dosha vikara and Rakta-pitta, Trina Panchamula are used along with milk.

Sushruta has included Brihat-Laghu-Kantaka-Valli and Trina Panchamula under Pancha Panchamula.

Madhyama Panchamula

Bala, Punarnava, Eranda, Mudgaparni, Mashaparni.

Properties: Kapha-vatahara.

Jeevana Panchamula

Abhiru, Veera, Jeevanti, Jeevaka, Rishabhaka.

Properties: Chakshushya, Vrishya, Vata-pittahara.

Pancha Valkala

Vata, Udumbara, Ashwattha, Parisha and Plaksha are also called Pancha Kshirivriksha. As the bark is the useful part, these are also known as Pancha Valkala. Shirisha (or) Vetasa may be used in the place of Parisha.

Properties: Kashaya rasa, Shita virya, Grahi.

Indications: Vrana-shotha, Visarpa, Yoni roga.

Kshiratraya

Arka kshira, Vata kshira and Snuhi kshira which are considered as Kshiratraya are used in Marana-karma as described in Rasashastra. Ashmantha, Snuhi and Arkakshira are also mentioned as Kshiratraya.

Used in Vamana and Virechana.

Triphala

Harithaki, Vibhitaka and Amalaki are collectively called as Triphala. They are also called Phalatrika or Vara.

According to some, these three must be taken in equal quantities and some mention that one Harithaki, two Vibhitaka and four Amalaki phalas must be taken.

Properties: Kapha-pittahara, Deepaniya, Chakshushya.[2]

Indications: Vishama jwara, Prameha, Kushta.

Swalpa Triphala	-	Kashmari, Kharjura, Parushaka
Madhura Triphala	-	Draksha, Kashmari, Kharjura
Sugandha Triphala	-	Jatiphala, Pugiphala, Lavanga.

Trikatu

Shunthi, Pippali, Maricha are collectivety called as Trikatu. These are also called Katutrika or Tryushana or Vyosha.

Properties: Deepaniya.

Indications: Shwasa, Kasa, Gulma, Medoroga, Prameha, Shlipada, Pinasa.[3]

Trimada

Vidanga, Musta, Chitraka.

<u>Properties:</u> Grahi.

<u>Indications:</u> Krimi, Atisara.

Chaturushana

Shunthi, Pippali, Maricha, Pippalimula.

<u>Properties:</u> Deepaniya.

<u>Indications:</u> Shwasa, Kasa, Gulma, Prameha, Sthoulya, Shlipada.

Panchakola

Pippali, Pippalimula, Chavya, Chitraka and Nagara. These are used in Kola pramana (1/2 Karsha), so the group is known by the name Panchakola. These are also called Panchushana due to their Ushna virya property.[4]

<u>Properties:</u> Katu rasa, Katu vipaka, Ushna virya, Pachana, Deepana, Kapha-vatahara.

<u>Indications:</u> Gulma, Anaha, Pleeha, Udara-shula.

Shadushana

Pippali, Pippalimula, Chavya, Chitraka, Nagara, Maricha.

<u>Properties:</u> Ruksha, Ushna, Vishaghna.

Chaturbeeja

Methika, Chandrashura, Kalajaji, Yavani.[5]

<u>Properties:</u> Ushna virya, Vata-shamaka.

<u>Indications:</u> Parshwashula, Katishula, Ajirna, Adhmana. Vataroga.

Jeevaniya Gana

Jeevaka, Rishabhaka, Meda, Mahameda, Kakoli, Kshirakakoli, Mudgaparni, Mashaparni, Jeevanti, Yashtimadhu.

<u>Properties:</u> Madhura rasa, Sheeta virya, Jeevaniya, Balya, Vatahara.

<u>Indications:</u> Vatavyadhi, Shosha, Shukradosha, Karshya, Ojokshaya.

Ashta Varga

Jeevaka, Rishabhaka, Meda, Mahameda, Kakoli, Kshirakakoli, Vriddhi, Ruddhi. Bhavamishra suggests Vidari, satavani, Aswgandha and varahikanda as substitues respectively.[6]

Properties: Madhura rasa, Madhura vipaka, Shita virya, Guru guna, Vrishya, Brimhana, Balya, Jeevaniya, Vata-pittahara, Shukrala.

Indications: Shukra-kshaya, Ojokshaya, Prameha, Asthi-bhagna, Vataroga, Trishna, Jwara, Rakta-vikara.

Trijataka

Twak, Ela, Patraka.

Chaturjataka[7]

Twak, Ela, Patraka, Nagakeshara.

Properties: Ruksha, Teekshna, Laghu guna, Ushna virya, Kapha-vatashamaka, Pittakara, Deepana, Varnya, Vishaghna, Mukha-shodhaka.

Panchatikta

Guduchi, Nimbamula twak, Vasa, Kantakari, Patolapatra.

Properties: Pittahara.

Indications: Jwara, Kushta, Kasa, Shwasa.

Panchamla

Amlavetasa, Jambira, Matulunga, Naranga, Nimbuka.[8]

Properties: Deepana, Pachana.

Indications: Hridroga, Trishna, Arshas, Grahani, Shula.

Maha Panchavisha

Shringika, Kalakuta, Mustaka, Vatsanabhi, Saktuka.

Properties: Vyavayi, Vikashi, Vishaghna.

Upavisha

Arkakshira, Snuhikshira, Langali, Karavira, Gunja, Ahiphena, Dhattura, Vishatindukabeeja, Jayapala, Vijaya (bhanga) and Bhallataka are include, under upavisha.[9]

Properties: Vyavayi, Vikashi.

Indications: Shwasa, Kasa.

Jangama Dravya
(Drugs of Animal Origin)

Ksheerashtaka

Go, Mahisha, Aja, Ushtra, Avika, Ashwa, Hasti, Nari.[10]

Properties: Balya, Medhya, Vrishya.

Indications: Prameha.

Mutrashtaka

Khara, Ushtra, Ashwa, Go, Aja, Avika, Mahisha, Hasti.[11]

Properties: Ushna, Teekshna, Ruksha, Deepaniya, Krimighna, Vishaghna.

Indications: Krimi.

Pitta Panchaka

Mastya, Go, Ashwa, Mayura, Manushya.[12]

Properties: Deepaniya, Pachaniya.

Bhauma Ganas

(Drugs of Mineral Origin)

Lavana Panchaka

Saindhava, Sauvarchala, Vid, Samudra, Gudbhida.[13]

Properties: Deepana, Pachana.

Indications: Gulma, Ajeerna.

Ksharadwaya

Sarjakshara, Yavakshara.[14]

Ksharashtaka

Palasha, Sehunda, Apamarga, Chincha, Arka, Tilanala Kshara, Yava kshara, Sarjakshara.[15]

Properties & Indications: Gulma, Shula.

•

References

1. दशमूलं त्रिदोषघ्नं श्वासकासशिरोरुजः।
तन्द्राशोथज्वरानाहपार्श्वपीड़ाऽरुचीर्हरेत् ।। (भा. प्र.-गुडू.-41)
गणः श्वासहरो ह्येष कफपित्तानिलापहः।
आमस्य पाचनश्चैव सर्वज्वरविनाशनः।। (सु. सू.-38.71)
2. त्रिफला कफपित्तघ्नी मेहकुष्ठविनाशिनी।
चक्षुष्या दीपिनी चैव विषमज्वरनाशिनी।। (सु. सू.-38.57)
3. त्र्यूषणं कफमेदोघ्नं मेहकुष्ठत्वगामयान्।
निहन्याद्दीपनं गुल्मपीनसाग्न्यल्पतामपि।। (सु. सू.-38.59)
4. पिप्पलीपिप्पलीमूलचव्यचित्रकनागरैः ।
पञ्चभिः कोलमात्रं यत्पञ्चकोलं तदुच्यते।। (भा. प्र. नि., हरी.)
5. मेथिकाचन्द्रशूरश्चकालाजाजी यवानिका।
एतच्चतुष्टयं युक्तं चतुर्बीजमिति स्मृतम्।। (भा. प्र. नि. हरी.)

तच्चूर्णं भक्षितं नित्यं निहन्ति पवनामयम्।
अजीर्णशूलमाध्मानं पार्श्वशूलं कटिव्यथाम्।। (भा. प्र. नि. हरी.)

6. मेदाजीवककाकोली ऋद्धिद्वन्द्वेऽपि चासति।
वरीविदार्यश्वगन्धावाराहींश्च क्रमात्क्षिपेत्।।

7. त्वगेलापत्रकैस्तुल्यैस्त्रिसुगन्धित्रिजातकम्।
नागकेसरसंयुक्तञ्चातुर्जातकमुच्यते ।। (भा. प्र.)

8. अम्लवेतस, जम्बीर, लुङ्ग (मातुलुङ्ग), नारंग, निम्बुक। (रसतरंगिणी)
जम्बीर, नारंग, अम्लवेतस, तिन्तिडीक, बीजपूर। (राजनिघण्टु)

9. अर्कक्षीरं स्नुहीक्षीरं लाङ्गलीकरवीरकौ।
गुञ्जाहिफेनो धत्तूरः सप्तोपविषजातयः।। (राजनिघण्टु)
विषतिन्दुकबीजञ्च त्वहिफेनञ्च रेचकम्।
धत्तूरबीजं विजया गुञ्जा भल्लातकाह्वयः।।
अर्कक्षीरं स्नुहीक्षीरं लाङ्गली करवीरकम्।
समाख्यातो गणोऽयं तु बुधैरुपविषाभिधः।। (रसतरङ्गिणी)

10. आविक्षीरमजाक्षीरं गोक्षीरं माहिषञ्च यत्।
उष्ट्रीणामथ नागीनां वडवायाः स्त्रियास्तथा।। (च. सू.-1.107-108)

11. अविमूत्रमजामूत्रङ्गोमूत्रं माहिषञ्च यत्।
हस्तिमूत्रमथोष्ट्रस्य हयस्य च खरस्य च।। (च. सू.-1.95)

12. पित्तं पञ्चविधं मत्स्यगवाश्वनरबर्हिजम्। (रसार्णव)

13. सौवर्चलं सैन्धवञ्च विडमौद्भिदमेव च।
सामुद्रेण सहैतानि पञ्च स्युर्लवणानि च।। (च. सू.-1.90)

14. स्वर्जिका यावशूकश्च क्षारद्वयमुदाहृतम्। (भा. प्र. नि. हरी.-257)

15. पलाशवज्रिशिखरी चिञ्चाऽर्कतिलनालजाः।।
यवजः स्वर्जिका चेति क्षाराष्टकमुदाहृतम्। (भा. प्र. नि. हरी.-258-259)

13 DRAVYA SANGRAHANA AND SAMRAKSHANA

- Dravya : Namakarana-Paryaya (Basis of nomenclature and synonyms of drugs).
- Desha-Bhumi pravhibhaga (Country - Soil divisions)
- Sangrahaneeya Dravya-swarupa (Characteristics of drug to be collected)
- Sangrahana-vidhi (Methods of collection)
- Sangrahakala-vijnana (Knowledge of Drug collection)
  Avayava-bhed, Virya-bheda Sangraha (Collection according to part used and of Virya)
- Ahara-Jangama Samgrahana (Collection of food articles and drugs of animal origin)
- Samrakshana-vidhi (Preservation methods)
- Bheshajagara (Drug stores)
- Sangrihita dravya : Sushka & Ardra-vidhi (Preservation of collected drugs by dry and wet methods)
- Mana-paribhasha (Prachina-Arvachina)
  (Definitions of measurement Poutava, Druvaya, Payya mana—discussions according to ancient & modern perspective)

Dravya : Namakarana-Paryaya

(Basis of Nomenclature and Synonyms of Drugs)

Indentification of drugs can be known from cowherds, sages, hunters, and those who roam in the forests, as also those whose diet consists of roots or tubers.[1]

[1A]In Raja Nighantu seven factors are quoted as the basis of nomenclature and they are as follows:

Factor	*Meaning*	*Example*
1. Rudhi	Specific term	Kinhi – Apamarga Katwanga – Shyonaka Panchampacha – Daruharidra
2. Swabhava	Natural power	Nidrari – Kirata Mangalya, Subhadra – Shami

Factor	*Meaning*	*Example*
3. Deshyokta	Place of origin	Vaidehi – Pippali Malayaja – Chandana
4. Lanchana	Specific character	Chitra tandula – Vidanga Pancharaji phala – Patola
5. Upama	Similarity	Ajashringi, Varahikanda, Mayura-shikha, Kritamla, Jyotishmati
6. Virya	Potency	Ushna – Shunthi Sheeta – Bala
7. Lanchana	Miscellaneous	Analanama – Chitraka Sakrahwa – Indrayava

Nomenclature basing upon their appearance, nature, parts used, action, characteristics etc:

Factor	*Example*		
1. On basis of weight	Kola	-	Pippali
	Akshapala	-	Vibhitaka
2. Nodes	Shad granthi	-	Vacha
	Shata granthi	-	Durva
3. Historical importance	Koushika	-	Guggulu
	Vibihshana	-	Nala
	Chanakya	-	Muli
4. Latex	Pita dugdha	-	Swarnakshiri
	Payasya	-	Kshirakakoli
5. Spines	Deergha kantaka	-	Babbula
	Tikshna kantaka	-	Ingudi
6. Flowers	Pita pushpa	-	Atibala
	Visha pushpaka	-	Madana phala
	Tamra pushpa	-	Kovidara
7. Fruits	Kanta phala	-	Jeemutaka
	Sneha phala	-	Kantakari
	Amruta phala	-	Patola
8. Leaves	Tamra pallava	-	Rohitaka, Ashoka
	Vrutta patra	-	Padma
	Lekhayadala	-	Tala
9. Action on animals	Ashwamara	-	Karavira
	Kakaghna	-	Karanjabheda
	Krimighna	-	Vidanga

Desha-Bhumi Pravibhaga

(Country-Soil Division)

Desha has been classified into 3 types:

1. Jangala
2. Anupa
3. Sadharana

Jangala Desha

It is characterised as a place of sparse vegetation, having few or no hills or mountains, rivers and lakes etc. in or near about. It is a place which can be aptly described as dry, arid, windy, waterless and sparsely vegetated.

Anupa Desha

It is the reverse of Jangala desha. It can be characterised as a moist and water logged place densely vegetated, having large hills and mountains in it.

Sadharana Desha

This can be described as an environment possessing moderate vegetation, hills and mountains, sufficient rainfall and water supply.[2]

Though earth is also Panchabhautika, due to predominance of each Bhuta, it is of 5 types.

Parthiva Bhumi

Rocky area, with big trees having Shyava and Krishna coloured mud.

Jaliya Bhumi

Area with plenty of water resources, Snigdha, Sheeta gunas, Snigdha, Trina varieties, and delicate plants.

Agneya Bhumi

Soil with different colours lighter, mixed with plenty of stones and small trees.

Vayavya Bhumi

Soil with rough and ash coloured stones, lean and small trees (xerophytes).

Akashiya Bhumi

Soil is sandy with greyish or balckish colour. It consists of tasteless water, and dry trees.

Basing on Gandha (smell), Varna (colour) and Rasa (taste) Sushruta has classified Bhumi into six categories.

Sangrahaneeya Dravya Swarupa

(Characteristics of Drugs to be Collected)

1. **Prasashta Bhumi** (Ideal Soil)

Soil which is devoid of big stones, excess of water, unctuous, smooth, tight, blackish, whitish or reddish soil and grassy is the ideal soil for collection of a Dravya.

2. **Prashasta Dravya** (Ideal Dravya)

Dravya should be obtained from best soil, free from pests, poisons, weapons, severe sunlight etc. It must have single predominant taste well developed, and should be collected which is spread in the direction of north or east.[3]

Sangrahana Vidhi

(Methods of Collection of Drugs)

Drugs are required to be collected keeping in view the appropriate habitat (Desha-sampat), appropriate season (Kala-sampat) and their effective attributes (Guna-sampat). One should collect the various parts of these plants while facing towards the east or north after performing auspicious rites/rituals in a spirit of compassion, while living a pure life, while wearing white dress, after offering prayers to the Gods, Ashwinis, Cows and Brahmins, and while observing fast.[4]

Plants which grow on ant hills, filthy ground, marshy places, burial ground, barren and saline soils and open streets infested with insects do not serve any medicinal purpose. Plants affected by fire or cold are useless.

Sangrahakala Vijnana

(Time of Collection According to Part Used)

Avayawabheda Sangrahana[5]

Useful part	*Sushruta Samhita*	*Charaka Samhita*	*Raja Nighantu*
1. Mula	Pravrit	Grishma/Shishira	Sishira ritu
2. Patra	Varsha	Varsha/Vasanta	Sishira
3. Shakha	--	Varsha/Vasanta	--
4. Pushpa	--	Yatha ritu	Vasanta
5. Phala	Grishma	Yatha ritu	Vasanta
6. Saara	Vasanta	Hemanta	--

Useful part	*Sushruta Samhita*	*Charaka Samhita*	*Raja Nighantu*
7. Twak	Sharat	Sharat	–
8. Kanda	–	Sharat	Hemanta
9. Ksheera	Hemanta	Sharat	–
10. Panchanga	–	–	Sharat

Drug Collection basing on Karma[6]

Action	*Ritu*	*Bhuta dominance*
Vamana	Vasanta	Agni+Akasha
Virechana	Vasanta	Prithivi + Jala
Vasti, Nasya & other Karmas	Sharat	--
Samshamana	--	Akashabhuta

Virya Bheda Sangrahana (Collection According to Virya)[7]

Virya	*Oushadha*	*Ritu*	*Desha*
Ushna	Agneya	Sharat, Vasanta, Grishma	Vindhya ranges
Sheeta	Soumya	Varsha, Hemanta, Shisira	Himalaya

Jangama Dravya Sangraha[8]

Blood, hair, hoof - Young adults or Vayastha

Milk, urine, faeces - Jirnahara (after food is digested)

Relating to the collection of food articles, Sushruta has given the following instructions:

1. Fruits:

Ripened fruits only should be collected except Bilwa phala which is to be collected in unripen state. Draksha and Haritaki are collected in dry state.

2. Leafy Vegetables:

Hard, dry, infected by pests and unseasoned must not be collected.

3. Tubers:

Mature, seasonally harvested, wet and non infected must be collected. Mulaka must be collected in Sushka (dry state) avastha.

4. Rice Grains:

Drugs which are not exposed to cold or hot air, bugs, polluted soil, water etc. and not mixed with other food grains only must be collected.

Collection of Drugs According to Modern Aspect

The usual time for collection of leaves is when the flowers are just beginning to expand, or the flowering just arriving at its height. At this time it is reasonable to assume that the leaves are in the most healthy state and contain an optimum of the products of the plants metabolism and one can obtain the most desirable therapeutic action. As moisture decreases the constituents, they are collected in dry weather. Collection of flowers must always be made in fine, dry weather, because the petals which are damp when gathered become badly discoloured during drying.

Roots and rhizomes are usually collected when their tissues are fully stored with reserve foods, it being assumed that medical constituents will be almost abundant during this season. In temperate regions autumn is therefore the season for collection.

The time of collection of bark is usually spring or early summer, when the sap is rising in the stem and the cambium is active and therefore more easily torn than at other seasons. Gallas are collected after the escape of the gall wasp.

Samrakshana Vidhi
(Preservation methods)

The collected raw drugs should be systematically preserved in a room, where the atmosphere is not affected by smoke, rain, droughts or dampness (moisture). The material should be covered by pieces of linen and kept in earthen or china clay pots or wooden boxes, or hung on pegs after being well protected. Such a drug apartment which is situated in a clean and suitable place is always desirable.

Expiry Time for Ayurvedic Preparations

1. General preparations	:	Upto1 year
2. Churnas	:	Upto 2 months
3. Vati and Lehya	:	Upto 1 year
4. Taila and Ghrita	:	Upto 16 months
5. Dhatus and Asavas	:	Retains their properties for longer periods
6. Aushadhi (Annuals)	:	Loose their efficacy after a year

Modern Storage Methods

Drugs are maintained in a sound condition by adopting proper methods of storage and a study of the causes of deterioration enables one to perceive the general principles which must govern conditions of storage. It is clear that dryness is the most fundamental requirement, since no living organism can exist or develop without a minimum moisture. Mites are unable to develop in flour if the moisture content is maintained below 11% and moisture content below 9% prevents the growth of bacteria and fungi. Next to the moisture light and temperature should be controlled and the access to the drugs of spores and of living organisms must be prevented. These conditions may be satisfied by different means and the exact method adopted for any given drug may not necessarily be the same in all circumstances. Well closed opaque containers fulfill most of the necessary conditions. A dry atmosphere is maintained by the use of dessicating agent, such as quick lime. The ill effects produced by light can be largely prevented by the use of amber glass bottles.

The fact that a raised temperature facilitates the production of dry atmosphere may lead one to over look the other deleterious changes that heat may produce for it is often necessary to store articles in a cool place as well as in a dry atmosphere. A low temperature is also useful to prevent the development of spores and eggs which, generally speaking, are unable to develop unless the temperature is higher than about 10°C. For this reason cold storage in some form of refrigeration is a valuable means of preventing the development of living organisms in all kinds of drugs. It enables one to store large stocks of substances which are particularly prone to attack.

Bhesajagara
(Drug Stores)

According to Vagbhata—The drug stores should be located either in the eastern or northern quarter, in a secret place and equipped with pots, lids, bags, racks and almirahs in which drugs are to be stored (Ashtangasamgraha, Sut.8)[9]

Samgrihita Dravya Samrakshana

The collected herbs can be preserved either by dry method or wet method.

Dry Method:

The herbs are to be pressed between blotting papers and if not dried can be exposed to sunlight. The dried specimen should be pasted on the herbarium sheet.

Wet Method:

The green drugs can be preserved in jars containing 5-10% of formalin solution and the solution should be changed periodically. Copper sulphate is also added in smaller quantities to give it the blue colour. Specimens which are preserved by this method are not useful for processing the medicines. The drugs can be preserved in one of the liquid medium like Kanji, honey, oil and ghee. Green herbs which are preserved in air-tight containers can be used for processing formulations.

Mana Paribhasa

Process of recording length, weight and volume is known as Mana (or) measurement.[10] Mana is of two types: (1) Kalinga (2) Magadha and Magadha is considered to be the best mana.[11]

In old treatise Mana is of 3 types:

1. Poutava : Weight measurement
2. Druvaya : Volume measurement
3. Payya : Length measurement.

1 (a). Poutava mana of Charaka

6 Vamshi	=	1 Marichi
6 Marichi	=	1 Sarshapa
8 Sarshapa	=	1 Tandula
2 Tandula	=	1 Dhanyamasha
2 Dhanyamasha	=	1 Yava (1/2 Ratti)
4 Yava	=	1 Andika (2 Ratti)
4 Andika	=	1 Mashaka (8 Ratti)
3 Mashaka	=	1 Shana (24 Ratti = ¼ Tola)
2 Shana	=	1 Kola (48 Ratti = ½ Tola) or Dramkshana
2 Kola	=	1 Karsha (96 Ratti = 1 Tola = 11.5gm.) (Suvarna/Aksha)
2 Karsha	=	1 Shukti = 2 Tola
2 Shukti	=	1 Pala = 4 Tola (Mushti or Bilwa or Prakuncha)
2 Pala	=	1 Prasruta = 8 Tola
2 Prasruta	=	1 Kudava = 16 Tola (Anjali)

2 Kudava	=	1 Manika = 32 Tola
2 Manika	=	1 Prastha = 64 Tola
4 Prastha	=	1 Adhaka = 256 Tola (Kamsa)
4 Adhaka	=	1 Drona = 1024 Tola (Ghata)
2 Drona	=	1 Shurpa = 2048 Tola (Kumbha)
2 Shurpa	=	1 Khari = 4096 Tola (Bhari or Goni)
32 Shurpa	=	1 Vaha = 65,536 Tola
100 Pala	=	1 Tulaa = 400 Tola = 4.670 kg.

1 (b). Poutava mana of Sushruta & Sharngadhara

30 Pramanus	= 1 Vamshi=0.035 mg
6 Vamshi	= 1 Marichi = 0.21 mg
3 Marichi	= 1 Rajika = 1.25 mg
3 Rajika	= 1 Sarshapa = 4 mg.
8 Sarshapa	= 1 Yava = 32 mg
4 Yava	= 1 Gunja/Ratti = 125 mg
6 Ratti	= 1 Mashak = 750 mg.
4 Mashaka	= 1 Sana = ¼ Tola = 3 gm.
2 Sana	= 1 Kola = ½ Tola = 6 gm.
2 Kola	= 1 Karsha = 1 Tola = 12 gm.
2 Karsha	= 1 Shukti = 2 Tola = 24 gm.
2 Shukti	= 1 Pala = 4 Tola = 48 gm.
2 Pala	= 1 Prasruti = 8 Tola = 2Pala = 96 gm.
2 Prasruti	= 1 Kudava = 16 Tola = 4 Pala = 192 gm.
2 Kudava	= 1 Manika or Sharava = 32 Tola = 8 Pala = 384 gm
2 Sharava	= 1 Prastha = 64 Tola = 16 Pala = 786 gm.
4 Prastha	= 1 Adhaka = 256 Tola = 64 Pala = 3072 gm.
4 Adhaka	= 1 Drona = 1024 Tola = 256 Pala = 12.288 Kg.
2 Drona	= 1 Shurpa = 2048 Tola = 512 Pala = 24.576 Kg.
2 Shurpa	= 1 Droni = 4096 Tola = 1024 Pala = 49.152 Kg
4 Droni	= 1 Khari = 16384 Tola = 4096 Pala = 196.608 Kg.
2000 Pala	= 1 Bhara = 8000 Tola = 96.00 Kg.
100 Pala	= 1 Tula = 400 Tola=4.8 Kg

Quadraple Formula of Sharngadhara

4 Masha	=	1 Tanka (Shana)
4 Tanka	=	1 Aksha (Karsha)
4 Aksha	=	1 Bilva (Pala)
4 Bilva	=	1 Kudava
4 Kudava	=	1 Prastha
4 Prastha	=	1 Adhaka
4 Adhaka	=	1 Rashi (Drona)
4 Drona	=	1 Goni
4 Goni	=	1 Khari

Poutava Mana of Sushruta

12 Dhanyamasha	=	1 Suvarnamasha
16 Suvarnamasha	=	1 Suvarna (Karsha)
19 Nishpava	=	1 Dharana
2 Dharana	=	1 Karsha

Afterwards, the measurements increase by four folds as Pala, Kudava, Prastha, Adhaka and Drona.

100 Pala	=	1 Tulaa
200 Pala	=	1 Bhara.

Note: This measurement is meant for dry drug. In case of wet, double quantity is accepted.

Kalinga Mana

12 Goura sarshapa	=	1 Yava
2 Yava	=	1 Gunja
3 Gunja	=	1 Valla
8 Gunja	=	1 Masha
4 Masha	=	1 Shana
6 Masha	=	1 Gadyana
10 Masha	=	1 Karsha
4 Karsha	=	1 Pala
4 Pala	=	1 Kudava

2. Druvya Mana of Sushruta:

8 Bindus	=	1 Shana
32 Bindu	=	1 Shukti
64 Bindu	=	1 Panishukti

Bindu = Fluid or liquid obtained after inserting index finger upto 2nd inter phalangeal joint.[12]

3. Payya mana

1 Angula	=	Length of the Thread parred through 8 yavas
12 Angula	=	1 Bitashti (9 inches)
21 Angula	=	1 Aratni (16 1/2 inches)
2 Bitashti	=	1 Hasta (18 inches)
Vyama	=	4 Hands (6 feet)

Metric Weights & Measurements (Modern Methods)

Length:

10 Millimetres	=	1 Centimetre
10 Centimetres	=	1 Decimetre
10 Decimetres	=	1 Metre
10 Metres	=	1 Decametre
10 Decametres	=	1 Hectametre
10 Hectametres	=	1 Kilometre

Volume:

1000 cu Millimetres	=	1 cu Centimetre
1000 cu Centimetres	=	1cu Decimetre
100 cu Decimetres	=	1 cu Metre

Weight:

10 Milligrams	=	1 Centigram
10 Centigrams	=	1 Decigram
10 Decigrams	=	1 Gram
10 Grams	=	1 Decagram
10 Decagrams	=	1 Hectogram
10 Hectograms	=	1 Kilogram
100 Kilograms	=	1 Quintal
10 Quintals	=	1 Ton

Capacity:

10 Millilitres	=	1 Centilitre
10 Centilitres	=	1 Decilitre
10 Decilitres	=	1 Litre
10 Litres	=	1 Decalitre
10 Decalitres	=	1 Hectolitre
10 Hectolitres	=	1 Kilolitre

Area:

12 Inches	=	1 Foot
3 Feet	=	1 Yard

22 Yards	=	1 Chain
10 Chains	=	1 Furlong
8 Furlongs	=	1 Mile
640 Acres	=	1 Sq. Mile
1000 Sqm	=	1 Acre (4840 Sq. yards)
2.47 Acres	=	1 Hectare
247 Acres	=	1 Sq.Km.

Research Carried out About Collection of Medicinal Plants

Medicinal plant collected during periods or seasons show varied alkaloid content, the abstract of such research is given below.

The plants were cultured on specially prepared raised beds 15 cm. high and 5cm. long having 3 tier layers, lowermost of black-cotton soil, middle layer of river sand and raw manure and upper layer—most of black cotton soil, sand and dung mixture (1:1:1). Each tier is of 5cm. thickness. Pieces of rhizomes were planted on different days as per lunar calendar. Growth of plants recorded in 10 replicates with one control was set in during experimentation. The plants were periodically taken out weighed and analysed for active principles.

Chemically analysis was carried as per methods outlined in Paech-Tracey (1955). Osmotic pressure of cell-sap within xylem vessels by specially designed mercury manometers and pressure gauze. Soil temperature was recorded by feues thermometers. Micro-climate data of the surrounding area was collected from local agricultural observatory.

It is observed that percentage of oil within the rhizome vary with intensity of lunar phases and highest percentage could be obtained on full moon days. **(Effects of Phases of Moon on the Growth and Active Principles of Acorus calamuṣ (Bach.), As reported by C.R. Karnick. Published in the Journal Nagarjun-June, 1977).**

Plants were grown on different phases of the moon and on Pushya-nakshatras. Total % percentage of alakaloid was estimated in accordance with the method outlined in Paech & Tracey (1955).

Total constituents, osmotic pressure in Sap (root) and plant growth have relatively high during full moon phase when compared to new moon phase. The maximum growth was seen during the month of October and chemical constituents were found to be high in percentage during this month.

Observation shows that moon rays have a profound effect on the cell-sap within the plants which in turn affect the transpiration, root-pressure and presence of active principles.

So much so, results obtained in clinical trails show that the incidence of recurrence of disease wanes if drugs are properly administered and proper care is taken to understand the underlying Ayurvedic principles. **(Effect of Lunar Phase-days on the Growth and Active Constituents of Medicinal Plants – Series I: Adhatoda vasica Needs. (Adulsa), As reported by C.R. Karnick. Published in the Journal Nagarjun-June, 1977).**

Experimental trials of medicinal plants charged with 'Mantras' or high energized resonance and responses to various ailments are recorded.

Effect of 'Gayatri mantra'—*"Om bhur bhuvah svah tat-savitur-varenyam bhargo devasya dheemahi dhiyo yo nah prochodayat"* on Tulasi (Ocimum sanctum Linn) and its therapeutic effect on patients suffering from stomach-ache, fevers, colic was studied.

The plants in question was charged with 'Gayatri mantra' for 10 days continuously during early mornings between 7 a.m. to 8 a.m. The plants were taken out on the tenth day and the five parts of the plant (i.e. Panca-anga, viz. roots, stems, leaves, flowers and fruits) were powdered into drug and given to the patients on empty stomach with black cow's milk.

The Lakshmana plant was charged with the Mantra *"Om Sri Keshwaya namah"* continuously for 120 days. The plants were taken out on a "Guru-pushya Naksatra" day and 5 parts (Panca-anga) were dried and powdered. A colloidal gel was prepared in a double distilled water and this fluid was sprayed in the left nostrils of the female patients on "Pushya Naksatra day". Spray contain 10 to 100 ppm. of drug, 0.5ml was only used. The urine was tested for steroidal hormones. The menstrual cycle of the females became regular and the presence of estrogens in the urine was found to be increased. The females were found mentally settled, the digestion increased and they could get sound sleep. Later it was observed that it helped in conception of the issues.

Effect of mantra *"Om Anataya namah"* on Tylophora indica Linn. and its effect on patients suffering from bronchial infections was studied. Drug prepared from five parts (Panca-anga) of the plant were administered to patients and the results obtainird have been encouraging. **(Effect of Mantras on Plants, As reported by C.R. Karnick, Published in the Journal Ancient Science of Life, 1983)**

•

References

1. गोपालास्तापसा व्याधा ये चान्ये वनचारिणः।
मूलाहाराश्च ये तेभ्यो भेषजव्यक्तिरिष्यते।। (सु. सू.-36.8)
ओषधीर्नामरूपाभ्यां जानते ह्यजपा वने।
अविपाश्चैव गोपाश्च ये चान्ये वनवासिनः।। (च. सू.-1.121)
नामानि क्वचिदिह रूढितः प्रभावाद्देश्योत्त्या क्वचिदिह लाञ्छनौपमाभ्याम्।
वीर्येण क्वचिदितराह्वयादिदेशाद् द्रव्याणामिह सप्तधोदितानि।।
(रा. नि.-13)
एकं तु नाम प्रथितं बहूनामेकस्य नामानि तथा बहूनि।
द्रव्यस्य जात्याकृतिवर्णवीर्यरसप्रभावादिगुणैर्भवन्ति।।
नामश्रुतं केनचिदेकमेव तेनैव जानाति स भैषजं तु।
अन्यस्तथाऽन्येन तु वेत्ति नाम्ना तदैव चान्योऽथ परे हि कश्चित्।।
बहून्यतः प्राकृतसंस्कृतानि नामानि विज्ञाय बहूंश्च पृष्ट्वा।
दृष्ट्वा च संस्पृश्य च जातिलिङ्गैर्विद्याद्भिषग्भेषजमादरेण।। (ध. नि.-9.11)
2. अल्पोदकद्रुमो यस्तु प्रवातः प्रचुरातपः।
ज्ञेयः स जाङ्गलो देशः स्वल्परोगतमोऽपि च।।
प्रचुरोदकवृक्षो यो निवातो दुर्लभातपः।
अनूपो बहुदोषश्च समः साधारणो मतः।। (च. वि.-3.47-48)
बहूदकनगोऽनूपः कफमारुतरोगवान्।
जाङ्गलोऽल्पाम्बुशाखी च पित्तासृङ्मारुतोत्तरः।
संसृष्टलक्षणो यस्तु देशः साधारणो मतः।। (शा. पू. ख.-1.64-65)
3. 'तत्र यानि कालजातान्युपागतसम्पूर्णप्रमाणरसवीर्यगन्धानि कालातपाग्निसलिलपवन-जन्तुभिरनुपहतगन्धवर्णरसस्पर्शप्रभावाणि प्रत्यग्राण्युदीच्यां दिशि स्थितानि।'
(च. क.-1.10)
4. मंगलाचारः कल्याणवृत्तः शुचिः शुक्लवासाः सम्पूज्य देवता अश्विनौ गोब्राह्मणांश्च प्राङ्मुखः उदङ्मुखो वा गृह्णीयात् । (च.क. 2)

5. 'तेषां शाखापलाशमचिरप्ररूढं वर्षावसन्तयोर्ग्राह्यं, ग्रीष्मे मूलानि, शिशिरे वा शीर्णप्ररूढ-पर्णानां, शरदि त्वक्कन्दक्षीराणि, हेमन्ते साराणि, यथर्तुपुष्पफलमिति।'
(च. क.-1.10)
6. शरद्यखिलकार्यार्थं ग्राह्यं सरसमौषधम्।
विरेक-वमनार्थं च वसन्तान्ते समाहरेत्।। (शा. पू. ख.-1.7-8)
7. आग्नेया विन्ध्यशैलाद्याः सौम्यो हिमगिरिर्मतः।
अतस्तदौषधानि स्युरनुरूपाणि हेतुभिः।। (शा. पू. ख.-1.61-62)
8. जाङ्गमानां वयःस्थानां रक्तरोमनखादिकम्।
क्षीरमूत्रपुरीषाणि जीर्णाहारेषु संहरेत्।। (सु. सू.-36.16)
9. प्रशस्तायां दिशि शुचौ भेषजागारमिष्यते। (सु. सू.-36.17)
प्लोतमृद्भाण्डफलकशङ्कुविन्यस्तभेषजम्। (सु. सू.-36.17)
10. 'मीयतेऽनेन इति मानम्'
पौतवं द्रुवयं पाय्यमिति मानार्थकं त्रयम्। (अमरकोश 2.9.85)
'तुलाद्यैः पौतवं मानं' (हेमचन्द्र)
'द्रुवयं कुडवादिभिः' (हेमचन्द्र)
'पाय्यं हस्तादिभिः' (हेमचन्द्र)
11. कालिङ्गं मागधं चैव द्विविधं मानमुच्यते।
कालिङ्गान्मागधं श्रेष्ठं मानं मानविदो विदुः।। (शा. पू. खं.-1.43)
12. प्रदेशिन्यङ्गुलीपर्वद्वयान्मग्नसमुद्धृतात्।
यावत्पतत्यसौ बिन्दुः..............................।। (अ. हृ. सू.-20.9-10)
तस्य प्रमाणमष्टौ बिन्दवः प्रदेशिनीपर्वद्वयनिःसृता प्रथमा मात्रा, द्वितीया शुक्तिः, तृतीया पाणिशुक्तिः। (सु. चि.-40.28)

•

14

DRAVYA SHODHANA

- Dravya Ashuddhi (Impurities of drugs)
- Dravya Shodhana (Purification of drugs)
- Dravya Krittrimata (Adulteration)

Dravya Ashuddhi
(Impurities of Drugs)

Acharyas of Ayurveda have advocated certain precautions to be observed while collecting the drugs and suggested various methods to separate certain physical impurities (mud etc.) and to detoxicity the poisonous chemical contamination.

According to Sushruta

1. Organic impurities
   - i. Natural
   - ii. Artificial
2. Inorganic impurities
   - i. Natural
   - ii. Artificial

Rasashastra classified the Dravya ashuddhi as

1. Naisargika
   - i. Physical
   - ii. Natural
2. Yaugika
   - i. Chemical
   - ii. Natural
3. Oupadhika
   - i. Chemical
   - ii. Artificial

According to Dravyaguna Vijnana

1. Physical
   - i. Natural
   - ii. Artificial
2. Chemical
   - i. Natural
   - ii. Artificial

Dravya Shodhana
(Purification of Drugs)

The process of removing impurities and increasing the potency and efficacy of a substance is called Shodhana.[1]

There are 8 common procedures of purification. They are as follows:

1. Bhavana

This is a process in which the powdered drugs are soaked or triturated in some liquid for a specific period.

Eg: Hingula in Nimbu swarasa for 3-7 times.

2.Swedana

The process of boiling the drug by suspending in liquids is called Swedana.

Eg: Guggulu in Godugdha or Triphala kashaya.

3. Avapa

This is a process in which some substance is added to the liquified metals.

Eg: Addition of Apamarga kshara to the liquified Vanga.

4. Nirvapa

In this process, metallic drugs are heated and suddenly dipped in liquids.

Eg: Heated copper leaves dipped in Amla drayvas.

5. Mardana

Grinding or pounding the drugs is known as Mardana.

Eg: Mercury (Parada) is grinded with Lashuna kalka and Suddha jala.

6. Patana

Distillation and sublimation.

Eg: Mercury (Parada) after Mardana is heated in Valuka yantra.

7. Bharjana

Frying the drug in the pan with (or) without other substances before powdering is called Bharjana.

Eg: Dry Pippali is fried before powdering, wet Hingu is fried in ghee.

8. Kshalana

Process of washing the drugs to remove impurities is Kshalana.

Eg: Tubers are washed to remove mud.

<u>Purification of some of the drugs</u>

1. Vishamushti

Seeds are tied in a cloth and subjected to sudation and thereafter fried in Goghrita after removing seed coat.

2. Jayapala

Seed coat is removed and subjected to sudation for one Prahara and the process is repeated for 3 times.

3. Dattura

Seeds subjected to sudation in Godugdha for one Prahara and cleaned with Ushna jala.

4. Gunja

Seeds are powdered and subjected to sudation for 1-2 Prahara is Godugdha or Kanjilka.

5. Bhanga

Leaves are subjected to Bharjana in Goghrita or to mild heat.

6. Ahiphena

Ahiphena should be subjected to Mardana for one day in Goghrita.

Dravya krittrimata

(Adulteration)

Adulteration occurs when a drug is scare or when the price of drug is normally high, though there may be no scarcity. The adulterant must be some material which is both cheap and fairly available in large quantities.

Methods of Adulteration:

1. Manufacture of substitutes—Materials are artificially manufactured so as to simulate the general form and appearance of various drugs. Eg: Artificial invert sugar for honey.

2. Substitution of inferior commercial varieties. Eg: Provence Senna (Cassia auriculata) used to adulterate Senna.

3. Substitution of exhausted drugs—Some drugs are used in very large amounts for the manufacture of preparations after which the vegetable residue retain very much the appearance of the original material. Eg: Preparation of volatile oils from cloves and cardamom. Removal of colouring matter and recolouring by artificial dyes is done with saffron.

4. Substitution of superficially similar but cheaper natural substances, usually having no relation of the genuine articles. Eg: clove stalks and mother cloves are often mixed with cloves.

5. Addition of worthless heavy materials. Eg: Pieces of limestone in Hingu (Asafoetida) and lead shot pieces in Ahipena (opium).

6. Addition of synthetic principles to fortify inferior products such as adding citral to oil of lemon.

7. The presence of adventitious matter naturally occurring with drug if in excessive amount also constitutes an adulteration.

8. For powdered materials, generally powdered waste products of a suitable colour and density are used. Eg: Powdered olive stones to drugs like powdered liquorice or pepper.

Detection of adulteration fall in to two main sections:

i. Establishment of the identify of the adulterant.
ii. Determination of the quality of the drug.

Establishment of identity:

a. Gross morphology
b. Histology and microscopical morphology
c. Microscopical linear measurements
d. Solubilities
e. Qualitative chemical tests
f. Physical constants such as specific gravity, viscosity, refractive index for oils etc.
g. Ultraviolet light.

Determination of quality:

a. Process of assay for alkaloid, resin, volatile oil, glycoside etc.
b. Yield to solvents
c. Ash
d. Crude fibre

In Ayurvedic literature the references are available indicating Grahya-Agrahya lakshanas of certain substances like Shilajita, Pravala, Mukta which help us for establishing geneunity of the drug. The author of Rajanighantu has described certains tests to identify the artificial or adulterated Kasturi (musk). Adulteration which is in practice among certain Ayurvedic drugs are mentioned below.

1. Chitramula	:	Badaramula (or) Amalaki mula twak.
2. Chavya	:	Maricha mula.
3. Kayaphala	:	Instead of its fruit, stem bark or Kumbhi twak are used.
4. Hingu	:	Unctuous powder is stained with yellow colour.
5. Shilajita	:	It may be prepared artificially by mixing, Gomutraghana, Triphala-ghana, Lauha-raja, Kachu, Surekshara, Kanyasara, citric acid etc.
6. Madhu	:	Artificially prepared from jaggery.
7. Yashtimadhu	:	Gunja root.
8. Guduchi sattwa	:	Rice flour + lime.
9. Dasamoola	:	Only bark/Aerial parts of some plants.
10. Vansalochana	:	Artificial silicon like substance.

Are the Ayurvedic Purificatory Procedures Rational ?

Ayurvedic texts described certain purificatory procedures (Shodhana) for certain poisonous drugs before incorporating them into formulations. In recent researches it was observed that the ancient purificatory procedures can significantly reduce the toxicity of poisonous substances and one such example is quoted below.

The crude drug root of aconite contains about 1.4 percent of total alkaloids whereas the root treated with cow's urine contains only 1.27 percent alkaloid. Treatment with cow's urine and exposure to sunlight have brought about a partial change of the toxic alkaloids i.e., aconitine and pseduo-aconitine into far less poisonous substances benzyl-aconitine and veratsoyl (Kirtikar & Basu).

●

References

1. 'मलविच्छित्तयोर्यत्तु शोधनं तदिहोच्यते।' (रसतरङ्गिणी-2.52)

●

15

BESHAJA PRAYOGA VIJNANA

- Prashasta Bheshaja (Characteristics of a good drug)
- Bheshaja-prayoga (Usage of drug)
- Prayojya Anga (Parts used)
- Dravya-samyoga-virudha (Incompatability of drugs)
- Aushadhi yoga (Drug formulations)
- Dravya Matra-nirupana (Discussion on the quantity and posology of drug)
- Anupana-vyavastha (Vehicle)
- Bhaishajya kala (Time of administration)
- Bhaishajya Prayoga-marga (Routes of medication)
- Aushadhi Vyavasthapatra Lekhana (Knowledge of prescription writing)

Prashasta Bheshaja
(Characteristics of Good Drugs)

Bheshaja is one of the Chatushpadas. Bheshaja (medicament) should be prepared in many forms and by different processes. They should possess many valuable properties. The constituents (herbs) with which they are manufactured should be grown in proper soil, fully matured and gathered in a proper season, having regard to the principles and rules prescribed for their collection, curing and storage, and prepared suitably as specified for each disease. The following four characteristics are mentioned for Bheshaja in the classical texts of Ayurveda.[1]

1. Yogyata	:	Must be eligible for medicaments.
2. Bahuta	:	Availability in abundant quantity.
3. Aneka Vidha Kalpana	:	Available in various forms or Kalpana.
4. Sampat	:	Possess all the properties like Rasa, Guna, Virya, Vipaka and Karma in optimum quantity.

As far as possible only fresh drugs or plants should be used in medicine, the exceptions are Vidanga (Embelia ribes), Pippali (Piper longum), jaggery, coriander, ghee and honey.

Bheshaja Prayoga
(Usage of Drug)

While administering the drug one has to consider the various factors like part used, incompatibility, dosage, vehicle and time of administration etc. When two drugs having similar potencies are combined the final effect of the Aushadha gets increased which is called 'synergism'. When the drug is soaked in Swarasa, the power of the drug is enhanced.

Nomenclature of Aushadha yogas is based on—

1. Main drug Eg: Ashwagandhadi lehya
2. Inventor's name Eg: Bhaskara lavana
3. Similarity with other item Eg: Rasa parpati.
4. Main action Eg: Swhasakuthara, Rechaka vati etc.

Prayojya Anga
(Part Used)

Oudbhida Dravya:[2]

1. Mula (root) Eg: Bilva
2. Twak (bark) Eg: Aswattha
3. Sara (heart wood) Eg: Khadira
4. Niryasa (resin) Eg: Guggulu
5. Nala (tubes) Eg: Kamala
6. Swarasa (juice)
7. Pallava (tender leaves) Eg: Jambu
8. Kshara (alkalies) Eg: Apamarga
9. Kshira (latex) Eg: Snuhi
10. Phala (fruit) Eg: Haritaki
11. Pushpa (flower) Eg: Dhataki
12. Bhasma (ash) Eg: Triphala
13. Taila (oil) Eg: Eranda
14. Kantaka (spines) Eg: Shalmali
15. Patra (leaf) Eg: Talisha
16. Shrunga (terminal bud) Eg: Vata
17. Kanda (tubers/rhizome) Eg: Surana
18. Praroha (areial root) Eg: Vata

Jangama Dravya[3]

1. Madhu (honey)	6. Rakta (blood)
2. Gorasa (milk products)	7. Mamsa (meat)
3. Pitta (bile)	8. Vit (faeces)
4. Vasa (lard)	9. Mutra (urine)
5. Majja (bone marrow)	10. Charma (skin)
11. Shukra (semen)	14. Shringa (horns)
12. Asthi (bone)	15. Nakha (nails)
13. Snayu (ligaments)	16. Khura (hoofs)

Dravya Samyoga-Viruddha
(Incompatibility of Drugs)

Those substances, which cause the increase of Dosas in the body but do not expel them out (of the body) are known as Viruddha, and so they remain antagonistic to the Dhatus (tissues).

Even naturally, imcompatability happens by the combination of substances in respect of their strength of qualities, of unequal or equal proportions or both, or by different processes of cooking.

Milk is incompatable along with Kulattha, Panasa fruit with Matsya; boiled curds, mixtures of equal quantities of honey and ghee, water of alkaline regions, partaking flour made into thick solution with water at night; and Yavaka (small variety of barely) are all incompatibles.

The use of incompatable foods will produce boils, swelling, toxicity, abscess, tumours of the abdomen, tuberculosis; loss of vigour, strength, memory, sense perceptions and intellect; fever, haemorrhagic diseases, the eight Mahagadas (dreaded diseases) and even death just like poison.[4]

<u>Notes:</u> The eight dreaded diseases are Vatavyadhi (disease of the nervous system), Ashmari (renal calculus), Kushta (leprosy and other skin diseases), Meha (Urinary abnormalities), Udara, (enlargement of the abdomen), Bhagandara (fistula-in-ano), Arshas (haemorrhoids) and Grahani (disease of the duodenum).

Usage of two or more combination of Dravyas is Samyoga. It may be Hitakara (or) Ahitakara. The Ahitakara samyoga is called Viruddhata. This is of 3 types—

1. Mana-viruddha : Madhu and Ghrita in equal quantities.

2. Guna-viruddha	:	Rasa – Madhura and Lavana. Virya – Matsya and Dugdha.
3. Karma-viruddha	:	Kutaja + Danti.

According to Charaka, Viruddhatwa is of 18 types—

1. Desha	:	Dependent on area. Eg: Usage of Ruksha dravyas in Jangala desha.
2. Kala	:	Dependent on time. Eg: Usage of Ruksha dravya in winter.
3. Agni	:	Dependent on digestion. Eg: Over eating in Agnimandya.
4. Matra	:	Dependent on dose. Eg: Honey and ghee in equal ratios.
5. Satmya	:	Depends on habit. Eg: Habituated to pungent and hot foods and consuming sweet and cold substance.
6. Dosha	:	Depends on humors. Eg: In Vata-prakruti Vata-vriddhi.
7. Samskara	:	Depends on procedure. Eg: Peacock meat fried in castor oil.
8. Virya	:	Depends on potency. Eg: Ushna dravya + Sheeta dravya.
9. Koshta	:	Depends on GIT. Eg: Mild laxative in severe constipation.
10. Avastha	:	Depends on the conditions. Eg: Giving Vata-vardhakas to a exhausted person.
11. Parihara	:	Depends on Parihara. Eg: Consuming pork and then hot water immediately.
12. Krama	:	Eg: Consuming food without proper cleaning.
13. Upachara	:	Eg: Consuming ghee and then cold water.
14. Paka	:	While cooking. Eg: Over roasted rice.

15. Samyoga	:	Combination. Eg: Milk and sour substances.
16. Hritvirodha	:	Distaste. Eg: Consuming foods having distaste.
17. Sampat	:	Dependent on quality–Vikrit rasa-dravya sevana.
18. Vidhi	:	Dependent on eating procedures. Eg: Not eating alone or laughing & speaking while eating.

Aushadi Yoga

In the Ayurvedic therapeutics either single drug or compound formulations are mainly prescribed.

The recipes are named after the principal ingredients and not after the ingredients having secondary therapeutic value. These ingredients like alcohol, however, follow the effects of the principal drugs used in the recipe.

Sometimes the drugs of secondary nature have antagonistic potency. Even then they do not contradict the effects of the principal drug. If these drugs of secondary nature are similar in potency as that of the principal drugs, then the recipe becomes all the more effective therapeutically.

Eg. Principal drugs like Danti, etc. have strong action, and meat-soup etc. are added to the recipes of Danti are mild in action. Ela, etc., are cardiac tonics. When added to emetic drugs like Madana, they are likely to reduce the emetic effect.

Drugs of antagonistic potency are added to a recipe in order to impart desirable colour, taste, touch and smell. Such addition also helps to effectively cure the diseases.

Emetic and purgative recipes (therapies) are administered for the treatment of several diseases. But the disease cannot be fully cured simply by emesis or purgation. Therefore, in emetic and purgative recipes, some other drugs, even those having opposite potencies, are added so that the recipe as a whole becomes effective to cure the disease.

In addition to adding to the potency of the recipe, it is necessary to impregnate the ingredients of a recipe with the juice or decoction of other drugs. When properly impregnated, even a small quantity of the drug becomes exceedingly effective. Therefore, ingredients of a recipe should be impregnated with the juice or decoction of other ingredients having identical potency.

By virtue of appropriate Samyoga (addition of ingredients), Vishlesha (elimination of ingredients), Kala (appropriate time of administration) and Samskara (processing) even a small quantity of a drug may produce more powerful effects, and otherwise even a recipe in large quantity may produce very mild effects.

If a drug is added with ingredients having identical potency, then the effect of the recipe taken even in small quantity becomes more powerful. Similarly, if a drug is added with ingredients having opposite potency then the effect of the recipe taken even in large quantity becomes milder. In certain cases, the milder effect of the recipe is necessary in order to make it suitable to the requirements of the nature of Kostha (nature of bowel).

In the same way, the effects of Vishlesha (elimination of ingredients), Kala (time of administration) and Samskara (processing) can be explained and illustrated.

The roots of Danti and Dravanti should be smeared with the paste (of the powder) of Pippali and honey, and covered with Kusha. The bundle should then be smeared with mud and fomented with steam. Thereafter, the roots should be taken out and dried in the sun. By the exposure to the heat of the fire and sun, the Vikashi attribute (toxic effect which causes looseness of joints) is removed. Because of the effects of the heat of fire and sun-rays, Danti and Dravanti do not produce much of adverse effects.

The nomenclature of a Yoga is given basing on the important drug (e.g. Ashwagandhadi lehya), inventor's name (eg. Bhaskara lavana), indication (e.g. Shwasakuthara, Shulakuthara) and the appearance of the processed drug (eg. Rasaparpati) etc.

Dravya Matra Nirupana

(Discussion on the Quantity and Posology of Drug)

Chakrapani in his book Chakradutta mentions that there is no fixity of a dose of drugs. It should be decided according to Doshas, digestive fire (Agni), strength (Bala), age, disease, drugs and bowels (Koshtha). However, in respect of fatty preparations (Ghrita, Taila etc.), decoctions (Kwatha), juces etc. high, medium and low doses are one Pala (40 gm.), three Karshas (30 gm) and two Karshas (20 gm) respectively.

Matra is decided according to the following considerations:

1. Ayu : According to Sharngadhara,[5]

Child of 1 month	-	1 Ratti
Upto 1 year	-	1 Ratti every month (1.5 gm)
Upto 16 years	-	16 gms (One Masha every year)
Upto 70 years	-	Same dose

After 70 years-decrease at the rate of one Masha every year.

This dosage schedule is meant for Kalka and Churnas and for Kwatha the quantity should be 4 times to it.

Eg: upto 70 years = 64 ml.

2. Bala (strength)
3. Linga (sex)
4. Agni (Jatharagni)
5. Dosha
6. Vyadhi
7. Koshta
8. Dravya
9. Prakrutika asahishnuta
10. Abhyasa
11. Sattva
12. Desha
13. Kala
14. Kalpa

According to modern aspect, Matra is as follows:

Dose of a drug is defined as the quantity of drug required to be given at a time to produce desired effect. The dose is influenced by many factors such as—Age and weight of the patient.

Generally children require smaller doses than adults. Child dose can be calculated by Young's formula,

$$\frac{\text{Age of child}}{\text{Age of child} + 12} \text{xAdult dose}$$

A child above the age of 12 years receives adult dose. After the drug is completely absorbed, the blood concentration will depend upon the blood volume of the patient. Since blood volume has a fixed relation with the lean body weight (fat free body), the dose is often correlated with body weight to give comparable blood levels of a drug.

Sex:

Adult females usually require smaller dose than of males. This is probably because females have slightly less blood volume compared to their fat due to the presence of more fat.

Severity of a disease:

Dose varies with the severity of disease. Dose should be increased as per the severity but there are certain exceptions. In iron deficiency anaemia, dose of iron salt administered orally will remain the same irrespective of severity.

State of health and nutrition:

Debilitated and anaemic people are given smaller dose.

Pathological state:

Smaller doses are indicated if the organs of bio-transformation or excretion of a drug are diseased.

Eg: Morphine should be given in smaller doses to patients suffering from liver diseases.

Tolerance:

Patient may develop tolerance to the effect of drug if administered repeatedly and in such a situation larger dose should be given.

Anupana Vyasvastha

(Vehicle)

The liquid that is consumed along with drug or after the intake of drug is called Anupana.[6]

Just as the oil spreads quickly when put into water, so also the quick absorption and spread of the medicine is facilitated due to the addition of Anupana.

An after-drink (Anupana) tones up the body, gives satisfaction, invigorates, causes plumpiness, gives a feeling of contentment, makes the food move downwards easily, breaks the hard materials of the food, makes them soft, moistens them, helps for easy digestion and distribution to all the parts of the body.

After drink is to be avoided by those who are suffering from diseases of the parts of the body above the shoulders, dyspnoea, cough, excess salivation, hiccup, hoarseness of voice, injury to the chest and those who are indulging in too much of singing and speaking. For such persons, the after drink disturbs the stomach and chest, increases the moisture of the food in the throat and causes watery discharges from the tissues, indigestion, vomiting and other diseases.

After taking such a drink, person should not indulge in speaking, singing, walking long distances and sleeping.

Persons who are suffering from accumulation of moisture in the body, polyurea, diseases of the throat, eyes and ulcers should not take a after drink.

As an Anupana (after-drink, liquid to be taken after meals) water is the best because it is the chief source of all the tastes, it is accustomed to all living beings and possesses the properties of sustaining of life etc. It should be taken cold, after consuming curds, honey, barley, wheat and all other foods which cause burning sensation during digestion and in Sharat (autumn) and Grishma (summer) seasons. It should be taken hot, after consuming foods prepared from corn flour and such other substances which are hard to digest.

According to disease condition,

1. Vata rogas	:	Snigdha & Ushna padarthas
2. Pitta rogas	:	Madhura & Shitala
3. Kapha rogas	:	Ruksha & Ushna
4. Kshaya (Dhatu)	:	Mamsa rasa (soups)
5. Exhausted by various reasons	:	Kshira (milk)
6. Krisha (lean person)	:	Sura (beverage)
7. Sthula (obese)	:	Madhu (honey)
8. Agnimandya (loss of appetite)	:	Madya (alcohol)

According to 'Vaidyajivana' Anupanas indicated in various Vyadhis are:

	Roga	*Anupana*
1.	Shula	Hingu, Ghrita
2.	Jeerna jwara	Pippali, Madhu
3.	Vata-vyadhi	Rasona, Ghrita
4.	Shwasa	Trikatu+Madhu
5.	Prameha	Triphala+Sharkara
6.	Jwara	Musta+Parpataka
7.	Grahani	Takra (butter milk)

8.	Visha	Gold
9.	Chardi	Laja
10.	Atisara	Kutaja
11.	Raktapitta	Vasa
12.	Arshas	Chitramula
13.	Krimi	Vidanga

Bhaishajya Kala
(Time of Administration)

According to Charaka:

If the Apana-vayu is vitiated, then the medicine should be given before food. If the Samana-vayu is vitiated, then the medicine should be given during the meal. If Vyana-vayu is vitiated then the medicine should be given after the morning meal. If Udana-vayu is vitiated, then the medicine should be given after the meal. If Prana-vayu is vitiated, then the medicine should be given along with each morsel of food or in between morsels of food. In asthma, cough and morbid thirst, the medicine should be given at short intervals frequently. To the patient suffering from hiccup, medicine should be given before and after food by adding to the light articles of food. In anorexia, medicine should be mixed with various types of delicious food.

As regards the time with reference to the disease (Vyadhi), the patient suffering from fever should be given Peya (thin gruel), Kasaya (decoctions), mediciated milk, medicated Ghee and purgation therapy consecutively at an interval of six days after observing the duration (number of the days of suffering) of the disease.

Gushada Jirna-linga: Appearance of hunger, proper evacuation of stool and urine, lightness of the body and purity (of eructation)—these are the signs of proper digestion of the drugs as well as diet.

According to Sharngadhara

Medicines are generally administered in the morning specially so the Kashayas (decoctions). Sunrise, the time of midday meal, night meal, frequent intervals, and bed-time—these are the five suitable times for the administration of medicines.[7]

In diseases of Kapha and Pitta and for the purpose of Vamana (emesis), Vireka (purgation) and Lekhana (scarification) medicines should be administered in the mornings. This is the first period for the administration of medicines.

In diseases of Apanavata, medicines are given just before mid-day meal, in cases of Aruchi (anorexia) they should be given mixed with morsels of food, in disorders of Samanavata, for Agni-dipana (kindling of digestion) medicines are best given in the middle of the meal, in disorders of Vyanavata, end of the meal is best; in diseases like Hikka (hiccough), Akshepaka (convulsions) and Kampa (tremors) both times (before and after meals). This is the second period for the administration of medicines.

In disorders of Udanavata and disease like Swara-bhanga (hoarseness) etc, medicines are given between each morsel of night meal; in disorders of Pranavata it should be after the meal. This is the third period.

In diseases like Thrisna (thirst), Chardi (vomiting), Hikka (hiccough), Shwasa (dyspnoea) and Gara (homicidal poisoning) medicines are to be given at frequent intervals or along with food. This is the fourth period.

In diseases of the head and for Lekhana (curetting action), Brimhana (strengthening and fattening action), Pachana (digestive action) and Shamana (palliative action) medicines should be given on empty stomach at night. This is the fifth period.

According to Chakrakapni Dutta

The times of administration of medicines are eleven in number such as—without food, before meals, during meals, after meals, mixed with food during its preparation itself, in between meals (of afternoon and night), at the commencement and end of the meals, often (frequently) irrespective of meals, mixed or along with one morsel, in between such morsels and at night (bed time).

Charaka[8]	***Vagbhata***	***Sharngadhara***
1. Bhaktadau	1. Abhakta	1. Suryodaya
2. Bhaktamadhya	2. Pragbhakta	2. Divasa bhojana
3. Muhurmuhuh	3. Madhya-bhakta	3. Sayam bhojana
4. Samudga	4. Adho-bhakta	4. Muhurmuhuh
5. Bhaktha samyuta	5. Sama-bhakta	5. Nishi
6. Sagrasa	6. Antara-bhakta	
7. Grasantara	7. Samudga	

Charaka	*Vagbhata*	*Sharngadhara*
8. Nishi	8. Muhurmuhuh	
	9. Sagrasa	
	10. Grasantara	
	11. Nishi	

The frequency of drug administration is mainly determined by its biological half life. Biological half life of a drug is the time required for the blood level to drop down to 50% of the initial peak level. If the blood level of the drug is to be maintained half the initial (loading) dose will have to be given at intervals equal to its biological half life. In certain instances biological half life of a drug has no relation to frequency of administration. Tranquillising effect of reserpine appears long after its administration and is still present after all reserpine is eliminated from the body. Twice a day administration of reserpine is therefore enough to maintain the effect though the biological half life is only 4 hours. Certain drugs are administered on empty stomach, before meals and after meals also.

Intake of food in the condition of undigested drug or that of drug in case of indigestion of food does not alleviate the disease, instead it gives rise to other diseases. Vayu normalised in its course, general normalcy, hunger, thirst, feeling of well-being, lightness and clarity of the sensation and eructation are indicative signs of complete digestion of the drugs. Feeling of exhaustion, burning sensation, lassitude, giddiness, fainting, headache, restlessness and loss of strength indicate the complete digestion of the drug. Drug which is administered on empty stomach becomes more potent and alleviates the disease without delay but children, old people, women and delicate persons suffer from complications like depression and debility.

Bhaishajya Prayoga-marga
(Routes of Medication)

The Aushadha for reaching its Adhishtana must be administered by different routes. According to Charaka, in Amashaya rogas, drug must be administered through mouth, in Shirogata rogas through nose and in Pakwashayagata rogas it must be administered through Guda (anus).

Bhaishajya-marga is of two types according to the variety of treatment.

1. Antharparimarjana
2. Bahirparimarjana

<u>I. Antah Parimarjana</u>

1. Mouth	:	Vamana, Virechana
2. Guda	:	Vasti, Varti
3. Nasika	:	Nasya karma
4. Mutra-marga	:	Uttara vasti
5. Yoni-marga	:	Uttara vasti

<u>II. Bahih Parimarjana</u>

1. Twak	:	Abhyanga, Sweda, Murdhataila
2. Netra	:	Aschyotana, Anjana, Putapaka etc.

Routes of administration influence the absorption and excretion of the drugs. The following are the channels of administration.

1. Oral Route

This is the most commonly employed route for drug.
Eg: Pills, powders, capsules.

2. Sub-lingual Administration

Rapid onset of absorption and quick termination of drug's effect.

3. Enema

Administration of medicines in a liquid form into the rectum is called enema. It is of 2 types:

<u>a. Evacuation enema:</u> The quantity of fluid administered at a time is about 600 ml. Eg: Soap water enema.

<u>b. Retention enema:</u> The quantity of fluid administered is usually 100-120ml. The fluid containing the drug is retained in the rectum so that drug may act systematically after absorption through the mucous membrane. Eg: Paraldehyde enema for production of basal anaesthesia.

4. Parental

<u>a. Inhalation:</u> Drugs given by this route are quickly absorbed and produce rapid local and systemic effects. Drugs may be administered as solid particles as nebulized particles from solution or in the form of vapour.

<u>b. Injection:</u> This method is also imperative in the case of

drugs likely to be decomposed in the gut and absorbed in an inactive form.

Varieties: Intradermal, subcutaneous, intramuscular, intravenous, intraarterial, Intrathecal, Intraperitoneal, intraarticular.

5. Iontophoresis

Galvanic current is used for bringing about the penetration of drugs into deeper tissues.

6. Inuction

Drugs rubbed into the skin can get absorbed and produce their systemic effect. Eg: Nitrate ointment in angina pectoris, subcutaneous implantation of solid pellets. Eg: Synthetic oestrogens.

A drug may exert different effects when given by different routes:

rug	*Route*	*Action*
1. Magnesium Sulphate	Oral	Purgative
2. Magnesium Sulphate	Intravenous	Anti-convulsant
3. Hypertonic Magnesium Sulphate	Rectum	Reduces intracranial tension

Aushadhi Vyavasthapatra Lekahana

(Knowledge of Prescription Writing)

The prescription is an order to a chemist to supply certain drugs in a particular form to a patient to be used as directed.

The details of prescription are usually written in the following order:

1. The superscription, or heading which consists of the sign R_j, which originally representing the eye of hours and later an invocation to Jupiter, now stands for the initial of 'Recipe' — Take of.

2. The inscription, which designates—

a. The ingredients

b. The quantity of each required.

The names of the ingredients should be written each on a separate line, followed by the quantity ordered and the last item should be the solvent or diluent.

This part of the prescription usually consists of—

a. The basis or principal active ingredient.

b. The adjuvants or that which assists its action.
c. The corrigens or that which corrects its operation.
d. The vehicle or excipient which imparts an agreeable form.

The abbreviation 'aa' for ana meaning of each, is used to avoid repetition of same quantity.

3. The subscription, which gives directions to the dispenser as to:

a. The form of the remedy.
b. Instructions relating to its preparation.
c. Quantity to be sent and manner of sending.

4. The signature (from signature-let it be labelled) consisting of direction to the patient which are to be written on the lable.

The directions to the patient to be written on the lable should answer the questions — how much, how often, when and in what manner the substances to be taken or applied.

5. The patient's name — this part of the prescription is better written on the top.

6. The name or initials of the prescriber and the date on which the prescription was written.

●

References

1. बहुता तत्र योग्यत्वमनेकविधकल्पना।
सम्पच्चेति चतुष्कोऽयं द्रव्याणां गुण उच्यते।। (च. सू.-9.7)
2. मूलत्वक्सारनिर्यासनालस्वरसपल्लवाः ।
क्षाराः क्षीरं फलं पुष्पं भस्मतैलानि कण्टकाः।।
पत्राणि शुङ्गाः कन्दाश्च प्ररोहाश्चौद्भिदो गणः।। (च. सू.-1.74-75)
अतिस्थूलजटा याः स्युस्तासां ग्राह्यास्त्वचो बुधैः।।
3: मधूनि गोरसाः पित्तं वसा मज्जाऽसृगामिषम्।
विण्मूत्रचर्मरेतोऽस्थि स्नायुशृङ्गनखा खुराः।
जङ्गमेभ्यः प्रयुज्यन्ते केशा रोमानि रोचनाः।। (च. सू.-1.69-70)

4. षाण्ढ्यान्ध्यवीसर्पदकोदराणां विस्फोटकोन्मादभगन्दराणाम्।
मूर्च्छामदाध्मानगलग्रहाणां पाण्ड्वामयस्यामविषस्य चैव।।
किलासकुष्ठग्रहणीगदानां शोथाम्लपित्तज्वरपीनसानाम्।
सन्तानदोषस्य तथैव मृत्योर्विरुद्धमन्नं प्रवदन्ति हेतुम्।।
(च. सू.-26.102-103)

5. बालस्य प्रथमे मासि देया भेषजरत्तिका।।
अवलेही कृतैकैव क्षीरक्षौद्रसिताघृतैः।
वर्धयेत्तावदेकैकां यावद्भवति वत्सरः।।
माषैर्वृद्धिस्तदूर्ध्वं स्याद्यावत्षोडशवत्सरः।
ततः स्थिरा भवेत्तावद्यावद्वर्षाणि सप्ततिः।।
ततो बालकवन्मात्रा ह्रासनीया शनैः शनैः।
मात्रेयं. कल्कचूर्णानां कषायाणां चतुर्गुणा।। (शा. पू. ख.-6.44-52)

6. 'अनु सह पश्चात् वा पीयते इति अनुपानम्।'
सर्वेषामनुपानानां माहेन्द्रं तोयमुत्तमम्। (सु. सू.-46.439)
रोचनं बृंहणं वृष्यं दोषसङ्घातभेदनम्।
तर्पणं मार्दवकरं श्रमक्लमहरं सुखम्।।
दीपनं दोषशमनं पिपासाच्छेदनं परम्।
बल्यं वर्णकरं सम्यगनुपानं सदोच्यते।। (सु. सू.-46.442-443)

7. ज्ञेयः पञ्चविधः कालो भैषज्यग्रहणे नृणाम्।
किञ्चित् सूर्योदये जाते तथा दिवसभोजने।।
सायन्तने भोजने च मुहुश्चापि तथा निशि। (शा. पू. ख.-2.2-3)

8. भैषज्यकालो भक्तादौ भक्तमध्ये मुहुर्मुहः ।
सामुद्गं भक्तसंयुक्तं ग्रासे ग्रासान्तरे निशि । (च.चि.-30)

●

16
History of Dravyaguna

- Pracheena kala – Veda & Dravyaguna (Seeds of Dravya-guna)
- Madhyama kala
- Adhunika kala

Ayurvedic classics divided the entire subject of Ayurveda (Science of life) into eight branches otherwise known as Ashtanga Ayurveda. Though the classification which commanded a lot of recognition and respect for several centuries, it was the author of Rajanighantu (approx. 17th century A.D.) who modified the classification and included Dravyaguna for the first time as one of the eight branch of Ayurveda.

History of Ayurveda is broadly divided into the following periods:

Prachina kala	-	4000 BC – 7 AD
Madhyama kala	-	8 AD – 15 AD
Adhunika kala	-	16th AD onwards

Pracheena Kala

In the Vedic literature the drug classification was described elaborately. In the Purusha-sukta of Rigveda all the substances are divided into Sashana (Chetana) and Anashana (Achetana). Medicinal plants are classified such as Apushpa (without flowers), Sapushpa (with flowers), Phalini (with fruit) and Aphalini (without fruits).

In Rigveda, the synonym 'Vanina' is given to Vanaspatya. Certain drugs are retaining the same nomenclature described in Vedas.
Eg: Ashwattha, Udumbara.

Some of the names have been distorted.
Eg: Kashmarya for Kasamarya.

Discussing about numerical expression of plants historians concluded that 67, 81, 89 herbs were described in Rigveda, Yajurveda and Atharvaveda respectively. Fundamental principles of drug action have been discussed briefly in the Vedic literuature. Dwidha viryavada was also proposed regarding the concept of drug action.

Rasayana, Vajeekarana, Nidra-janana, Kasahara, Balya, Deepana, Rakshoghna, Kesha-vardhana, Vishaghna are some of the pharmacological actions discussed in Vedas. Out of 18 Puranas many a single drug claims are mentioned in Agnipurana.

Charaka, Sushruta and Vagbhata (Ashtanga Sangraha & Ashtanga Hridaya) agree on the point that Ayurveda is the Upanga/ Upaveda of Rigveda or Atharvaveda consisting of eight parts. The Chinese traveller I. Tsing (671-695AD) knew those eight parts of Indian medicine and opined that these eight parts (arts) of Ayurveda existed originally in eight books and at a later stage brought together into a single book i.e. Samhita. The total number of Sanskrit names of herbs are about 1270, 1100 and 1150 in Sushruta Samhita, Charaka Samhita and Ashtanga Hridaya respectively.

The exercise of inclusion of new drugs into Ayurvedic Materia Medica started during 9th century and Vrinda, the author of Siddhayoga incorporated a new drug namely Parasika yavani (a drug imported from Persia) and at a later stage the authors of Dhanwantari Nighantu and Paryaya-ratna-mala introduced opium, Bhanga in their works. During the 15th century Bhavaprakasha incorporated Dwipantara vacha into Ayurvedic medicine and Narahari of Rajanighantu introduced another new drug namely Jhandu.

Samhita Kala

Charaka Samhita

In the Sutrasthana, first chapter, drugs are classified according to the source and in the same chapter another classification basing on Doshas i.e., Dosha-prashamana, Dhatu-pradushana and Swastahitha is given. In the 4th chapter, drug classification basing on pharmacological actions (into 50 groups) is described and in the 27th chapter Ahara dravyas are classified into 12 Vargas. Agrya oushadhis are mentioned in the 25th chapter.

Sushruta Samhita

Sushruta described Ahara and Aushadha dravyas in different Vargas. Ahara dravyas are mentioned in Sutrasthana 45 & 46 chapters and Aushadha dravyas are classified in to 44 groups and included them in 38 & 39 chapters. He has also enumerated celestial (Divya) plants like Soma with their geographical distribution. He introduced two Vargas i.e. Dhatu varga and Ratna varga.

Ashtanga Sangraha

Vagbhata mentioned 50 groups enumerated by Charaka in 14 & 15 chapters of Sutrasthana. Twenty five Vargas of Sushruta are described in the 18th chapter. He specifically introduced some Ganas namely Padmaka, Asana, Vatsakadi, Trijataka, Chaturjataka, Madhyama and Jeevaniya panchamulas, Panchakola etc. Ahara dravyas are described in 6 & 7 chapters. The description of Lavana, Kshara, Dhatu, and Ratna are collectively discussed in the chapter 26th (Vividhoushadha Vijnaniya).

Astanga Hridaya

Vagbhata followed Sushruta and described 33 groups in the 15th chapter of Sutrasthana. Regarding Ahara dravyas, Drava-ahara dravyas are descrbed in 5 Vargas and Anna dravyas in 7 Vargas. Charaka's Ganas were not quoted by Vagbhata of Ashtanga Hridaya.

Madhyama Kala

Ashtanga Nighantu

Ashtanga Nighantu is the work of Vahatacharya who is considered to be different from the author of Ashtanga Sangraha and Ashtanga Hridaya since some new drugs were mentioned in this Nighantu. Jejjata (9th AD), Chakrapani dutta (11th AD) and the author of Paryaya-ratna-mala (9th AD) have mentioned this work by which one can conclude that the Nighantu was written during 8th century AD. In this Nighantu only Paryayas (synonyms of various drugs) are mentioned.

Paryayaratnamala:

Indrakarasunu Madhava was the author of this book. Sarvananda (13th AD) quoted about Paryayaratnamala in his work. The drugs namely Ahiphena, Bhanga mentioned in Dhanwantari Nighantu and Rasaratna Samuchchaya (10th AD) are described in this work. This work may be placed between 8th-9th A.D.

The synonyms of various drugs were also mentioned in this work.

Dhanwantari Nighantu

According to the opinion of most of the scholars this Nighantu is considered to be the oldest and foremost Nighantu with the details pertaining to pharmacological and therapeutic profiles about the drugs. Since the manuscripts available in different libraries indicate about the mentioning of Ahiphena, Bhanga, Jayapala etc; it can be safely concluded that this work belongs to medieval period. The author of this book is Mahendra Boghika. As per the external evidence this work was quoted by the commentator of Amarakosha namely Kshiraswamy (11 AD) and Hemadri and Arunadutta (13 AD); This work may be placed between 10-13 AD. The drugs are described in 7 Vargas namely Guduchyadi, Shatapushpadi, Chandanadi, Karaviradi, Amradi, Suvarnadi and Mishrakadi.

Dravyaguna Samgraha

Chakrapani Dutta (11th AD) described mainly Ahara dravyas under 15 Vargas. In the beginning of this work the fundamental principles i.e., Rasa, Guna, Virya, etc. were discussed.

Shodhala Nighantu

Shodhala, the author of this Nighantu followed Dhanwantari Nighantu and described the contents in 27 Vargas. Among these Vargas Lakshmanadi varga is considered to be most important. The author followed Ashtanga Hridaya to describe Rasa, Guna, Virya, Vipaka etc. He is famous for his brevity about the pharmacological and therapeutic implication of drugs. Sharngadhara (13 AD) and Madanapala (14 AD) followed Shodhala in their works. Basing on this evidence Shodhala can be placed between 10-13 AD. His another work is Gada-nigraha. Ahiphena and Bhanga were referred in Gada-nigraha but these drugs were not mentioned in Shodhala Nighantu.

Madhava Dravyaguna

Madhava, the author of this work followed Shodhala and was quoted by Shivakosha (17 AD), Shivadasa Sen (15 AD), Adhamalla (14 AD) and Bopadeva (13 AD) and hence it can be presumed that he belongs to 13 AD. It consists of 29 Vargas. First and last Vargas are written elaborately. The drugs namely Jayapala, Bhanga, Aniphena were described in this book.

Siddhamantra

Keshava has described the drugs in 8 Vargas on Dosha basis i.e., Vataghna varga, Pittaghna varga, Kaphaghna varga, Vata-pittaghna varga, Kapha-vataghna varga, Kapha-pittaghna varga, Doshaghna varga and Doshala varga. In general, the actions of drugs on Doshas are described by their Rasadi gunas. But the author described Rasa, Guna, Virya, Vipaka of drugs basing on their action on Doshas. Keshava was the court physician of King Singhana (1210-1247) and can be placed during early part of 12th century AD. Bopadeva has written the famous commentary by the name Prakasha-vyakhya.

Hridayadeepaka Nighantu

The synonyms alone have been described for the drugs described in Ashtanga Hridaya and the work was named as Hridayadeepaka by Bopadeva. He is the son of Keshava, the author of Siddhamantra and the court scholar of king Mahadeva (1200-1270). He has written commentaries on Siddhamantra and Sharngadhara Samhita.

Nighantu-shesha:

This work was written by Hemachandra Suri, belonging to Jain religion during 12 AD. It consists of six Khandas and deals mainly with the synonyms of the drugs.

Madanadi Nighantu:

This glossary was written by Chandranandana during 10-11 cent. AD and also known as 'Guna Nighantu'. The content of the book was developed based on Ganas described in Ashtanga Hridaya.

Madanapala Nighantu:

The king of Tika dynasty Sri Madanpala has written this Nighantu during 1374 A.D. The drugs are described in 13 Vargas. Bhanga, Ahiphena, Jayapala, Parasikayavani, Chowhara, Sulaemani kharjura, Amritaphala, Grinjana, Madhukarkati etc. are some of the drugs mentioned in this Nighantu. In some of printed copies, Yashada drug was mentioned but Acharya Priyavrat Sharma opines that Yashada was not mentioned by Madanapala.

Kaiyyadeva Nighantu

It is also known as 'Pathyapathya Vibodhaka' and was written by Kaiyyadeva. This Nighantu consists of 9 Vargas and opium was not described in it. In Vihara varga the disease Shitapitta was described. Historians opine that this Nighantu was written during 1425-1451 AD.

Adhunika Kala

Rajanighantu

Rajanighantu is also known as 'Nighanturaja' and 'Abhidhana Chudamani'. The author Narahari in the introductioin clearly acknowledged the consulted works by him while preparing this Nighantu namely Dhanwantari Nighantu, Madanapala Nighantu, Halayudha, Amarakosha etc. The names of the drugs were mentioned in Sanskrit, Prakruta, Kannadi, Andhra, Marathi and other regioinal languages. The drug Jhandu which was introduced into India during 16th century was mentioned by the author and basing on this point the Nighantu can be considered as the work of 17th AD. Pita karaveera, Mayaphala are some of the drugs specially mentioned in this Nighantu. The credit of including Dravyaguna among 8 specialities of Ayurveda should be given to this author. Total subject was delt in 23 Vargas.

Bhavaprakasha

Bhavamishra is the author of this Samhita and he was the son of Latakana Mishra. The entire work is divided into 3 Khandas (section) and in the first Khanda various drugs including basic concepts were described in 24 Vargas. He has introduced a new drug namely Dwipantaravacha (Madhusnuhi) and described a new disease known as Phirangi. Yashada is enumerated among Saptha-dhatus. He belongs to 16th AD.

Rajavallabha

Narayana Dasa (1760) has redacted the Nighantu written by Vaidya Rajavallabha. Drugs being utilised during the daily regimen (Dinacharya) was discussed from Dravyaguna perspective and the entire subject matter was divided into six chapters. As the Shlokas mentioned in Madanpala Nighantu and Bhavaprakasha Nighantu were copied as it is, this can be considered as the 17th century work.

Nighanturatnakara

Vishnu Vasananadeva Godabole (Vasudeva) has written this Nighantu during 1867. It is a bilingual work written with Sanskrit Shlokas and the commentary in Marathi language. First section of the book deals with Dravyaguna, Rasashastra, Arka-prakasha and second section enumerates Nidana and Chikitsa of various diseases. Peetakaraveera, Akharakarbha, Pudina, Sitaphala, Karpura taila are some of drugs described in this Nighantu.

Shaligrama Nighantu

Lala Shaligrama completed this book in the year 1896. Several imported drugs have been included in the first section among 23 Vargas. This Nighantu is considered to be the last Nighantu of 19th century. 'Shaligrama-Aushadha-Shabda-Sagara' is considered as another work of the same author.

Nighantu Adarsha

Bapalal Vaidya, a versatile scholar with rich experience in the identification of medicinal plants has written Nighantu Adarsha according to the botanical classification. He is the first person to include not only Nirkuti for the synonyms of medicinal plants but also more number of Amayika-prayoga (therapeutic uses) of herbs. His knowledge regarding controversial drugs is exemplary and he authored several articles and a book namely 'Some Controversial Drugs in Indian Medicine' on this aspect. Nighantu Adarsha is being considered as the best book on subject of Dravyaguna during 20th century. It is published in two languages Gujarati and Hindi.

Shivakosha

Shviadutta Mishra has written this book consisting of 540 Shlokas and the drugs are described in alphabetical order. This book is also known as 'Nanarthoushadhi Kosha'. According to P.K. Gode the period of the author was determined as 1625- 1700 A.D.

Dravyaguna Shataka

Trimall Bhatt the author of Dravyaguna Shataka belongs to 17th century. This work consists of 15 Vargas and 102 Shlokas. Food substances were mainly described in this work and Madanapala was quoted while describing the drugs. He has also written another book namely 'Yoga Tarangini'.

Vaidyavatamsa

Lolimbraja (17 AD) has written a small book consisting of 57 verses. Under leafy vegetables Ashwabala was described.

Ayurveda Vijnana

Vinodalal Sen (19 AD) has written this in four parts and in Dravya-sthana several drugs viz. Rumimastagi, Salama-mishri, Syamaparni (tea), Sheetabija (isabgol) etc. were described.

Siddha Bheshaja Maninala

Krishna Rama Bhatta of Jaipur completed this work in 1886. Drugs are described in 18 Vargas and drugs like Mamira, Kasini etc. were mentioned. He has advocated to administer pure mercury at the dose of Shana (4 gms) or Ardhashana (2 gm) in the management of Shula.

Sandigdha Nirnayas

Bhagiratha Swamy published this work during 1936 from Kolkata. In this book he described controversial drugs in detail.

Vanoushadhi Darpana

Kaviraj Viraja Charana Gupta published first part in the year 1908 and second part during 1909. Drugs were described with the Benegali vernacular and Latin names.

Dravyaguna Vijnana

Acharya Yadavji Trikamji has written this book in two volumes. First volume consists of fundamental principes of Dravyaguna and the second volume deals with the details about various drugs from botanical perspective.

Acharya Priyavrat Sharma has written another book with the same title consisting of 5 volumes. He has enumerated drugs basing on the pharmacological actions.

His other works on Dravyaguna are 'Dravyaguna-kosha', 'Dravyaguna-sutram', 'Priya Nighantu', 'Classical uses of Medicinal Plants', 'Namrupjnanam' etc.

Dr. C.L. Yadav of Varanasi has also written a book named Dravyaguna Vijnana as per the CCIM syllabus.

Vanoushadhi Darshika

Thakur Balwant Singh, a botanist while working at Banaras Hindu University has made good efforts in sorting out controversies among Ayurvedic herbs and enumerated his field experiences in this book. His other works are 'Bihar ki Vanaspatiya', 'Prarambhika Udbhida Shastra' and 'Glossary of Vegetable Drugs in Brihattrayi'.

Dr. K. Nishteswar of Vijayawada has written two books namely Dravyaguna Moulika Siddhanta and Dravyaguna Prayoga Vijnanam (Co-authored by K. Arunee kumar) according to CCIM syllabus in Telugu language (published during 1986 and 1987) and these two books gained reputation as the most standard reference books on the subject of Dravyaguna by the student cammunity of Andhra Pradesh.

Vanaspati Shastra

Jayakrishna Indraji Thakur has written Vanaspati Sastra in 1910, who is considered to be an expert in the field of drug identification.

Pharmacographia India

William Dymock, Warden and Hooper in 1890 edited and published the volume which consists of research results of ancient Indian medicinal plants carried out by them.

Indian Medicinal Plants

Kirtikar and Basu published it in 1913 with the line diagrams of many plants. This book is published in four parts.

Another book having same title has been written by Dr. Prakash Paranjpe of Pune consisting of coloured photographs and detailed description of 140 prominent drugs.

Indian Materia Medica

It is written by K.N.Nadkarni and published in 1908 in two parts. In the first part, 2871 herbs are described and the second volume consists of information about animal products and mineral drugs.

Indigenous Drugs of India

Col. R.N. Chopra has published it in 1954. During the post independence era, he is considered to be the first person to carry out intensive research on medicinal plants of India.

Dictionary of Economic Products of India

George Watt published it during 1908 consisting of economic products in an alphabetic order.

SECOND PAPER

Part - A

Detail Study of 122 Dravyas

1
VATSANĀBHA

Aconitum ferox Wall. Family : Ranunculaceae

Chief Characters :

1. Perennial shrub grows upto 2m. height.
2. Simple leaf.
3. Racemose inflorescence.
4. Blue coloured flowers.
5. Fruit - follicle.

Synonyms : Kshweda, Garala, Amrita.

Properties : Rasa - Madhura; Guna - Laghu, Ruksha, Tikshna, Vyavayi, Vikasi; Virya - Ushna and Vipaka - Katu.

Pharmacological Actions : Vata-kapha hara, Rasayana, Vishahara, Balya, Grahi, Madakari, Brimhana, Yogavahi.

Indications : Kushta, Madhumeha, Agnimandya, Shwasa, Kasa, Sannipata jwara, Plihodara, Shotha, Apachi.

Therapeutic Uses :

1. Headache : Yastimadhu 1 gm and aconite 250 gm are pounded finely and put into the nostril at the dose of a mustard seed. This recipe reduces all types of headache (B.P.)
2. Scorpion bite : The paste of the root as an external application relieves pain due to scorpian bite.
3. Shoola : Powder of pippali, pippalimoola and vatsanabha should be taken in equal quantity mixed with honey. (R.R.S.)

Parts Used : Root.

Preparations & Dosage : Powder 60-125 mg.

Specific Formulations : Anandabhairava, Tribhuvanakeerti rasa, Sanjeevani vati.

सिन्दुवारसदृक्पत्रो वत्सनाभ्याकृतिस्तथा ।
यत्पार्श्वेन तरोर्वृद्धिर्वत्सनाभः स भाषितः ।। भा०प्र०

2
ATIVIṢĀ

Aconitum heterophyllum Wall. Cat   Family : Ranunculaceae

Chief Characters :

1. Perennial shrub grows upto 1-3 feet height.
2. Simple leaf, alternate phyllotaxy.
3. Racemose inflorescence, blue coloured flowers.
4. Fruit - follicle.

Synonyms : Sisubhaishajya, Gunavallabha, Bhangura, Shukla-kanda.

Gana :

Charaka : Arshoghna, Lekhaniya.
Sushruta : Pippalyadi, Vachadi, Mustadi.

Properties : Rasa - Tikta, Katu; Guna - Laghu, Ruksha; Virya - Ushna and Vipaka - Katu.

Pharmacological Actions : Kaphapitta hara, Deepana, Pachana, Grahi, Vishaghna.

Indications : Atisara, Chardi, Krimi, Kasa, Jwara. Balaroga and Mushikavisha.

Therapeutic Uses :

1. Rat poision : The paste of ativisha taken with honey is efficacious in rat poisoning. (S.S.)
2. Children's diseases : In case of cough, fever and vomiting ativisha is given singly with honey or combined with karkata shringi and pippali also. (A.H.)
3. Diarrhoea : Ankota (3 parts) and ativisha (1 part) mixed together is taken with rice water. It checks all abdominal disorders. (V.S.)

Parts Used : Root (tuber).

Preparations & Dosage : Churna 1-3 gms.

Specific Formulations : Bala chaturbhadra, Ativishadi churna.

विषा त्वतिविषा विश्वा शृङ्गी प्रतिविषाऽरुणा ।
शुक्लकन्दा चोपविषा भङ्गुरा घुणवल्लभा ॥
विषा सोष्णा कटुस्तिक्ता पाचनी दीपनी हरेत् ।
कफपित्तातिसारामविषकासवमिकृमीन् ॥ भा०प्र०

3

GUḌŪCĪ

Tinospora cordifolia Willd. Miers ex Hook f. et. Thoms.

Family : Menispermaceae

Chief Characters :

1. Perennial climber.
2. Simple leaf, alternate phyllotaxy.
3. Green & yellow coloured flowers, unisexual flowers.
4. Racemose inflorescence.
5. Fruit - drupe.

Synonyms : Madhuparni, Chinnaruha, Chinnodbhava, Amruta, Vatsadani, Kundali, Jivanti, Tantrika, Soma, Somavalli, Chandrahasa, Vayastha, Mandali, Devanirmita, Vishalya, Rasayani, Chakralakshanika.

Gana :

Charaka : Vayahsthapana, Dahaprashamana, Trishna nigrahana, Truptighna, Stanya shodhana.

Sushruta : Guduchyadi, Patoladi, Aragwadhadi, Kakolyadi.

Properties : Rasa - Tikta, Kashaya; Guna - Guru, Snigdha; Virya - Ushna and Vipaka - Madhura.

Pharmacological Actions : Tridoshahara, Rasayana, Grahi, Deepaniya, Medhya, Chakshusya.

Indications : Pandu, Kamala, Jwara, Daha, Trishna, Kushta, Prameha, Vatarakta, Krimi, Chardi, Kasa.

Therapeutic Uses :

1. Fever : Guduchi juice alone checks vishama jwara. Decoction of cold infusion of guduci checks fever caused by vata. (S.S.)
2. Jaundice : Paste of guduchi leaves with butter milk relieves jaundice. (B.P.)
3. Vatarakta : Decoction of guduci, eranda and vasa mixed with castor oil controls generalised vatarakta. (S.G.)

4. Vata located in heart : For this one should take guduchi and maricha pounded together with hot water in morning. (B.S.)

Parts Used : Stem starch, Leaf.

Preparations & Dosage : Decoction 50-100 ml; Churna 3-6 gm; Sattwa 1-2 gm.

Specific Formulations : Samshamani vati, Amritarista.

गुडूची मधुपर्णी स्यादमृताऽमृतवल्लरी ।
छिन्ना छिन्नरुहा छिन्नोद्भवा वत्सादनीति च ॥
जीवन्ती तन्त्रिका सोमा सोमवल्ली च कुण्डली ।
चक्रलक्षणिका धीरा विशल्या च रसायनी ॥
चन्द्रहासा वयःस्था च मण्डली देवनिर्मिता ।
गुडूची कटुका तिक्ता स्वादुपाका रसायनी ॥
सङ्ग्राहिणी कषायोष्णा लघ्वी बल्याग्निदीपनी ।
दोषत्रयामतृड्दाहमेहकासांश्च पाण्डुताम् ॥
कामला कुष्ठवातास्रज्वरकृमिवमीन् हरेत् । भा०प्र०

Research Studies: Oral administrations of the aqueous and alcoholic extracts of the plant caused reduction in fasting blood sugar in rabbits and rats. The bitter fractions of the aqueous extract caused in significant reduction in blood sugar level, it inhibited the adrenaline induced hyperglycaemia significantly. (Gupta et al, IJNR. 55.7 : 733)

The effect of aqueous extract of T- cardifolia stem caused. reduction of blood sugar in alloxan induced hyperglycaemic rats and rabbits in dose of 400 mg/kg. body weight. (Raghunathan & Sharma, 1969)

The drug has further proved to be effective as anti-rheumatic and diuretic (Sisodia & Laxminarayana 1966) as well as having anti-inflammatory properties (Rai and Gupta 1966). They have further carried out experimental evaluation of the drug for dissolution of Urinary calculii. In 22 rats, the stone formation was induced by implanting zinc pellets into the bladder. The deposition of the secondary salts over the zing pellets was inhibited by the aqueous extracts of T. cordifolia. (I.J.p.p. 10 : 12, 2 : 21)

4

PĀṬHĀ

Cissampelos pariera **Linn.** Family : Menispermaceae

Chief Characters :

1. Perennial herb grows upt 6 mts. height.
2. Simple leaf, alternate phyllotaxy.
3. Green coloured flowers.
4. Cyamose inflorescence - male flowers.
5. Racemose inflorescence - female flowers.
6. Fruits - drupe.

Synonyms : Prachinna, Papachelika, Ambashta, Ekashthila, Rasa, Pathika, Vartiktika.

Gana :

Charaka : Jwarahara, Sandhaniya, Stanya shodhana.

Sushruta : Mustadi, Aragwadhadi, Pippalyadi, Ambashtadi.

Properties : Rasa - Tikta; Guna - Laghu, Tikshna; Virya - Ushna and Vipaka - Katu.

Pharmacological Actions : Vatakaphahara, Balya, Vishaghna, Grahi.

Indications : Shoola, Jwara, Chardi, Gulma, Atisara, Vrana, Krimi, Kandu, Kushta, Hridroga, Daha, Shwasa.

Therapeutic Uses :

1. Fever : Juice of patha root taken in morning for three days checks fever with rigor. (V.D.)
2. Diarrhoea : Powder of patha root should be taken with curd. (B.P.)
3. Piles : (a) Patha combined with any one of duralabha, bilva, yavani and shunthi relieves piles. (C.S.)
   (b) Buttermilk added with patha act as carminative and relieves constipation. (A.H.)

Parts Used : Root, Rhizome.

Preparations & Dosage : Decoction 50-100 ml.; Powder 1-3 gm.

Specific Formulation : Shaddharana yoga.

पाठाऽम्बष्ठाऽम्बष्टकी च प्राचीना पापचेलिका ।
राकाऽष्ठीला रसा प्रोक्ता पाठिका वरतिक्तिका ॥
पाठोष्णा कटुका तीक्ष्णा वातश्लेष्महरी लघुः ।
हन्ति शूलज्वरच्छर्दिकुष्ठातीसारहृद्रुजः ॥
दाह-कण्डू-विष-श्वास-कृमि-गुल्म-गर-व्रणान् ॥ भा०प्र०

5
DĀRUHARIDRĀ

Berberis aristata DC. Family : Berberidaceae

Chief Characters :

1. Evergreen shrub.
2. Simple leaf, oval shaped leaves.
3. Yellow coloured flowers.
4. Compund corymb inflorescence.
5. Fruit - berry.

Synonyms : Peetadru, Darvi, Katankateri, Pachampacha, Parnini, Peeta, Peetadaru, Peetakarna, Haridru, Parjanya, Parjini.

Gana :

Charaka : Arshoghna, Kandughna, Lekhaniya.
Sushruta : Haridradi, Mustadi, Lakshadi.

Properties : Rasa - Tikta, Kashaya; Guna - Laghu, Ruksha; Virya - Ushna and Vipaka - Katu.

Pharmacological Actions : Kaphapittahara, Chedaniya, Rasayana, Varnya.

Indications : Prameha, Kandu, Kushta, Visarpa, Karnaroga, Netraroga, Vrana, Shweta pradara, Kamala, Pandu, Shotha, Mukharoga.

Therapeutic Uses :

1. Jaundice : One suffering from jaundice should take in the morning cooled decoction of darvi with honey. (C.D.)
2. Leucorrhoea : Decoction of daruharidra mixed with honey should be taken followed by intake of rice-water. (G.N.)
3. Prameha : Darvi and amalaki juice mixed with honey alleviate prameha. (V.M.)

Parts Used : Root, Stem, Fruit.

Preparations & Dosage : Decoction 50-100 ml;, Rasanjana 1-3 gm.; Fruit 5-10 gm.

Specific Formulations : Darvyadi kwatha, Darvyadi taila.

दार्वी दारुहरिद्रा च पर्जन्या पर्जनीति च ।
कटङ्कटेरी पीता च भवेत्सैव पचम्पचा ॥
सैव कालीयक: प्रोक्तस्तथा कालेयकोऽपि च ।
पीतद्रुश्च हरिद्रुश्च पीतदारु च पीतकम् ।
दार्वी निशागुणा किन्तु नेत्रकर्णास्यरोगनुत् ॥ भा०प्र०

Research Studies: Berberine, an alkaloid obtained from the plant Berberis aristata, has been claimed to be effective in the treatment of certain diarrhoeas. The drug has been shown to inhibit the cholera toxin induced inflammation in rats and is claimed to be useful in the treatment of Cholera (PPT). Berberine in dilution of 1 in 80,000 is toxic to Leishmania tropica, and it has been used sucessfully in oriental sore. It helps to expel the malaria parasites into the peripheral circulations and acts as a provocative agent in the diagnosis of malaria. (PMMT)

6
AHIPHENA

Papaver somniferum Linn. Family : Papaveraceae

Chief Characters :

1. Annual shrub, grows upto 1 mtr. height.
2. Oval shaped leaves.
3. White or red coloured flowers.
4. Fruits - porous capsule.

Synonyms : Aphuka, Khasaphalaksheera.

Gana :

Upavisha (R.R.S.)

Properties : Rasa - Tikta, Kashaya; Guna - Laghu, Ruksha, Sukshma, Vyavayi, Vikasi; Virya - Ushna and Vipaka - Katu.

Pharmacological Actions : Kaphahara, Vatapittakara, Grahi, Madakari, Avrishya (seeds), Dhatu soshaka, Sukra stambhaka, Vajikarana.

Indications : Kasa, Atisara, Jwara, Shoola, Darunaka.

Therapeutic Uses :

1. Diarrhoea : Intake of 125 mg. (one ratti) of ahiphena alongwith goat's milk relieves diarrhoea. (B.R.)
2. Dandruff : The seeds pounded with milk and applied destroy dandruff. (S.G.)

Parts Used : Latex, Seeds, Fruit.

Preparations & Dosage : Powder 3-5 gm.; Latex 30-125 mg.

Specific Formulations : Ahiphenasava, Nidrodaya vati, Karpuradi rasa, Akarakarabhadi taila.

उक्तं खसफलक्षीरमाफूकमहिफेनकम् ।
आपूकं शोषणं ग्राही श्लेष्मघ्नं वातपित्तलम् ।
तथा खसफलोद्भूतवल्कलप्रायमित्यपि ॥ भा०प्र०

7
VARUṆA

Crataeva religiosa Forst F. Family : Capparaceae

Chief Characters :

1. Deciduous tree grows upto 15mts. height.
2. Trifoliate compound leaf, alternate phyllotaxy.
3. Light yellow coloured flowers.
4. Corymb inflorescence.
5. Fruit - berry.

Synonyms : Varana, Setu, Kumaraka, Tiktasaka.

Gana :

Sushruta : Tiktavarga, Varunadi, Vata samshamana.

Properties : Rasa - Tikta, Kashaya, Madhura, Katu; Guna - Laghu, Ruksha; Virya - Ushna and Vipaka - Katu.

Pharmacological Actions : Kaphavatahara, Deepana, Pittala, Bhedana.

Indications : Ashmari, Vidradi, Gulma, Krimi, Gandamala, Mutra kricchra, Vatarakta.

Therapeutic Uses :

1. Calculus : Intake of decoction of varuna (root-bark) added with its paste, dissolves calculus. (V.M.)
2. Gandamala : Decoction of varuna root taken with honey destroys gandamala of chronic origin. (V.M.)
3. Abscess : Decoction of root of Varuna should be taken. It controls the unripe abscess. (Y.R.)

Parts Used : Bark.

Preparations & Dosage : Decoction 50-100 ml.

Specific Formulations : Varunadi taila, Varunadi ghrita, Kanchanara guggulu.

वरुणो वरण: सेतु तिक्तशाक: कुमारक: ।
वरुण: पित्तलो भेदी श्लेष्मकृच्छ्राश्ममारुतान् ॥
निहन्ति गुल्मवातास्त्रकृमींश्चोष्णोऽग्निदीपन: ।
कषायो मधुरस्तिक्त: कटुको रूक्षको लघु: ॥ भा०प्र०

Research Studies: Some of the fraction of C. nurvala showed promising anti-inflammatory and anti-arthritic activities. It has been found to produce prolonged hypotension of gradual onset. (CCRIMH. Annual report , 1972-73)

8
TUVARAKA

Hydnocarpus wightiane Blome   Family : Flacourtiaceae

Chief Characters :

1. Evergreen tree grows upto 15mts. height.
2. Simple leaf, alternate phyllotaxy.
3. White coloured flowers, racemose inflorescence.
4. Unisexual flowers.
5. Fruit - berry.

Synonyms : Kushtaha, Alasakapaha, Katukapittha, Kushtavairi.

Properties : Rasa - Tikta, Katu; Guna - Tikshna, Snigdha; Virya - Ushna and Vipaka - Katu.

Pharmacological Actions : Kaphavata shamaka, Deepana, Grahi, Rasayana, Rechana.

Indications : Kushta, Krimi, Kandu, Prameha, Netraroga.

Therapeutic Uses :

1. Rasayana : Seeds of tuvaraka act as good rasayana when taken regularly. (A.H.)
2. Pakshma kopa : Bathing the eye with tuvaraka oil relieves pakshama kopa. (S.S.)
3. Night Blindness : Tuvaraka fruit pulp, rocksalt, srotanjana should be burnt in a closed sarava (puta process) and tuvaraka oil should be added to it. It should be used as collyrium. It cures kacha, neeli, timira, naktandya and other eye disorders. (S.S.)

Parts Used : Fruit pulp, Seed, Oil.

Preparations & Dosage : Seed powder 1-3 gm.; Oil 10 ml.

Specific Formulations : Tuvaraka lepa, Tuvarasti vataka, Tuvarakadi taila.

तुवरस्तु वरश्चोष्णो रसे पाके च तिक्तक: ।
कफव्रणकृमिमेहकुष्ठज्वरविनाशन: ।
आनाहमर्श: शोफश्च नाशयेदिति ते जगु: ।। नि०र०

Research Studies: Recent research has confirmed the antileprotic action of Chaulmogra oil. It was found to inhibit the growth of leprosy germs when tested in the foot pads of mice. Many tuberculoid leprosy causes in which there is extensive nerve damage seems to improve with chaulmogra oil much faster than dapsone.

9
NĀGAKEŚARA

Mesua ferrea Linn. Family : Guttiferae

Chief Characters :

1. Tree grows upto 20mts. height.
2. Simple leaf, opposite phyllotaxy.
3. White coloured flowers.
4. Fruit - berry.

Synonyms : Kanchanahwaya, Nagapushpa, Champeya, Kesara, Nagakinjalka.

Gana :

Sushruta : Eladi, Priyangwadi, Vachadi.

Properties : Rasa - Tikta, Kashaya; Guna - Laghu, Ruksha; Virya - Ushna and Vipaka - Katu.

Pharmacological Actions : Kaphapittahara, Pachana, Grahi, Pramadi, Vishahara.

Indications : Raktarsha, Raktapradara, Atisara, Chardi, Jwara, Trishna, Kushta, Visarpa, Kandu.

Therapeutic Uses :

1. Bleeding piles : By regular use of nagakeshara with butter and sugar, the bleeding from piles is checked. (C.S.)
2. Leucorrhoea : Nagakeshara, should be taken with buttermilk for three days with a diet of buttermilk in order to check leucorrhoea. (B.S.)
3. Haemorrhage : Powder of nagakeshara with sugar is an excellant drug for checking haemorrhage. (B.S.)

Parts Used : Stamens, flowers.

Preparations & Dosage : Powder 1-3 gm.

Specific Formulations : Kesaradi Kashaya, Eladi chruna.

नागपुष्पः स्मृतो नागः केशरो नागकेशरः ।
चाम्पेयो नागकिञ्जल्कः कथितः काञ्चनाह्वयः ॥
नागपुष्पं कषायोष्णं रूक्षं लघ्वामपाचनम् ।
ज्वरकण्डूतृषास्वेदच्छर्दिहृल्लासनाशनम् ।
दौर्गन्ध्यकुष्ठवीसर्पकफपित्तविषापहम् ॥ भा०प्र०

Research Studies: The seed oil has shown to potentiate bronchodilator activity of isoprenaline both in vitro and in vivo experiments. The activity was located in the phenolic compounds isolated from the seed oil. (Annual report, 1975-76. CCRIMH)

10
ŚĀLA

Shorea robusta Gaertn. Family : Dipterocarpaceae

Chief Characters :

1. Tree grows upto 30m. height.
2. White flowers, panicle inflorescence.
3. Simple leaf, alternate phyllotaxy.
4. Fruit - indehiscent capsule.

Synonyms **:** Salasara, Dhupavriksha, Sarja, Karsya, Aswakarna, Sasyasambhara.

Gana **:**

Charaka : Vedhana sthapana, Kashaya skandha.

Sushruta : Salasaradi, Raudhradi.

Properties : Rasa - Kashaya, Madhura; Guna - Ruksha; Virya - Sheeta and Vipaka - Katu.

Pharmacological Actions : Kaphapittahara, Sthambhana, Varnya, Vrana shodhana, Vrana ropana, Swedana.

Indications : Kushta, Kandu, Prameha, Vrana, Krimi, Asthibhagna, Bradhna, Vidradhi, Badhirya, Yoni roga, Karna roga.

Therapeutic Uses :

1. Prameha : Shala, kampillaka and mustaka (10gm. each) mixed with honey, amalaka juice and haridra should be taken. (S.S.)
2. Small Pox : Sarjarasa, pounded with the juice of shigru leaves should be applied locally. (V.D.)

Parts Used : Bark, Rala (Gum resin), Flowers.

Preparations & Dosage : Bark decoction 50-100ml.; Rala powder 1-3gm.

Specific Formulations : Salasaradi churna, Sarjarasa malahara, Salasaradi kwatha, Atasyadi lepa.

Bhavamishra mentions Ajakarana or Sarjana as another variety of Shala and it is identified as Vateria indica (Dipterocarpaceae). Similarly Aswakarna is a separate plant and the plant Dipterocarpus alatus is considered as its source.

शालस्तु सर्जकार्श्याश्वकर्णका: शस्यशम्बर: ।
अश्वकर्ण: कषाय: स्याद् व्रणस्वेदकफक्रिमीन् ।
ब्रघ्नविद्रधिबाधिर्ययोनिकर्णगदान् हरेत् ॥ भा०प्र०

11
BALĀ

Sida cordifolia Linn. Family : Malvaceae

Chief Characters :

1. Annual shrub, grows upto 1m. height.
2. Yellow flowers.
3. Simple leaf, alternate phyllotaxy.
4. Fruit - capsule.

Synonyms : Bala : Vatya, Vatyalika, Vatyalaka.
Nagabala : Gangeruki, Hrashwagavedhuka, Jhasha,
Atibala : Rishyaprokta, Kankatika.
Mahabala : Peetapushpa, Sahadevi.

Gana :

Charaka : Balya, Brimhaniya, Prajasthapana.

Sushruta : Vata samshamana.

Properties : Rasa - Madhura; Guna - Laghu, Snigdha, Picchala; Virya - Sheeta and Vipaka - Madhura.

Pharmacological Actions : Vatapittahara, Balya, Grahi, Brimhana, Vrishya, Prajasthapana.

Indications : Raktapitta, Kshaya, Prameha, Mutratisara.

Therapeutic Uses :

1. Pradara : Root of bala mixed with honey is taken with milk. (C.D.)
2. Vatavyadhi : Oil prepared from bala (root-paste) decoction, milk and oil should be used for drinking, bathing and snuffing. It alleviates all vata vyadhis. (V.S.)

Atibala : (Abutilon indicum G. Don.)

1. Dysuria : Decoction of root of atibala alleviates all types of mutrakrichchra (dysuria). (C.D.)

Parts Used : Root, Seed.

Preparations & Dosage : Juice 10-20 ml.; Powder 3-6 gm.

Specific Formulations : Balarishta, Ksheerabala taila, Candanabala lakshadi taila, Baladi ghrita, Baladi kwatha.

बलावाट्यालिका वाट्या सैव वाट्यालकाऽपि च ।
महाबला पीतपुष्पा सहदेवी च सा स्मृता ॥
ततोऽन्याऽतिबला ऋष्यप्रोक्ता कङ्कतिका च सा ।
गाङ्गेरुकी नागबला झषा ह्रस्वगवेधुका ॥
बलाचतुष्टयं शीतं मधुरं बलकान्तिकृत् ।
स्निग्धं ग्राही समीरास्रपित्तास्रक्षतनाशनम् ॥
बलामूलत्वचश्चूर्णं पीतं सक्षीरशर्करम् ।
मूत्रातिसारं हरति दृष्टमेतन्न संशय: ॥
हरेन्महाबला कृच्छ्रं भवेद्वातानुलोमिनी ।
हन्यादतिबला मेहं पयसा सितया समम् ॥ भा०प्र०

Research Studies: In an experimental study the rasayan drugs namely bala, atibala, mahabala and bhumibala have been screened for their immuno-enhancing properties. Animals of drug treated group showed statistically an enhanced production of anti 'S' typhi 'O' antibodies. Abutilon indicum (Atibala) was the best drug in augmenting antibody production. (Dixit S.P. et al, JRIMYH, Vol. xiii, No 3, Sept. 1978)

12
NĀGABALĀ

Sida humilis Willd. Family : Malvaceae

Chief Characters :

1. Annual shrub, grows upto 1m. height.
2. Simple leaf, alternate phyllotaxy.
3. Yellow flowers, bisexual flowers.
4. Fruit - schizocarp.

Synonyms : Vishwadeva, Bhumi bala.

Properties : Rasa - Madhura, Kashaya; Guna - Guru, Snigdha, Picchila; Virya - Sheeta and Vipaka - Madhura.

Pharmacological Actions : Vatapittahara, Rasayana, Balya, Grahi.

Indications : Mutrakriccha, Vrana, Rajayakshma, Kasa, Shwasa, Hridroga, Kshaya, Raktapitta.

Therapeutic Uses :

1. Hridroga : Powder of nagabala root should be used with milk. It relieves heart disease, cough and dyspnoea. (C.D.)
2. Rajayakshma : One should use the powder of nagabala mixed with ghee and honey in morning. It alleviates consumption. (G.N.)
3. Sadyo vrana : The wound should be irrigated with the juice of nagabala root. It alleviates pain immediately. (S.G.)

Parts Used : Root.

Preparations & Dosage : Decoction 50-100 ml.; Root bark powder 3-6 gm.

Acharya Priyavrat Sharma opines that Grewia hirsuta Vahl. (Gulsakari) should be considered as Nagbala. Prof. K.C. Chunekar quotes the following plants as Nagabala :

1. Sida humilis Cav. (S. Veronicaefolia Lam.)
2. Sida Spinosa Linn.
3. Grewia hirsuta Vanb.

Bapalal Vaidya opines that Nagabala is a synonym of Gangeruki and the plant Grewia populifolia (G. Lenax) as the source of Nagabala and considers Sida humilis as Bhumibala.

गङ्गेरुकी नागबला झषा ह्रस्वगवेधुका । भा०प्र०
गाङ्गेरुकी मधुराम्ला कषायोष्णा गुरुस्तथा ॥
कटुस्तिक्ता च वातघ्नी व्रणपित्तविकारजित् । ध०नि०
बलया नागबला गुर्वी रक्तपित्तक्षयपहा ।
वृष्या रसायनी तस्याझन्तकफलवत् फलम् । कै०नि०

13
ŚĀLMALĪ

Bombax ceiba Linn. Family : Bambacaceae

Chief Characters :

1. Tree, consists of thorns all over the stem.
2. Compound leaf, alternate phyllotaxy.
3. Red flowers, bisexual.
4. Fruit - loculicidal capsule.

Synonyms : Mocha, Picchila, Raktapushpa, Sthirayu, Kantakadhya, Purani, Tulini.

Gana :

Charaka : Purisha virajaneeya, Shonita sthapana, Vedana sthapana, Kashaya skandha.

Sushruta : Priyangwadi.

Properties : Rasa - Madhura, Kashaya; Guna - Laghu, Snigdha, Kashaya; Virya - Sheeta and Vipaka - Madhura.

Pharmacological Actions : Vatapittahara, Rasayana, Balya, Vrishya, Grahi, Sleshamala.

Indications : Pravahika, Atisara, Raktapitta, Pradara, Vatarakta.

Therapeutic Uses :

1. Menorrhagia : Vegetables of shálmali flowers cooked with ghee and rocksalt checks bleeding. (B.P.N.)
2. Burning sensation in feet : Application of the paste of shalmali bark removes burning sensation of feet. (R.M.)
3. Freckles (Vyanga) : Sharp thorns of shalmali powder with milk should be applied to face. It makes the face handsome and smooth. (V.M.)

Parts Used : Root, Flower, Thorn, Gum resin.

Preparations & Dosage : Decoction 5-10 ml.; Gum resin 1-3 gm.; Flower juice 10-20 ml.

Specific Formulations : Gangadhara churna, Shalmali ghrita.

शाल्मलिस्तु भवोन्मोचा पिच्छिला पूरणीति च ।
रक्तपुष्पा स्थिरायुश्च कण्टकाढ्या च तूलिनी ॥
शाल्मली शीतला स्वाद्वी रसे पाके रसायनी ।
श्लेष्मला पित्तवातास्रहारिणी रक्तपित्तजित् ॥ भा०प्र०

14
GOKṢURA

Tribulus terrestris Linn. Family : Zygophyllaceae

Chief Characters :

1. Shrub, procumbent spreads upto 1m. length.
2. Paripinnate compound leaf.
3. Yellow flowers, bisexual flowers.
4. Fruit - septicidal capsule.

Synonyms : Trikantaka, Svadamstra, Ikshugandhika, Swadukantaka, Palankasha, Kshuraka, Gokantaka, Vanashringata.

Gana :

Charaka : Mutra virechaniya, Sothahara, Krimighna.

Sushruta : Vidharigandhadi, Veeratarvadi, Laghupanchamoola.

Properties : Rasa - Madhura; Guna - Guru, Snigdha; Virya - Sheeta and Vipaka - Madhura.

Pharmacological Actions : Vatapittashamaka, Deepana, Vastishodhana, Rasayana, Vrishya.

Indications : Ashmari, Prameha, Mutrakriccha, Hridroga, Shwasa, Kasa, Arshas.

Therapeutic Uses :

1. Dysuria : Decoction of whole plant of gokshura mixed with honey and sugar should be taken. It alleviates the disorders of dysuria. (B.S.)
2. Calculus : Powder of the seeds of gokshura mixed with honey and taken with sheep milk for a week breaks calculus. (S.S.)
3. Sosha : Powder of gokshura fruits and aswagandha mixed with honey is taken with milk. It alleviates consumption and cough. (R.M.)

Parts Used : Fruit, Root.

Preparations & Dosage : Fruit powder 3-6gm.; Decoction 50-100 ml.

Specific Formulations : Gokshura guggulu, Gokshuradi churna, Dasamularista, Gokshuradi kwatha.

गोक्षुरः क्षुरकोऽपि स्यात्त्रिकण्टः स्वादुकण्टकः ।
गोकण्टको गोक्षुरको वनशृङ्गाट इत्यपि ॥
पलङ्कषा श्वदंष्ट्रा च तथा स्यादिक्षुगन्धिका ।
गोक्षुरः शीतलः स्वादुर्बलकृद्बस्तिशोधनः ॥
मधुरो दीपनो वृष्यः पुष्टिदश्चाश्मरीहरः ।
प्रमेहश्वासकासार्शः कृच्छ्रहृद्रोगवातनुत् ॥ भा०प्र०

Research Studies: Gujral et al investigated the diuretic effect of decoction of fruit in rats and found a moderate diuretic activity as compared to urea.

Karandikar et al found the watery extract of Gokshura to possess similar diuretic activity like urea both in rats and dogs. They concluded that diuresis was due to high potassium content of the extract. Chopra and Nadkarni have reported it on sporadic clinical trials, with liquid extracts as diuretic with same positive result. (ARIM). Aqueous and alcoholic extracts of Gokshura caused hypotension in two species of animals viz. rat and dog had depressant effect on the respiration in rats.

15
CĀṄGERĪ

Oxalis corniculata Linn. Family : Oxalidaceae

Chief Characters :

1. Perennial shrub grows upto 1m. height.
2. Trifoliate compound leaves, alternate phyllotaxy.
3. Yellow flowers.
4. Spike inflorescence.
5. Fruit - capsule.

Synonyms : Amlapatrika, Chatuschada, Chukrika, Dantasata, Amlalonika, Ashmantaka, Kusali, Sephari.

Properties : Rasa - Amla, Kashaya; Guna - Laghu, Ruksha; Virya - Ushna and Vipaka - Amla.

Pharmacological Actions : Kaphavatahara, Deepana, Grahi, Ruchya.

Indications : Grahani, Atisara, Arshas, Kushta.

Therapeutic Uses :

1. Piles : Curry prepared from the leaves of trivrit, danti, cangeri and citraka fried in ghee and oil mixed with curd should be given. (C.S.)
2. Grahani roga : Ghrita cooked with the paste of pippalyadi group, cangeri juice and curd is useful in grahani. (S.S.)
3. Scorpion poisoning : Rocksalt mixed with cangeri is rubbed on the spot of sting. (G.N.)

Parts Used : Panchanga (Whole plant).

Preparations & Dosage : Juice 5-10 ml.

Specific Formulation : Cangeri ghrita.

चाङ्गेरी चुक्रिका दन्तशठाम्बष्ठाम्ललोणिका ।
अश्मन्तकस्तु शफरी कुशली चाम्लपत्रकः ॥
चाङ्गेरी दीपनी रुच्या रूक्षोष्णा कफवातनुत् ।
पित्तलाऽम्ला ग्रहण्यर्शः कुष्ठातीसारनाशिनी ॥ भा०प्र०

Research Studies: The petroleum ether, benzene and chloroform extract showed significant analgesic, antipyretic and anti inflammatory activity. The petroleum ether extract also had some diuretic effect. (Annual report, 1975-76. CCRIMH)

16

NIMBŪKA

Citrus medica Var. acida. Family : Rutaceae

Chief Characters :

1. Big shrub.
2. Unifoliate compound leaf, alternate phyllotaxy.
3. Small white flowers..
4. Fruit - pericarp is very thick, hesperdium.

Synonyms : Nimbu, Nimbuka, Nimbooka, Dantasata.

Properties : Rasa - Amla, Katu; Guna - Laghu, Tikshna; Virya - Ushna and Vipaka - Amla.

Pharmacological Actions : Vatakaphahara, Deepana, Pachana, Chakshusya.

Indications : Agnimandhya, Gulma, Chardi, Krimi, Shoola, Vishuchi, Vataroga, Udara, Aruchi, Baddaguda.

Therapeutic Uses :

1. Amlapitta : Juice of jambeera is useful in amlapitta. (C.D.)
2. Masurika : Intake of jaggery soaked with the juice of jambeera with milk controls affection in the initial phase of masurika. (V.M.)

Parts Used : Fruit

Preparations & Dosage : Juice 3-6 ml.

Specific Formulation : Jambeeradi panaka.

निम्बूकमम्लं वातघ्नं दीपनं पाचनं लघु ॥

× × ×

निम्बुकं कृमिसमूहनाशनं तीक्ष्णमम्लमुदरग्रहापहम् ।
वातपित्तकफशूलिने हितं कष्टनष्टरुचिरोचनं परम् ॥
त्रिदोषवह्निक्षयवातरोगनिपीडितानां विषविह्वलानाम् ।
मन्दानले बद्धगुदे प्रदेयं विषूचिकायां मुनयो वदन्ति ॥ भा०प्र०

17
BILVA

Aegle marmelos Linn. Cors. Family : Rutaceae

Chief Characters :

1. Medium & deciduous tree grows upto 7mts. height.
2. Trifoliate compound leaves, alternate phyllotaxy.
3. Green flowers, panicle inflorescence.
4. Fruit - drupe.

Synonyms : Malooraha, Sriphala, Shandilya, Shailusha.

Gana :

Charaka : Sothahara, Arshoghna, Asthapanopaga.
Sushruta : Varunadi, Ambustadi.

Properties : Rasa - Kashaya Tikta; Guna - Laghu, Ruksha; Virya - Ushna and Vipaka - Katu.

Pharmacological Actions : Vatakaphahara, Deepana, Pachana, Grahi, Balya.

Indications : Sotha, Atisara, Grahani.

Therapeutic Uses :

1. Diarrhoea : Intake of bilva with jaggery checks diarrhoea with blood. Relieves pain due to ama and constipation and alleviates disorders of bowels. (C.D.)
2. Grahani roga : Paste of tender fruit of bilva mixed with shunthi powder and jaggery alleviates severe grahani roga if the patient is kept on the diet of buttermilk. (C.D.)
3. Vomiting : Cooled decoction of bilva added with honey should be taken in the three types of vomiting. (Y.R.)

Parts Used : Root, Leaf, Fruit, Bark.

Preparations & Dosage : Powder 3-6gm.; Juice 10-20 ml.

Specific Formulations : Dasamoolarishta, Jeerakabilwadi lehya, Bilwadi vati.

बिल्वः शाण्डिल्यशैलूषौ मालूरश्रीफलावपि ।
श्रीफलस्तुवरस्तिक्तो ग्राही रूक्षोऽग्निपित्तकृत् ॥
वातश्लेष्महरो बल्यो लघुरुष्णश्च पाचनः ॥ भा०प्र०

18
GUGGULU

Balsamodendron mukul Hook. Family : Burseraceae

Chief Characters :

1. Small tree grows upto 4 m. height.
2. Imparipinnate compound leaf, alternate phyllotaxy.
3. Pink flowers, unisexual flowers.
4. Male and female flowers appears on same plant.
5. Fruit - drupe.

Synonyms : Koushika, Pura, Palankasha, Devadhupa, Jatayu, Mahishaksha, Khumbholukhalaka.

Gana :

Charaka : Samjna sthapana.

Sushruta : Eladi.

Properties : Rasa - Katu, Tikta; Guna - Laghu, Ruksha, Tikshna, Vishada, Sukshma, Sara, Snigdha, Picchala; Virya - Ushna and Vipaka - Katu.

Pharmacological Actions : Tridoshahara, Deepana, Brimhana, Vrishya (Nava), Lekhana (Purana), Rasayana, Balya.

Indications : Medoroga, Prameha, Kushta, Ashmari, Sosha, Pidaka, Granthi, Apachi, Gandamala, Arshas, Krimi, Amavata.

Therapeutic Uses :

1. Sciatica : Rasna 40 gm. and guggulu 200 gm. are pounded with ghee and made into pills. Intake of it alleviates sciatica. (C.D.)
2. Krostukasirsha : In this disease, guggulu or guduchi with triphala decoction should be taken. (C.D.)
3. Wound : Guggulu should be used with triphala decoction in wounds, skin diseases, sinus and fistula in ano. (G.N.)

Parts Used : Gum Resin.

Preparations & Dosage : Gum Resin 2-4 gm.

Specific Formulations : Yogaraj guggulu, Simhanada guggulu, Kaishora guggulu, Chandraprabha vati, Arogyavardhani rasa.

गुग्गुलुर्देवधूपश्च जटायुः कौशिकः पुरः ।
कुम्भोलूखलकं क्लीबे महिषाक्षः पलङ्कषः ॥
महिषाक्षो महानीलः कुमुदः पद्म इत्यपि ।
हिरण्यः पञ्चमो ज्ञेयो गुग्गुलोः पञ्च जातयः ॥
भृङ्गाञ्जनसवर्णस्तु महिषाक्ष इति स्मृतः ।
महानीलस्तु विज्ञेयः स्वनामसमलक्षणः ॥
कुमुदः कुमुदाभः स्यात्पद्मो माणिक्यसन्निभः ।
हिरण्याख्यस्तु हेमाभः पञ्चानां लिङ्गमीरितम् ॥
महिषाक्षो महानीलो गजेन्द्राणां हितावुभौ ।
हयानां कुमुदः पद्मः स्वस्त्यारोग्यकरौ परौ ॥
विशेषेण मनुष्याणां कनकः परिकीर्त्तितः ।
कदाचिन्महिषाक्षश्च मतः कैश्चिन्नृणामपि ॥
गुग्गुलुर्विशदस्तिक्तो वीर्योष्णः पित्तलः सरः ।
कषायः कटुकः पाके कटू रूक्षो लघुः परः ॥
भग्नसन्धानकृद् वृष्यः सूक्ष्मः स्वर्यो रसायनः ।
दीपनः पिच्छिलो बल्यः कफवातव्रणापची: ॥
मेदोमेहाश्मवातांश्च क्लेदकुष्ठाममारुतान् ।
पिडिकाग्रन्थिशोफार्शो गण्डमाला कृमीञ्जयेत् ॥
माधुर्याच्छमयेद्वातं कषायत्वाच्च पित्तहा ।
तिक्तत्वाद् कफजित्तेन गुग्गुलुः सर्वदोषहा ॥
स नवो बृंहणो वृष्यः पुराणस्त्वतिलेखनः ।
स्निग्धः काञ्चनसाकाशः पक्वजम्बूफलोपमः ॥
नूतनो गुग्गुलुः प्रोक्तः सुगन्धिर्यस्तु पिच्छिलः ।
शुष्को दुर्गन्धकश्चैव त्यक्तप्रकृतिवर्णकः ॥
पुराणः स तु विज्ञेयो गुग्गुलुर्वीर्यवर्जितः ।
अम्लं तीक्ष्णमजीर्णं च व्यवायं श्रममातपम् ॥
मद्यं रोषं त्यजेत्सम्यक् गुणार्थी पुरसेवकः ॥ भा०प्र०

<u>Research Studies:</u> The oleoresin present in the plant was found to be a highly potent anti-inflammatory agent, as compared to the hydorcortisone butazolidin against Brownlee's formaldehyde induced arthritis in albino rats (Gujrat et al 1960). It has been proved to be a potent hypocholestrolemic hypo lipidaemic, anti-atherosclerotic agent both in clinical as well as in experimental studies. (Satyvathi 1966, Tripathi 1966, Dwarakanath and Satyavathi 1970, Arora et al 1973 and Gupta et al 1974) The oral administration of fraction A of petroleum ether

extract of gum Guggulu brought about a significant reduction in serum cholesterol and serum total lipids over a treatment period of 21 days and the results compare favourably with in the effect of clofibrate on serum lipids (Kuppurajan et al 1978 PID). The diuretic activity of oleo-resin was reported by Gujral et al. At the dose of 0.25mg/100 gm of rat weight. The oleo resin elicited moderate degree of diuretic action. (JIMA 25,49,195)

19
TEJOHVA

Zanthoxylum alatum Roxb. Family : Rutaceae

Chief Characters :

1. Small tree, consists of thorns.
2. Compound leaf, alternate phyllotaxy.
3. Green flowers, panicle inflorescence.
4. Pink coloured ripen fruit.

Synonyms : Tejovati, Tejaswini, Tumburu, Sourabha, Vanaja.

Gana :

Charaka : Sirovirechana, Katuskandha.

Properties : Rasa - Katu, Tikta; Guna - Laghu, Ruksha, Tikshna; Virya - Ushna and Vipaka - Katu.

Pharmacological Actions : Kaphavatahara, Deepana, Pachana, Kanthya.

Indications : Mukharoga, Kantharoga, Hikka, Agnimandhya, Udara, Krimi, Shwasa, Kasa, Hridroga, Arshas, Karnashoola, Akshiruja, Sirahshoola.

Therapeutic Uses :

1. Diarrhoea : Powder of bark of tejowathi is useful in diarrhoea.
2. Toothache : One should keep chewing tejovati fruit and twak powder to alleviate toothache.

Parts Used : Bark, Fruit.

Preparations & Dosage : Powder 1-2 gm.

Specific Formulations : Tejovatyadi ghrita, Tambwadi churna.

तेजस्विनी तेजवती तेजोह्वा तेजनी तथा ।
तेजस्विनी कफश्वासकासास्यामयवातहृत् ।
पाचन्युष्णा कटुस्तिक्ता रुचिवह्निप्रदीपिनी ।। भा०प्र०

20
NIMBA

Azadirachta indica A. Juss. Family : Meliaceae

Chief Characters :

1. Big tree grows upto 12-16 m. height.
2. Compound leaf, opposite phyllotaxy.
3. Small white flowers, panicle inflorescence.
4. Fruit - drupe.

Synonyms : Arishta, Hinguniryasa, Pichumarda, Sarvatobhadra, Pichumanda, Tiktaka, Paribhadra.

Gana :

Charaka : Kandughna, Tiktaskandha.

Sushruta : Aragwadhadi, Guduchyadi, Lakshadi.

Properties : Rasa - Tikta, Kashaya; Guna - Laghu; Virya - Sheeta and Vipaka - Katu.

Pharmacological Actions : Kaphapittahara, Grahi, Deepana, Ahridya, Netrya (Leaf), Bhedana (Fruit).

Indications : Kushta, Krimi, Jwara, Vrana, Kasa, Chardi, Aruchi, Hrillasa, Shwasa, Prameha, Gulma, Arsha, Trishna.

Therapeutic Uses :

1. Kustha : One who takes haritaki and nimba or nimba and amalaka for a month is relieved from all types of kustha. (G.N.)
2. Krimi : Intake of juice of nimba mixed with honey acts as an excellent anthelmintic. (H.S.)
3. Jaundice : One suffering from jaundice should take nimba mixed with honey in the morning. (C.D.)

Parts Used : Fruit, Leaf, Bark, Seed, Oil.

Preparations & Dosage : Bark powder 2-4 gm.; Leaf juice 10-20 ml.; Oil 5-10 drops.

Specific Formulations : Nimbadi churna, Nimbarista, Nimba haridra khanda.

निम्बः स्यात्पिचुमर्दश्च पिचुमन्दश्च तिक्तकः ।
अरिष्टः पारिभद्रश्च हिङ्गुनिर्यास इत्यपि ॥

निम्बः शीतो लघुर्ग्राही कटुपाकोऽग्निवातनुत् ।
अहृद्यः श्रमतृट्कासज्वरारुचिकृमिप्रणुत् ।
व्रणपित्तकफश्छर्दिकुष्ठहृल्लासमेहनुत् ॥
निम्बपत्रं स्मृतं नेत्र्यं कृमिपित्तविषप्रणुत् ॥
वातलं कटुपाकश्च सर्वारोचककुष्ठनुत् ।
निम्बफलं रसे तिक्तं पाके तु कटुभेदनम् ॥
स्निग्धं लघूष्णं कुष्ठघ्नं गुल्मार्शः कृमिमेहनुत् ॥ भा०प्र०

Research Studies: Recently, Neem oil has been reported to be an effective spermicidal agent in rats, rhesus monkeys and humans. It has also been found to have anti-implantation effect when applied intravaginally. The female albino rats treated orally and allowed to complete the term 80 % of animals did not deliver, indicating foetal resorption and 80% antifertility activity (IJMR, Jan 1986 pp 89-92). Influence of Azadirachta indica (Neem) leaf extract on the immunotoxicity of stress and xenobiotics in experimental animals.

Anti hyperglycaemic activity of Neem leaf extract in streptozotocin induced non insulin-dependent Diabetes mellitus. (Indian Journal of Pharmacology 29/1 Feb. 1997.)

21
JYOTIṢMATĪ

Celastrus paniculatus Willd. Family : Celastraceae

Chief Characters :

1. Big shrub, climber.
2. Simple leaf, alternate phyllotaxy.
3. Green and yellow coloured flowers.
4. Panicle inflorescence.
5. Fruit - loculicidal capsule.

Synonyms : Supingala, Katabhi, Tejaswini, Peetataila, Vega, Lata, Jyotishka, Kanguni, Paravatapadi, Panya, Pinya, Kakandani.

Gana :

Charaka : Sirovirechanopaga.

Sushruta : Adhobhagahara, Sirovirechana.

Properties : Rasa - Katu, Tikta; Guna - Tikshna; Virya - Ushna (Anushna) and Vipaka - Katu.

Pharmacological Actions : Kaphavatahara, Deepana, Medhya, Sara, Vamini, Buddhiprada, Smritipada.

Indications : Udara, Gulma, Kushta, Vatavyadi.

Therapeutic Uses :

1. Udara : Jyotishmati seed oil when taken alongwith milk for seven days cures sannipatodara. (V.S.)
2. Amenorrhoea : By intake of fried jyotishmati leaves with sour gruel induce menstruation. (C.D.)
3. Leucorrhoea : Jyotishmati oil processed in apamarga kshara for seven times and when used as an ointment alleviates leucorrhoea. (Y.R.)

Parts Used : Seed, Leaf, Oil.

Preparations & Dosage : Powder 1-2 gm.; Oil 5-15 drops.

Specific Formulations : Jyotishmati taila.

ज्योतिष्मती स्यात्कटभी ज्योतिष्का कङ्गुनीति च ।
पारावतपदीपिण्या लता प्रोक्ता ककुन्दनी ॥
ज्योतिष्मती कटुस्तिक्ता सरा कफसमीरजित् ।
अत्युष्णा वामनी तीक्ष्णा वह्निबुद्धिस्मृतिप्रदा ॥ भा०प्र०

22
KARKAṬAŚṚṄGĪ

Pistacia intergerrima Stew-ex. Brordis.

Family : Anacardiaceae

Chief Characters :

1. Tree grows upto 12m height.
2. Compound leaf, coriaceous leaves.
3. Leaf petiole & leaf consists of gall. The insect which forms the gall is known as Aphis.
4. Unisexual red flowers on separate trees, paniculate inflorescence.
5. Fruit - drupe.

Synonyms : Srungi, Ajasrungi, Vakra, Kulira vishanika, Chakra, Karkatakhya.

Gana :

Charaka : Kasahara, Hikkanigrahana

Sushruta : Kakolyadi.

Properties : Rasa - Kashaya, Tikta; Guna - Laghu, Ruksha; Virya - Ushna and Vipaka - Katu.

Pharmacological Actions : Kaphavatahara, Deepana, Grahi, Vrishya.

Indications : Shwasa, Kasa, Hikka, Aruchi, Jwara, Chardi, Trishna, Urdhwavata.

Therapeutic Uses :

1. Cough : The powder of karkatashringi should be licked with oil in vataja kasa. (C.S.)
2. Asthma : Powder of karkatashringi and seeds of radish mixed with honey and ghee alleviates swasa in children. (V.S.)
3. Vomiting : In order to check vomiting caused by kapha karkatashringi mixed with musta should be given. (C.S.)
4. Aphrodisiac : The male who takes paste of karkatashringi mixedwith milk and maintains on diet of cereals with sugar, ghee and milk participates like a bull in the sex. (A.H.)

Parts Used : Gall.

Preparations & Dosage : Powder 1-3 gm.

Specific Formulations : Bala chaturbhadra, Shrungyadi churna, Chyavanaprasha.

शृङ्गी कर्कटशृङ्गी च स्यात्कुलीरविषाणिका ।
अजशृङ्गी च चक्रा च कर्कटाख्या च कीर्तिता ॥
शृङ्गी कषाया तिक्तोष्णा कफवातक्षयज्वरान् ।
श्वासोर्ध्ववाततृट्कासहिक्काऽरुचिर्वमीन् हरेत् ॥ भा०प्र०

23
BHALLĀTAKA

Semecarpus anacardium Linn. Family : Anacardiaceae

Chief Characters :

1. Deciduous tree grows upto 15m. height.
2. Simple leaf, alternate phyllotaxy.
3. Green coloured flowers, panicle inflorescence.
4. Fruit - berry.

Synonyms : Arushkara, Agnimukhi, Sophakrit, Viravriksha, Arushka, Agnika, Bhalli.

Gana :

Charaka : Deepaniya, Bhedaniya, Kushtaghna, Mutrasangrahana.

Sushruta : Nyagrodhadi, Mustadi.

Properties : Rasa - Katu, Tikta, Kashaya; Guna - Laghu, Snigdha, Tikshna; Virya - Ushna and Vipaka - Madhura.

Pharmacological Actions : Vatakaphahara, Deepana, Bhedana, Medhya, Rasayana, Vrishya, Mutra sangrahana, Brimhana (Majja).

Indications : Arshas, Grahini, Gulma, Krimi, Kushta, Vrana, Sotha, Kaphaja rogas, Udara, Shwitra, Agnimadhya.

Therapeutic Uses :

1. Kushta : In kaphaja kushta, ghee prepared with bhallataka, haritaki and vidanga is efficacious and oil of bhallataka is useful for all varities of kushta. (S.S.)
2. Splenomegaly : Bhallataka, haritaki and jeeraka are mixed with jaggery and made into sweet bolus. It alleviates the disease even in its advanced stage. (V.M.)
3. Worms : Bhallataka taila mixed with vidanga in half quantity and heated in the sun should be taken. It acts as good anthelmintic.

Parts Used : Fruit.

Preparations & Dosage : Paste 3-6gm.; Oil 10-20 drops.

Specific Formulations : Bhallatakavati, Amrita bhallataki, Chincha bhallataka.

भल्लातकः कषायोष्णः शुक्रलो मधुरो लघुः ।
वातश्लेष्मोदरानाहकुष्ठाशोंग्रहणीगदान् ।
हन्ति गुल्मज्वरश्वित्रवह्निमान्द्यकृमिव्रणान् ॥ भा०प्र०

Research Studies: In the cases of Rheumatoid arthritis, it has shown significant response. Besides clinical improvement the ESR has been reduced and D-xylose absorption has also improved in whom it was impaired. In experimental study, its anti inflammatory effect has been observed (ARIM).

The marking nut contains K40. It is the accidental finding about the radio activity in the nut that initiated investigations about its chemotherapeutic value in cancer. Chloroform extract of whole nut is reported to give symptomatic relief in human cancer of the oesophagus and myeloid leukemia. (Indian Journal of Experimental Biology 1971 p. 399)

24
ŚIGRU

Moringa oleifera Lamk. Family : Moringaceae

Chief Characters :

1. Tree grows upto 10m. height.
2. Tripinnate compound leaf.
3. Panicle inflorescence
4. White coloured flowers.
5. Fruit - capsule.

Synonyms : Shobhanjana, Tikshna gandha, Mochaka, Akshiva.

Gana :

Charaka : Krimighna, Swedopaga, Shirovirechanopaga, Katuka skandha.

Sushruta : Varunadi, Shirovirechana.

Properties : Rasa - Katu, Tikta, Madhura; Guna - : Laghu, Ruksha, Tikshna; Virya - Ushna and Vipaka - Katu.

Pharmacological Actions : Kaphavatahara, Chakshusya, Hridya, Pittaraktakopaka, Avrishya (seeds), Sara, Shukrala, Grahi, Deepana, Vidahikara.

Indications : Vidradhi, Shotha, krimi, Kandu, Vrana, Apachi, Pleeha, Sirahshoola, Medoroga.

Therapeutic Uses :

1. Worms : Decoction of shigru and vidanga mixed with honey act as anthelmintic. (V.S.)
2. Ring worm : Paste of shigru root bark eradicates ring worm. (V.S.)
3. Calculi : Decoction of root of shigru is useful in calculi and gravel. (C.S.)
4. Splenomegaly : Intake of powder of pippali, rock salt and chitraka with decoction of shigru bark cures splenomegaly. (S.S.)

Parts Used : Root bark, Seed.

Preparations & Dosage : Root bark juice 10-20 ml.; Seed powder 1-3 gm.

Specific Formulations : Shigrutwagadi lepa, Shigrupushpa rasayan, Shighrawadi churna.

शोभाञ्जनः शिग्रुतीक्ष्णगन्धकाक्षीवमोचकाः ।
तद्बीजं श्वेतमरिचं मधुशिग्रुः सलोहितः ।
शिग्रुः कटुः कटुः पाके तीक्ष्णोष्णो मधुरो लघुः ॥
दीपनी रोचनो रूक्षः क्षारः तिक्तो विदाहकृत् ।
संग्राही शुक्रलो हृद्यः पित्तरक्तप्रकोपणः ॥
चक्षुष्यः कफवातघ्नो विद्रधिश्वयथुक्रिमीन् ।
मेदोऽपची विषप्लीहगुल्मगण्डव्रणान् हरेत् ॥
श्वेतः प्रोक्तगुणो ज्ञेयो विशेषाद् दाहकृद् भवेत् ।
प्लीहानां विद्रधिं हन्ति व्रणघ्नः पित्तरक्तहृत् ।
मधुशिग्रुः प्रोक्तगुणो विशेषाद्दीपनः सरः ॥
शिग्रुवल्कलपत्राणां स्वरसः परमार्त्तिहृत् ॥
चक्षुष्यं शिग्रुजं बीजं तीक्ष्णोष्णं विषनाशनम् ।
अवृष्यं कफवातघ्नं तन्नस्येन शिरोऽर्त्तिनुत् ॥ भा०प्र०

Research Studies: Powdered drug and the different extracts of the stem bark of Moringaptery gosperma Gaertn. (Shigru)were studied for their oedema supressent activity in albino rats. All the extracts showed peak oedema supressant activity with in 2 hrs of carrageenan injection. The methanolic extract showed significant (p) oedema supressant activity similar to that of indo methacin at the first hour of carrageenan injection. (Rao K.S., Mishra S.H., Indian drugs 1977. 43 (3). 146-8)

Aqueous and alcoholic extracts of root and flower showed antihepatotoxic activity in paracetamol induced toxicity in albinorats (Ind. Journal of Pharm. Sci, 1998, 60 (1) pp. 33-35)

25
PALĀŚA

Butea monosperma Lamk. Family : Fabaceae

Chief Characters :

1. Tree grows upto 10-16m. height.
2. Trifoliate compound leaf.
3. Orange red coloured flowers.
4. Racemose inflorescence.
5. Fruit - dry legume (one seeded).

Synonyms : Raktapushpa, Shamidwara, Kimshuka, Kshara sreshtha, Bramhopaneta, Vatapotha, Brahma vriksha.

Gana :

Sushruta : Rodhradi, Mushkakadi, Ambusthadi, Nyagrodhadi.

Properties : Rasa - Katu, Tikta, Kashaya; Guna - Laghu, Snigdha, Ruksha; Virya - Ushna, Sheeta (Flower) and Vipaka - Katu (Fruit), Madhura (Flower).

Pharmacological Actions : Vatakaphahara, Deepana, Grahi, Vrishya, Rasayana, Sara.

Indications : Krimi, Arshas, Grahani, Kustha, Gulma, Vrana, Bhagna, Udara, Prameha.

Therapeutic Uses :

1. Krimi (Worms) : Decoction of palasha seed or paste of the same with rice water should be taken. (S.S.)
2. Pumsavana : One leaf of palasha pounded with milk should be taken by the pregnant woman for begetting powerful son. (B.P.)
3. Contraceptive : Palasha seeds pounded finely and mixed with ghee and honey should be applied locally in vagina during ritukala. It acts as contraceptive. (G.N.)

Parts Used : Bark, Pushpa, Seed, Gum resin.

Preparations & Dosage : Seed powder 3-6 gm.; Flower powder 3-6 gm., Oleo resin 1-3 gm.; Decoction 50-100 ml.

Specific Formulations : Krimimudgara rasa, Palashabeejadi churna, Palashakshara ghrita.

पलाशः किंशुकः पर्णो यज्ञियो रक्तपुष्पकः ।
क्षारश्रेष्ठो वातपोथो ब्रह्मवृक्षः समिद्वरः ॥
पलाशो दीपनो वृष्यः सरोष्णो व्रणगुल्मजित् ।
भग्नसन्धानकृद् दोषग्रहण्यर्शः कृमीन् हरेत् ॥
कषायः कटुकः तिक्तः स्निग्धो गुदजरोगजित् ।
तत् पुष्पं स्वादु पाके तु कटुतिक्तं कषायकम् ॥
वातलं कफपित्तास्रकृच्छ्रजिद् ग्राहि शीतलम् ।
तृड्दाहशमकं वातरक्तकुष्ठहरं परम् ॥
फलं लघूष्णं मेहार्शः कृमिवातकफापहम् ।
विपाके कटुकं रूक्षं कुष्ठं गुल्मोदरप्रणुत् ॥ भा०प्र०

26
APARĀJITĀ

Clitoria ternatea Linn. Family : Fabaceae

Chief Characters :

1. Perennial shrub, climber.
2. Imparipinnate compound leaf, alternate phyllotaxy.
3. White and blue coloured flowers, Cyamose inflorescence.
4. Fruit - legume.

Synonyms : Asphota, Girikarni, Vishnukranta.

Gana :

Charaka : Sirovirechanopaga.

Properties : Rasa - Katu, Tikta, Kashaya; Guna - Laghu, Ruksha; Virya - Sheeta and Vipaka - Katu.

Pharmacological Actions : Tridoshahara, Chakshusya, Medhya, Vishahara, Kanthya, Amahara.

Indications : Kushta, Shoola, Shotha, Raktatisara, Vrana, Shwitra, Mutraroga, Apachi, Unmada, Raktavaha and Mahasrotaojanya vyadhi, Sarpavisha, Galaganda, Bhrama, Shwasa, Kasa and Daha etc.

Therapeutic Uses :

1. Shotha (Oedema) : Intake of the paste of girikarnika relieves oedema. (H.S.)
2. Pumsavana : One should use the pounded root of white flowered aparajita with ghee in morning keeping on controlled diet. (Y.R.)
3. Shwitra (Vitiligo) : The root of white girikarnika is pounded with cold water and applied thickly on the spot affected by vitiligo which disappears in a fortnight or a month if chronic. (R.M.)

Parts Used : Root bark, Seed.

Preparations & Dosage : Root bark powder 1-3gm.; Seed powder 1-2gm.

Specific Formulations : Aparajita churna, Garbhapala rasa.

आस्फोता गिरिकर्णी स्याद्विष्णुक्रान्ताऽपराजिता ।
अपराजिते कटू मेध्ये शीते कण्ठ्ये सुदृष्टिदे ॥
कुष्ठमूत्रत्रिदोषामशोथव्रणविषापहे ।
कषायकटुके पाके तिक्ते च स्मृतिबुद्धिदे ॥ भा०प्र०

27
MADHUYAṢṬI

Glycyrrhiza glabra Linn. Family : Fabaceae

Chief Characters :

1. Perennial shrub grows upto 1.5m. height.
2. Imparipinnate compound leaf, alternate phyllotaxy.
3. Pale violet coloured flowers, racemose inflorescence.
4. Fruit - follicle.

Synonyms : Madhuka, Kleetaka, Yashtimadhuka.

Gana :

Charaka : Jeevaniya, Sandhaniya, Varnya, Kanthya, Kandughna, Chardinigrahana, Shonitasthapana, Mutravirajaniya, Snehopaga, Vamanopaga, Asthapanopaga.

Sushruta : Kakolyadi, Sarivadi, Anjanadi.

Properties : Rasa - Madhura; Guna - Guru, Snigdha; Virya - Sheeta and Vipaka - Madhura.

Pharmacological Actions : Tridoshahara, Varnya, Kanthya, Vrishya, Keshya, Balya, Jeevaniya, Rasayana, Chakshusya, Shukrala.

Indications : Chardi, Trishna, Daha, Raktapitta, Vranashotha, Kshaya, Hridroga, Visha, Glani.

Therapeutic Uses :

1. Heart disease : Paste of madhuyashti and katuka should be taken with sugar and water. (C.S.)
2. Headaches : Yashtimadhu 1gm. and aconite 250 mg. are pounded finely and mixed with mustard powder. By inhalation, it relieves all types of headache. (B.P.)
3. Urticaria : Madhuka mixed with sugar should be used. (C.D.)
4. For promoting lactation : Cow's milk mixed with yashtimadhu and sugar promotes lactation. (V.D.)

Parts Used : Root.

Preparations & Dosage : Powder 3-5 gm.

Specific Formulations : Madhuyashti taila, Madhukadi ghrita.

यष्टीमधु तथा यष्टीमधुकं क्लीतकं तथा ।
अन्यत्क्लीतनकं तत्तु भवेत्तोये मधूलिका ॥
यष्टी हिमा गुरुः स्वाद्वी चक्षुष्या बलवर्णकृत् ।
सुस्निग्धा शुक्रला केश्या स्वर्या पित्तानिलास्रजित् ।
व्रणशोथविषच्छर्दितृष्णाग्लानिक्षयापहा ॥ भा०प्र०

Research Studies: Gujral and his associates (1957) have screened a large number of drugs for their anti-arthritic effect and claimed that Glycyrrhiza glabra was the maximum effective drug in their series. Malhotra and Ahuja have started investigating the efficacy of Glycyrrhizinic acid as Steroidal agent. (ARIM: 1970)

Crude liquorice contains two sources of anti-ulcer activity, one related to glycyrrhizin (a glycoside) and one that remains after glycyrrhizin is removed. Deglycurrhizied liquorice preparations do not cause fluid retention but appear to retain some ulcer healing effect. They antagonise muscle spasm experimentally. (Clinical Pharmacology-Laurence D.R. 1980)

28
YAVĀSA

Alhagi camelorum Fisch. Family : Fabaceae

Chief Characters :

1. Perennial shrub, branches are covered with spines.
2. Simple leaf.
3. Pink flowers
4. Fruit - legume.

Synonyms : Yasa, Duhsparsha,Dhanvayasa, Kunasakaha.

Properties : Rasa - Madhura, Tikta, Kashaya; Guna - Laghu; Virya - Sheeta and Vipaka - Katu.

Pharmacological Actions : Kaphapittahara, Deepana, Balya, Medohara.

Indications : Jwara, Daha, Chardi, Trishna, Kushta, Vatarakta, Visarpa, Kasa, Mada, Bhrama, Raktapitta.

Therapeutic Uses :

1. Epistaxis : Juice of yavasa root should be used as snuff to control epistaxis. (C.S.)
2. Cough : Smoking dried powder of yavasa immediately cures the cough. (V.H.)
3. Alcoholism : Decoction made of panchanga of yavasa should be given. (C.S.)

Parts Used : Panchanga, Yavasa sharkara.

Preparations & Dosage : Juice 10-20 ml.; Decoction 40-80 ml.; Yavasa sharkara 3-6 gm.

Bhavamishra describes Duralabha(Fogonia arabica Linn—Zygophyllaceae) and yavasa combinedly and attributes similar actions to both the drugs.

यासो यवासो दुःस्पर्शो धन्वयासः कुनाशकः ।
दुरालभा दुरालभ्या समुद्रान्ता च रोदिनी ॥
गान्धारी कच्छुराऽनन्ता कषाया हरिविग्रहा ।
यासः स्वादुः सरस्तिक्तस्तूवरः शीतलो लघुः ॥
कफमेदोमदभ्रान्तिपित्तासृक्कुष्ठकासजित् ।
तृष्णाविसर्पवातास्रवमिज्वरहरः स्मृतः ॥
यवासस्य गुणैस्तुल्या बुधैरुक्ता दुरालभा ॥ भा०प्र०

29
ŚĀLAPARṆĪ

Desmodium gangeticum Linn. D.C. Family : Fabaceae

Chief Characters :

1. Perennial shrub grows upto 2m. height.
2. Compound leaf, alternate phyllotaxy.
3. Blue flowers, racemose inflorescence.
4. Fruit - follicle.

Synonyms : Triparni, Deerghapatra, Vidarigandha, Sthira, Guha, Pivari, Soumya, Deergangi, Amsumati.

Gana : Charaka : Angamarda prashamana, Shothahara, Balya, Snehopaga, Madhura skandha.
Sushruta : Vidarigandhadi, Laghupanchamoola.

Properties : Rasa - Madhura, Tikta; Guna - Guru, Snigdha; Virya - Ushna and Vipaka - Madhura.

Pharmacological Actions : Tridoshahara, Balya, Vrishya, Brimhana, Rasayana.

Indications : Shotha, Jwara, Chardi, Atisara, Arshas, Krimi, Shwasa, Kasa.

Therapeutic Uses :

1. Hemicrania : Snuffing with shalaparni juice alleviates hemicrania. (G.N.)
2. Delayed labour : Application of paste of shalaparni root on navel, pelvis, vulva etc. facilitates easy delivary. (V.M.)
3. Diarrhoea : In this one should take shalaparni as a vegetable regularly. (C.S.)

Parts Used : Panchanga (Whole plant).

Preparations & Dosage : Decoction 50-100 ml.

Specific Formulations : Shaliparnyadi kwatha, Dasamularishta.

शालपर्णी स्थिरा सौम्या त्रिपर्णी पीवरी गुहा ।
विदारिगन्धा दीर्घाङ्गी दीर्घपत्रांऽशुमत्यपि ॥
शालपर्णी गुरुश्छर्दिज्वरश्वासातिसारजित् ॥
शोषदोषत्रयहरी बृंहण्युक्ता रसायनी ।

तिक्ता विषहरी स्वादुः क्षतकासकृमिप्रणुत् ॥ भा०प्र०

Research Studies: Desmodium gangeticum has been found to possess the branchodilator, vasopressor, cardiac stimulant effects similar to indirectly acting catecholamines. The alkaloid fraction of D. gangeticum was found to possess mild analgesic and antipyretic activities. (Annual report CCRIMH, 1974-75)

30
PṚŚNIPARṆĪ

Uraria picta Desv. Family : Fabaceae

Chief Characters :

1. Perennial shrub, grows upto 2m. height.
2. Paripinnate compound leaf.
3. Pale violet flowers, racemose inflorescence.
4. Fruit - legume.

Synonyms : Simhapucchi, Kroshtuvinna, Guha, Dhawani.

Gana : Charaka : Angamarda prashamana, Shothahara, Sandhaniya, Madhura skandha.

Sushruta : Vidarigandhadi, Haridradi, Laghupanchamoola.

Properties : Rasa - Madhura, Tikta; Guna - Laghu, Snigdha; Virya - Ushna and Vipaka - Madhura.

Pharmacological Actions : Tridoshahara, Vrishya, Grahi.

Indications : Jwara, Daha, Atisara, Kasa, Shwasa, Shotha, Asthibhagna, Trishna.

Therapeutic Uses :

1. Fracture : Powdered root of prishniparni taken with meat soup for three weeks units the fracture. (B.P.)
2. Vatarakta : Goat's milk cooked with prishniparni and added with sugar and honey should be used. (S.S.)
3. Bleeding piles : Cow's milk cooked with roots of bala and prishniparni's should be given. (C.S.)

Parts Used : Root.

Preparations & Dosage : Decoction 50-100 ml.

Specific Formulations : Dashamoolarishta, Dashamoola katutrayadi kwatha.

पृश्निपर्णी पृथक्पर्णी चित्रपर्ण्यहिपर्ण्यपि ।
क्रोष्टुविन्ना सिंहपुच्छी कलशी धावनिर्गुहा ॥
पृश्निपर्णी त्रिदोषघ्नी वृष्योष्णा मधुराऽसरा ।
हन्ति दाहज्वरश्वासरक्तातीसारतृड्वमीः ॥ भा०प्र०

31
KARAÑJA

Pongamia pinnata Linn. Mess. Family : Fabaceae
(Derris indica)

Chief Characters :

1. Tree grows upto 15m. height.
2. Paripinnate compound leaf, opposite phyllotaxy.
3. Light pink coloured flowers.
4. Panicle inflorescence.
5. Fruit - drupe.

Synonyms : Karanja, Naktamala, Chirabilwa.

Gana :

Charaka : Kandughna, Katuka skandha.

Sushruta : Aragwadhadi, Varunadi, Arkadi, Syamadi, Kapha-samshamana.

Properties : Rasa - Tikta, Katu, Kashaya; Guna - Laghu, Tikshna; Virya - Ushna and Vipaka - Katu.

Pharmacological Actions : Kaphavatahara, Deepana, Pachana, Krimighna.

Indications : Arshas, Kushta, Prameha, Visarpa, Gulma, Krimi, Dushtavrana, Yoniroga, Unmada.

Therapeutic Uses :

1. Piles : Tender leaves of karanja fried in the mixture of oil and ghee and added with parched grain flour should be given. It acts as carminative and laxative. (C.S.)
2. Kushta : On leprotic wounds oil of karanja should be applied. (S.S.)
3. Granthi-visarpa : Hot paste of karanja bark should be applied. (C.S.)
4. Intrinsic haemorrhage : Karanja seed should be taken with honey and ghee. (S.S.)

Parts Used : Bark, Leaf, Seed, Root-bark.

Preparations & Dosage : Decoction, Juice 10-20 ml.; Seed powder 1-3 gm.

Specific Formulations : Karanjadi taila, Karanjadi ghrita.

करञ्जो नक्तमालश्च करजश्चिरबिल्वकः ।
घृतपूर्णकरञ्जोऽन्यः प्रकीर्यः पूतिकोऽपि च ॥
स चोक्तः पूतिकरञ्जः सोमवल्कश्च स स्मृतः ।
करञ्जः कटुकस्तीक्ष्णो वीर्योष्णो योनिदोषहृत् ।
कुष्ठोदावर्तगुल्मार्शोव्रणक्रिमिकफापहः ॥
तत्पत्रं कफवातार्शकृमिशोथहरं परम् ।
भेदनं कटुकं पाके वीर्योष्णं पित्तलं लघु ॥
तत्फलं कफवातघ्नं मेहार्शःकृमिकुष्ठजित् ।
घृतपूर्णकरञ्जोऽपि करञ्जसदृशो गुणैः ॥ भा०प्र०

Research Studies: Alcoholic and aqueous extract of the fresh bark are reported to exhibit marked anti-bacterial activity against M. pyogenes var aureus. The oil and its active constituent karanjin possess anti-bacterial properties. Alcoholic extracts of the oil showed activity against both gram positive and gram negative organism such as Micrococcus pyogenes var aureus, M. Pyogenes var. albus, M. Pyogenes var. citrues, Bacillus subtilis, corynebacterium diphtherius, Salmonelia typhosa, S. paratyphi A and B, E. secherichia coli (ANON, 1969 Watt. 1972)

32
LATĀKARAÑJA

Caesalpinia bonduc Linn. Roxb. Family : Caesalpinaceae

Chief Characters :

1. Perennial shrub, thorny climber.
2. Bipinnate compound leaf.
3. Yellow flowers, racemose inflorescence.
4. Fruit - Follicle.

Synonyms : Puti karanja, Kantaka karanja, Vitapa karanja, Kuberaksha, Prakeerya, Karanji.

Properties : Rasa - Tikta, Kashaya; Guna - Laghu, Ruksha; Virya - Ushna and Vipaka - Katu.

Pharmacological Actions : Trisoshahara, Deepana.

Indications : Shoola, Grahani, Prameha, Kushta, Vishamajwara.

Therapeutic Uses :

1. Filariasis : Juice of putikaranja leaves should be taken. (S.S.)
2. Worms : Juice of putikaranja leaves should be taken with honey. (S.S.)
3. Pox : In the first stage of pox only one should take trikatu powder with juice of putikaranja leaves to alleviate the condition. (C.D.)

Parts Used : Seed, Leave, Root-bark.

Preparations & Dosage : Powder 1-3 gm.; Juice 10-20 ml.

Specific Formulations : Kuberakshadi vati, Vishamajwaragni vati, Krimi kuthara rasa (Yogaratnakara).

कुबेराक्षी यकृत्प्लीहवातघ्नी व्रणरोपणी ॥ भा०प्र०

Research Studies: Petroleum ether extract at a dose of 150mg/kg per oral produced some anti inflammatory effect against acute type of inflammation produced by carrageenine and 5-HT. (Annual report CCRIMH 1977-78)

Seed powder has been administered with doses of 2 gm three times daily for 15 days. There is 100% improvement in symptoms as well as iradication of EH from the stool. (JRIMYH 13 : 1, 1978)

Significant blood sugar lowering effect of C. bonducella was observed in glucose loaded and allozan and streptozotocin induced diabetic animals. (National Conferenceon Recent Trends in Spieces & Medicinal Plant Reaserch, Calcutta, WB, India, A-47,2-4 April 98)

33

KAPIKACCHŪ

Mucuna prurita Hook. Family : Fabaceae

Chief Characters :

1. Perennial shrub, grows upto 5-6 m. height.
2. Trifoliate compound leaf, rhomboid leaflets.
3. Pale violet coloured flowers.
4. Cyamose inflorescence.
5. Black coloured fruit with 5-6 seeds.

Synonyms : Atmagupta, Markati, Kandura, Langali, Vrishya, Ajada, Vyanga, Duhshparsa, Pravrishayami, Shukasimbi.

Gana :

Charaka : Balya, Madhura skandha, Vamanopaga, Purisha virajaneeya.

Sushruta : Vidarigandhadi, Vata samshamana.

Vagbhata : Durvadigana.

Properties : Rasa - Tikta, Madhura; Guna - Guru, Snigdha; Virya - Ushna and Vipaka - Madhura.

Pharmacological Actions : Vatapittahara, Balya, Brimhana, Vrishya, Kapha-pitta-asrahara, Vajikarana, Mutrala, Stanyajanana.

Indications : Vatavyadhi, Mutrakriccha, Krimi, Yoniroga, Klaibya, Atisara, Kashtartava, Dushtavrana, Raktapitta.

Therapeutic Uses :

1. Vatavyadhi : By taking decoction of seeds of kapikacchu for a month one regains the strength in arms. (C.D.)
2. Aphrodisiac : Wheat flour is mixed with powder of kapikacchu seeds and cooked with milk. Then it is mixed with ghee and eaten followed by intake of milk. (S.S.)
3. Worms : The hairs on the fruit of kapikacchu are put within pulp of jaggery and swallowed. After few hours medicine for virechana should be given. (Anubhuta)

Parts Used : Seed, Root, Hairs.

Preparations & Dosage : Seed powder 3-6 gm.; Root decoction 50-100 ml.; Hairs 125 mg.

Specific Formulations : Vanarigutika, Mashabaladi pachana.

कपिकच्छूरात्मगुप्ता वृष्या प्रोक्ता च मर्कटी ।
अजडा कण्डुरा व्यङ्गा दु:स्पर्शा प्रावृषायणी ॥
लाङ्गली शूलशिम्बी च सैव प्रोक्ता महर्षिभि: ।
कपिकच्छूर्भृशं वृष्या मधुरा बृंहणी गुरु: ॥
तिक्ता वातहरी बल्या कफपित्तास्त्रनाशिनी ।
तद् बीजं वातशमनं स्मृतं वाजीकरं परम् ॥ भा०प्र०

Research Studies: Mucuna pruriens (Kapikacchu) seed aqueous extract increased the twitch response of the rat diaphragm to direct and indirect stimulation. The blocking effects of king cobra venom and d-tubocurarine at the neuromuscular junction which are reversed on the rabbit jejunum and the guinea pig ileum, the extract produced dose dependent contration, which were ontagonized by atropine, suggesting involvement of muscoronic receptors (Fitoterapia. v. 68 (4) : p. 366-370, 1997).

Reappraisal of Dopaminergic aspects of Mucuna pruriens and comparative profile with c-dope on CVS and CNS in animals. M.P contributed to improve anti parkinsonism activity and creates tolerability in animals (Indian drugs V. 33 (9); p. 465-472, 1996)

34
ŚARAPUṄKHĀ

Tephrosia purpurea Linn. Family : Fabaceae

Chief Characters :

1. Perennial hurb grows upto 80 cm. height.
2. Paripinnate compound leaf, alternate phyllotaxy..
3. Red coloured flowers.
4. Racemose inflorescence.
5. Fruit - legume.

Synonyms : Pleeha shatru, Neelivrkshakruti.

Properties : Rasa - Tikta, Kashaya; Guna - Laghu, Ruksha, Teekshna; Virya - Ushna and Vipaka - Katu.

Pharmacological Actions : Kaphavatahara, Rasayana.

Indications : Yakrutpleeha roga, Shoola, Krimi, Kasa, Shwasa, Jwara, Gulma, Vrana, Raktavikara.

Therapeutic Uses :

1. Splenomegaly : Paste of sharapunka should be taken with butter milk. It removes the disoder. (V.R.)
2. Wound healing : Sharapunkha mixed with honey heals all types of wounds when anointed. (G.N.)
3. Rat poisoning : Powder of sharapunkha seeds should be taken with butter milk. (A.H.)
4. Prameha : Powder of sharapunkha seeds especially cures prameha. (V.S.)

Parts Used : Root, Alkali of panchanga.

Preparations & Dosage : Powder 3-6 gm.; Juice 10-20 ml.; Kshara-1-3 gm.

Specific Formulation : Sarapunkha-mooladikhadya.

शरपुङ्खः प्लीहशत्रुर्नीलीवृक्षाकृतिश्च सः ।
शरपुङ्खो यकृत्प्लीहगुल्मव्रणविषापहः ॥
तिक्तः कषायः कासास्रश्वासज्वरहरो लघुः । भा०प्र०

Research Studies: The benzene extract showed significant analgesic activity when compared with that of morphine, petroleum ether, ether and benzene extracts significantly potentiated pentobarbitone induced sleeping time when administered orally or intrapertonially to mice and albino rats. (Annual report 1976-77 CCRIMH)

Oral adminstration of the aqueous extract of seeds of T. purpurea (Sharpimkha) led to marked lowering of blood glucose levels in normal and alloxan induced diabetic rabbits. The hypoglycemic effect of the extract was comparable with that of tolbutamide in normal rabbits. In diabetic rabbits, the extract exerted 60-70% hypoglycemic effect as compared to tolbutamide. (IJMR., Vol 81, April 1985)

The MeOH extract of the seeds of Psoralea corylifolia (Bakuchi)was found to inhibit the aggregation of rabbit platelets induced by arachidonic acid, collagen, and platelet activating factor (Journal of Natural Products V. 59 (7) p. 671-672, 1996)

35
BĀKUCĪ

Psoralea corylifolia Linn. Family : Fabaceae

Chief Characters :

1. Annual shrub, grows upto 1 m. height.
2. Unifoliate compound leaf, alternate phyllotaxy.
3. Blue coloured flowers.
4. Racemose inflorescence.
5. Fruit - legume.

Synonyms : Somaraji, Avalguja, Suparnikha, Shashilekha, Soma, Somavalli, Putiphali, Kustaghni, Kalameshi.

Gana :

Charaka : Tikta skandha.

Properties : Rasa - Katu, Tikta, Madhura; Guna - Laghu, Ruksha; Virya - Ushna and Vipaka - Katu.

Pharmacological Actions : Kaphavatahara, Keshya, Twachya, Pittala, Hridya, Sara, Rasayana.

Indications : Kushta, Chardi, Shwasa, Kasa, Shotha, Prameha, Jwara, Pandu, Krimi.

Therapeutic Uses :

1. Kushta : Bakuchi should be taken with warm water and the patient be exposed to the sun keeping on milk diet. Thus he gets rid of the disease. (V.M.)
2. Vitiligo : Decoction of amalaka and khadira (heart wood) added with bakuchi powder should be used regularly to alleviate vitiligo. (V.S.)
3. Deafness : One should take powder of musali and bakuchi in treatment of deafness. (B.S.)

Parts Used : Seed, Seedoil.

Preparations & Dosage : Powder 1-3 gm.

Specific Formulations : Mahaneela taila, Khadirarista.

अवल्गुजो बाकुची स्यात्सोमराजी सुपर्णिका ।
शशिलेखा कृष्णफला सोमा पूतिफलीति च ॥
सोमवल्ली कालमेषी कुष्ठघ्नी च प्रकीर्त्तिता ।

बाकुची मधुरा तिक्ता कटुपाका रसायनी ।।
विष्टम्भहृद्धिमा रुच्या सरा श्लेष्मास्रपित्तनुत् ।
रूक्षा हृद्या श्वासकुष्ठमेहज्वरकृमिप्रणुत् ।।
तत्फलं पित्तलं कुष्ठकफानिलहरं कटु ।
केश्यं त्वच्यकृमिश्वासकासशोथामपाण्डुनुत् ।। भा०प्र०

Research Studies: Anthelminthic studies of aqueous, etherial, alcoholic extracts of bakuchi seeds were carried out in vitro and in vivo, in addition to the kymographic studies on cestodes, trematodes and nematodes. Alcoholic extract was found to be most potent in vitro as well as in vivo and temporary paralysing action was also recorded by these extracts on flat worms and round worms. (Nagarjuna vol xxi, No. 4, 1977)

The essential oil of P. corylifolia has a powerful effect against the skin streptococci so far as it is known D. corylifolia is the only drug has a dual action i.e., action on both rougets cells and the melanoblastic cells are not functioning properly and their stimulation by the oil leads them to form an exude pigment which gradually diffuses into the decolourised areas. (Chopra)

36
KĀÑCANĀRA

Bauhinia purpurea Linn. Family : Caesalpinaceae

Chief Characters :

1. Tree, grows upto 10 m. height.
2. Simple leaf.
3. Purple coloured flowers.
4. Corymb inflorescence.
5. Fruit - legume.

Synonyms : Kanchanaka, Sonapushpaka, Gandhari, Yugmapatraka, Kovidara, Marika, Kundali, Tamrapushpa, Ashmantaka, Swalpa kesari (Kovidara).

Gana :

Charaka : Vamanopaga.

Sushruta : Kashayavarga.

Properties : Rasa - Kashaya; Guna - Laghu, Ruksha; Virya - Sheeta and Vipaka - Katu.

Pharmacological Actions : Kaphapittahara, Grahi, Deepana, Mutrala, Vranaropana.

Indications : Raktapitta, Raktapradara, Kushta, Krimi, Guda bhramsha, Gandamala, Muktrakriccha, Arsha, Vrana, Kshaya, Masurika, Kasa.

Therapeutic Uses :

1. Gandamala : Decoction of kanchanara bark added with shunthi powder relieves gandamala. (S.G.)
2. Pox : Decoction of kanchanara bark added with swarna makshika bhasma is useful in small pox. (B.P.)
3. Piles : Powder of kanchanara root should be taken with butter milk. (A.H.)
4. Internal haemorrhage : Powder of kanchanara flowers should be taken with honey to alleviate it. (C.S.)

Parts Used : Bark, Flower.

Preparations & Dosage : Bark powder 3-6 gm.; Decoction 40-80 ml.; Flower juice 10-20 ml.

Specific Formulations : Kanchanara guggulu, Kanchanara gutika.

काञ्चनारः काञ्चनको गण्डारिः शोणपुष्पकः ।
कोविदारश्च मरिकः कुद्दालो युग्मपत्रकः ॥
कुण्डली ताम्रपुष्पश्चाश्मन्तकः स्वल्पकेशरी ।
काञ्चनारो हिमो ग्राही तूवरः श्लेष्मपित्तनुत् ॥
कृमिकुष्ठगुदभ्रंशगण्डमालाव्रणापहः ।
कोविदारोऽपि तद्वत्स्यात्तयोः पुष्पं लघु स्मृतम् ॥
रूक्षं संग्राहि पित्तास्रप्रदरक्षयकासनुत् ॥ भा०प्र०

Research Studies: The clinical studies have revealed that preparations of stem bark of Kanchanara enhance the effect of anti-tuberculosis drugs used in cases of tubercular cervical lymphandenitis (Dixit, 1967). Bhakuni et al, 1967 reported that the alcoholic extract of stem bark showed CNS activity. Besides producing hypothermia in mice, it also responded to amphetamine hyper activity test. Recently its used in the treatment of experimental goitre in rats has been reported. (Veena et al., 1975)

37
AŚOKA

Saraca asoca Roxb. Family : Caesalpinaceae

Chief Characters :

1. Tree, grows upto 8-10 m. height.
2. Compound leaf.
3. Green or scarlet coloured flowers.
4. Corymb inflorescence.
5. Fruit - legume.

Synonyms : Vanjula, Kankela, Madhupushpa, Hemapushpa, Raktapinda pushpa, Gandha pushpa, Nata, Tamrapallava, Pallava.

Gana :

Charaka : Vedanasthapana, Kashaya skandha.
Sushruta : Rodhradi.

Properties : Rasa - Kashaya, Tikta; Guna - Laghu, Ruksha; Virya - Sheeta and Vipaka - Katu.

Pharmacological Actions : Pittahara, Grahi, Varnya, Hridya, Vishahara.

Indications : Raktapradara, Shoola, Gulma, Adhmana, Apachi, Krimi, Daha, Trishna, Shosha.

Therapeutic Uses :

1. Raktapradara : Intake cold milk boiled with the decoction of ashoka bark. (B.R.)
2. Dysuria and Calculus : Powder of ashoka seeds should be taken with water. (C.D.)

Parts Used : Bark, Seeds, Flowers.

Preparations & Dosage : Bark decoction 50ml.; Seed powder 3-6 gm.

Specific Formulations : Ashokarishta, Ashokaghrita.

अशोको हेमपुष्पश्च वञ्जुलस्ताम्रपल्लवः ।
कङ्केलिः पिण्डपुष्पश्च गन्धपुष्पो नटस्तथा ॥
अशोकः शीतलस्तिक्तो ग्राही वर्ण्यः कषायकः ।
दोषापचीतृषादाहकृमिशोषविषास्रजित् ॥ भा०प्र०

<u>Research Studies:</u> Ashok stimulates the uterus making the contractions more frequent and prolonged without producing tonic contractions like ergot or pitutary. It should be therefore prove useful in all cases of uterine haemorrhage, where ergot is indicated viz, menorrhagia, metorrhagia postartum haemorrhage etc. Its effects are possibly produced through the sympathetic nervous system which is inhibitory to the intestine and generally motor to the uterus. (B.N. Ghosh, PMMT)

The alcoholic extract was found to have good oxytocic activity in rats, guniea pig, human beings and dogs.

The uterine response to the extract was found to be conditioned by hormonal environment and stage of gestation. The extract had spasmodic action on rabbit's intestine, which was completely blocked by pentolinium suggesting the presence of some ganglion stimulating substance. The extract has a cardiotonic action in frog and dog. (PID)

38
ŚIRĪṢA

Albizzia lebbeck Linn. Family : Mimosaceae

Chief Characters :

1. Tree grows upto 15 m. height.
2. Bipinnate compound leaf, alternate phyllotaxy.
3. Greenish yellow coloured flowers.
4. Head inflorescence.
5. Fruit - follicle.

Synonyms : Sukapushpa, Mridupushpa, Bhandeera, Bhandilo, Bhandi, Kapitana, Sukataru, Sukapriya.

Gana :

Charaka : Vishaghna, Vedanasthapana, Sirovirechana, Kashayaskandha.

Sushruta : Salasaradi.

Properties : Rasa - Kashaya, Tikta, Madhura; Guna - Laghu, Ruksha, Tikshna; Virya - Anushna and Vipaka - Katu.

Pharmacological Actions : Tridoshahara, Varnya, Vishahara, Vedanasthapana.

Indications : Kushta, Kandu, Visarpa, Kasa, Shwasa, Shotha, Vrana.

Therapeutic Uses :

1. Kushta : Paste of bark of shirisha used as an ointment alleviates kushta. (C.S.)
2. Krimi : Juice of shirisha and kinhi mixed with honey should be taken internally. (S.U.)
3. Insect bite : Decoction of shirisha (root, flowers, sprouts, bark and seeds) mixed with trikatu, salt and honey should be taken. It destroys insect poisoning. (S.S.)

Parts Used : Bark, Seeds, Leaf, Pushpa.

Preparations & Dosage : Powder 3-6 gm.; Juice 10-20 ml.; Decoction 50-100 ml.

Specific Formulations : Panchashirisha ghrita, Shirisharista, Mahashirisha agada.

शिरीषो भण्डिलो भण्डी भण्डीरश्च कपीतनः ।
शुकपुष्पः शुकतरुर्मृदुपुष्पः शुकप्रियः ॥
शिरीषो मधुरोऽनुष्णास्तिक्तश्च तुवरो लघुः ।
दोषशोथविसर्पघ्नः कासव्रणविषापहः ॥ भा०प्र०

Research Studies: Studies were conducted with the aqueous decoction of stem bark and flowers. Both the extracts were significantly effective (P<0. 01) against bronchospasm induced by micro-aerosals of histamine acid phosphate (1% solution) and acetylcholine chloride (1% solution) in guniea pig bronchi. In another study, Shirisha has shown a significant disodium chromogylcate like action on the mast cells. The bark decoction produced significant reduction in the blood sugar content of the fasting rats in acute studies as well as after one week of its administration. There was also a significant reduction in serum cholesterol and adrenal cholesterol content of these rats. (Annual reports,CCRAS 1975-80)

39
ĀRAGWADHA

Cassia fistula Linn. Family : Caesalpinaceae

Chief Characters :

1. Tree grows upto 8 m. height.
2. Bipinnate compound leaf.
3. Yellow coloured flowers.
4. Racemose inflorescence
5. Fruit - legume.

Synonyms : Raja vriksha, Kritamala, Chaturangula, Deergha-phala, Sampaka, Suvarnaka, Swarnabhushana, Swarnanga, Chaturghaphala.

Gana :

Charaka : Kushtaghna, Kandughna, Tiktaskandha.

Sushruta : Aragwadhadi, Syamadi, Sleshma samshamana.

Properties : Rasa - Madhura; Guna - Mridu, Guru, Snigdha; Virya - Sheeta, Ushna (Dhanwantari Nighantu) and Vipaka - Madhura.

Pharmacological Actions : Kaphapittahara, Samshramana.

Indications : Jwara, Hridroga, Vatarakta, Kushta, Prameha, Udavarta, Shoola, Udara, Kamala, Amavata, Sadhyovrana, Gandamala.

Therapeutic Uses :

1. Kushta : Leaves of aragvadha are pounded with sour gruel (Kanjika) and applied on the part in case of ringworm, kitibha, kushtha and sidhma. (V.S.)
2. Amavata : Leaves of aragvadha are fried with mustard oil and taken in evening followed by meal. It alleviates ama. (B.P.)
3. Jaundice : Aragvadha in the dose of 40 gm. should be taken with juice of sugarcane, it alleviates jaundice. (C.S.)

Parts Used : Fruit pulp, Root bark, Leaf, Flowers.

Preparations & Dosage : Fruit pulp 5-10 gm.; Root-bark decoction 50-100 ml., Flowers 5-10 gm.

Specific Formulations : Aragwadhadi taila, Aragwadhadi lehya.

आरग्वधो राजवृक्षः शम्पाकश्चतुरङ्गुलः ।
आरवेतो व्याधिघातः कृतमालः सुवर्णकः ॥
कर्णिकारो दीर्घफलः स्वर्णाङ्गः स्वर्णभूषणः ।
आरग्वधो गुरुः स्वादुः शीतलः स्रंसनोत्तमः ॥
ज्वरहृद्रोगपित्तास्रवातोदावर्तशूलनुत् ।
तत्फलं स्रंसनं रुच्यं कुष्ठपित्तकफापहम् ।
ज्वरे तु सततं पथ्यं कोष्ठशुद्धिकरं परम् ॥ भा०प्र०

Research Studies: The leaves stem bark and fruitpulp had antibacterial activity while the root bark exhibited no such effect. The fruitpulp had the maximum activity. Anti-fungal activity against the dermatophytes was seen with the acetone extracts of the root bark and stem bark. The root bark had the maximum activity (Lillykuty et al JRIIM Vol IV, No. 1)

40
KHADIRA

Acacia catechu Willd. Family : Mimosaeceae

Chief Characters :

1. Tree grows upto 10 m. height.
2. Bipinnate compound leaf, alternate phyllotaxy.
3. Yellow coloured flowers.
4. Spike inflorescence.
5. Fruit - legume.

Synonyms : Gayatri, Raktasara, Dantadhavana, somavalka, Kantaki, Bahushalya, Yajniya, Balapatra.

Gana :

Charaka : Kushtaghna, Udarda prashamana, Kashaya skandha.

Sushruta : Salasaradi.

Properties : Rasa - Kashaya; Guna - Laghu, Ruksha; Virya - Sheeta and Vipaka - Katu.

Pharmacological Actions : Pittakaphahara, Pachana, Medohara, Dantya.

Indications : Kushta, Krimi, Kandu, Kasa, Prameha, Shwitra, Vrana, Shotha, Pandu, Jwara.

Therapeutic Uses :

1. Kushta : In food and drinks, bath, fumigation and external applications vidanga, the anthelmintic and khadira, the antileprotic are outstanding. (C.S.)
2. Prameha : In sanairmeha, decoction of khadira and in madhumeha, decoction of khadira and kramuka are useful. (S.S.)
3. Diseases of teeth : Decoction of khadira root heals the diseases of teeth. (H.S.)

Parts Used : Bark, Khadira sara.

Preparations & Dosage : Powder 1-3 gm.; Decoction 50-100 ml.; Khadira sara 0.5-1 gm.

Specific Formulations : Khadirarishta, Khadira vati.

खदिरो रक्तसारश्च गायत्री दन्तधावनः ।
कण्टकी बालपत्रश्च बहुशल्यश्च यज्ञियः ॥
खदिरः शीतलो दन्त्यः कण्डूकासारुचिप्रणुत् ॥
तिक्तः कषायो मेदोघ्नः कृमिमेहज्वरव्रणान् ।
श्वित्रशोथामपित्तास्रपाण्डुकुष्ठकफान् हरेत् ॥ भा०प्र०

<u>Research Studies:</u> Hepatoprotective activity of Ethylacefate extract of Acacia catechu (Khadira/Kattha) is studied in rats. The extract of Kattha inhibited the carbontetrachloride induced liver damage in albino rats at 20 mg/Kg b.w. as assessed by the biochemical and histopathological values. (Indian Journal of Pharmacology 1997; 29; pp-426-428.)

41
HARĪTAKĪ

Terminalia chebula Retz. Family : Combretaceae

Chief Characters :

1. Tree grows upto 15 m. height.
2. Simple leaf, opposite phyllotaxy.
3. Green flowers.
4. Spike inflorescence.
5. Oval shaped fruits.

Synonyms : Pathya, Abhaya, Amrita, Vayastha, Kayastha, Putana, Hemavati, Avyatha, Chetaki, Vijaya, Rohini, Jeevati.

Gana :

Charaka : Jwaraghna, Arshoghna, Kasaghna, Prajasthapana.

Sushruta : Amalakyadi, Triphala, Parushakadi.

Properties : Rasa - Pancharasa (Lavana varjita kashaya rasa pradhana); Guna - Laghu, Ruksha; Virya - Ushna and Vipaka - Madhura.

Pharmacological Actions : Tridoshahara, Anulomana, Deepana, Medhya, Rasayana, Chakshusya, Brimhana, Prajasthapana.

Indications : Kushta, Prameha, Krimi, Sotha, Hridroga, Mutrakriccha, Ashmari, Klaibya, Shoola, Pandu, Kamala, Grahani, Vishama jwara, Tamaka shwasa, Kasa, Chardi, Vatarakta, Hikka, Netraroga, Santharpana janya roga.

Therapeutic Uses :

1. Arshas : Haritaki mixed with jaggery should be taken daily. It alleviates piles, constipation and indigestion. (B.P.)
2. Amavata : One suffering from amavata, sciatica and scrotal enlargement should take regularly haritaki with castor oil. (G.N.)
3. Vishama jwara : Haritaki taken with honey alleviates vishama jwara. (G.N.)
4. Kushta : Intake of three hundred Haritaki fruits in divided doses for a period of 40 days (Mandalam) relieves Kushta roga (Basavarjaeeyam).

Parts Used : Fruit.

Preparations & Dosage : Powder 3-6 gm.

Specific Formulations : Triphala churna, Abhayarishta, Citraka haritaki, Agastya haritaki, Vyaghri haritaki, Danti haritaki.

हरीतक्यभया पथ्या कायस्था पूतनाऽमृता ।
हैमवत्यव्यथा चापि चेतकी श्रेयसी शिवा ॥
वयस्था विजया चापि जीवन्ती रोहिणीति च ॥
विजया रोहिणी चैव पूतना चामृताऽभया ।
जीवन्ती चेतकी चेति पथ्याया: सप्तजातय: ॥
हरीतकी पञ्चरसाऽलवणा तुवरा परम् ।
रूक्षोष्णा दीपनी मेध्या स्वादुपाका रसायनी ॥
चक्षुष्या लघुरायुष्या बृंहणी चानुलोमिनी ।
श्वासकासप्रमेहार्श: कुष्ठशोथोदरक्रिमीन् ॥
चर्विता वर्द्धयत्यग्निं पेषिता मलशोधनी ।
स्विन्ना संग्राहिणी पथ्या भृष्टा प्रोक्ता त्रिदोषनुत् ॥ भा०प्र०

Research Studies: Haritaki showed reduction in serum lipid levels without reduction in body weight. (CCRIMH, Annual report, 74-75)

42
VIBHĪTAKA

Terminalia bellirica Family : Combretaceae

Chief Characters :

1. Big tree grows upto 20 m. height.
2. Simple leaf, opposite phyllotaxy.
3. Green and yellow flowers.
4. Spike inflorescence.
5. Fruit - drupe.

Synonyms : Karshaphala, Aksha, Kalidruma, Bhutavasaha, Kaliyugalaya.

Gana :

Charaka : Jwarahara, Virechanopaga.

Sushruta : Triphala, Mustadi.

Properties : Rasa - Kashaya; Guna - Laghu, Ruksha; Virya - Ushna and Vipaka - Madhura.

Pharmacological Actions : Kaphapittahara, Bhedana, Chakshusya, Keshya, Madakari (Phalamajja).

Indications : Kasa, Shwasa, Krimi, Trishna, Chardi, Swarabheda, Ashmari, Atisara.

Therapeutic Uses :

1. Cough and asthma : Only bibhitaka is sufficient in all types of cough and asthma. (A.H.)
2. Calculus : Seeds of bibhitaka are pounded and taken with wine. It removes defects of urine and breaks calculus. (S.S.)
3. Diarrhoea : Burnt fruit of bibhitaka mixed with salt checks diarrhoea even if severe. (B.S.)

Parts Used : Fruit.

Preparations & Dosage : Powder 3-6 gm.

Specific Formulations : Triphala churna, Lavangadi vati.

बिभीतकस्त्रिलिङ्गः स्यादक्षः कर्षफलस्तु सः ।
कलिद्रुमो भूतवासस्तथा कलियुगालयः ।।

बिभीतकं स्वादुपाकं कषायं कफपित्तनुत् ।
उष्णवीर्यं हिमस्पर्शं भेदनं कासनाशनम् ॥
रूक्षं नेत्रहितं केश्यं कृमिवैस्वर्यनाशनम् ।
बिभीतमज्जातृट्छर्दिकफवातहरी लघुः ।
कषायो मदकृच्चाथ धात्रीमज्जाऽपि तद्गुणः ॥ भा०प्र०

43
ĀMALAKĪ

Phyllanthus emblica Linn. Family : Euphorbiaceae

Chief Characters :

1. Tree grows upto 7-8 m. height.
2. Simple leaf.
3. Light green coloured flowers, male and female flowers occur on same branch or on two different branches.
4. Fruit - capsule.

Synonyms : Amrita, Amritaphala, Vayastha, Dhatri, Tishyaphala, Vrishya, Jatiphala rasa, Shiva, Sriphala, Dhatriphala.

Gana :

Charaka : Kasahara, Jwarahara, Kushtaghna, Vayah sthapana, Virechanopaga.

Sushruta : Parushakadi, Triphala.

Properties : Rasa - Pancha rasa (Lavanavarjita), Amlapradhana; Guna - Guru, Ruksha, Sheeta; Virya - Sheeta and Vipaka- Madhura.

Pharmacological Actions : Tridoshahara, Chakshusya, Vrishya, Rasayana, Vayahsthapana, Deepana.

Indications : Prameha, Kushta, Atisara, Arshas, Shoola, Somaroga, Shweta pradara, Rakta pradara, Mutrakriccha, Raktapitta, Timira, Netrakopa.

Therapeutic Uses :

1. Prameha : Amalaki and haridra are the best remedies for prameha. (A.H.)
2. Pradara : The paste of amalaki seeds mixed with sugar and honey should be taken with water or powder or juice of amalaki should be administered with honey. (C.S.)
3. Dysuria : Amalaki taken with jaggery is rejuvenating, promotes semen and alleviates exertion, raktapitta, colic, burning sensation and dysuria. (V.M.)

Parts Used : Fruit.

Preparations & Dosage : Juice 10-20 ml.; Powder 3-6 gm.

Specific Formulations : Chyavanaprasha lehya, Dhatrilauha.

वयस्यामलकी वृष्या जातीफलरसं शिवम् ।
धात्रीफलं श्रीफलं च तथामृतफलं स्मृतम् ।
त्रिष्वामलकमाख्यातं धात्री तिष्यफलाऽमृता ॥
हरीतकीसमं धात्रीफलं किन्तु विशेषत: ।
रक्तपित्तप्रमेहघ्नं परं वृष्यं रसायनम् ॥
हन्ति वातं तदम्लत्वात् पित्तं माधुर्यशैत्यत: ।
कफं रूक्षकषायत्वात् फलं धात्र्यास्त्रिदोषजित् ॥ भा०प्र०

Research Studies: The inhibitory activity of the Phyllanthus embiica leaf extract against human polymorphonuclear leucocytosis (PNN) and platelet function was studied. The results showed that the leaves have inhibitory activity on PNNs and platelets, which confirm its anti-inflammatory and antipyretic properties. (Indian Journal of Physiology & Pharmacology V. 42 (2) : p. 299-302, 1998)

44
LAVAṄGA

Syzygium caryophyllum Gaertn. Family : Myrtaceae

Chief Characters :

1. Small tree.
2. Simple leaf, opposite phyllotaxy.
3. White flowers.
4. Cyamose inflorescence.
5. Fruit - berry, dry fruit.

Synonyms : Devakusuma, Divyagandha, Grahanihara, Srisanjnaka, Sriprasuna.

Properties : Rasa - Tikta, Katu; Guna - Laghu, Snigdha; Virya - Sheeta and Vipaka - Katu.

Pharmacological Actions : Kaphapittahara, Deepana, Pachana, Ruchya, Chakshusya.

Indications : Trishna, Chardi, Shoola, Adhmana, Grahani, Hikka, Kasa, Shwasa, Rajayakshma.

Therapeutic Uses :

1. Thirst : Clove water is useful in thirst and nausea. (V.H.)
2. Pain : Paste of lavanga pounded in warm water should be applied externally. (V.M.)

Parts Used : Flower, Oil.

Preparations & Dosage : Power 1-2 gm.; Oil 1-3 drops.

Specific Formulations : Lavangadi vati, Avipattikara churna, Lavanga chatuhsama, Lavangodaka, Lavangadi chruna.

लवङ्गं देवकुसुमं श्रीसंज्ञं श्रीप्रसूनकम् ।
लवङ्गं कटुकं तिक्तं लघु नेत्रहितं हिमम् ॥
दीपनं पाचनं रुच्यं कफपित्तास्त्रनाशकृत् ।
तृष्णां छर्दि तथाऽऽध्मानं शूलमाशु विनाशयेत् ।
कासं श्वासं च हिक्काञ्च क्षयं क्षपयति ध्रुवम् । भा०प्र०

Research Studies: Eugenol, an active principle of clove (lavanga) is an effective secratogogue in rats, causing dose dependent augmentation of gastric secretion. (Indian Journal of Pharmacology V. 29/1, Feb. 1997)

45
JAMBŪ

Syzygium cumini Linn. Family : Myrtaceae

Chief Characters :

1. Evergreen tree, grows upto 6-20 m. height.
2. Simple leaf, opposite phyllotaxy.
3. White flowers.
4. Panicle inflorescence.
5. Fruit - berry.

Synonyms : Phalendra, Surabhipatra, Kokileshta, Pikabhaksha, Nandi, Rajajambu, Mahaphala.

Gana :

Charaka : Mutra sangrahaniya, Mutra virajaniya, Chardi-nigrahana.

Sushruta : Nyagrodhadi.

Properties : Rasa - Kashaya, Madhura, Amla; Guna - Laghu, Ruksha; Virya - Sheeta and Vipaka - Katu.

Pharmacological Actions : Kaphapittahara, Vatakara, Grahi, Mutra sangrahaniya, Rechana, Vishtambi.

Indications : Chardi, Atisara, Raktapitta, Shwasa, Kasa, Daha, Krimi, Madhumeha, Vrana.

Therapeutic Uses :

1. Vomitting : One should take cooled decoction of the tender leaves of jambu and amra mixed with honey. (C.S.)
2. Diarrhoea : Juice extracted from the pounded leaves of jambu, amra and amalaki should be mixed with goat's milk and honey. It checks diarrhoea mixed with blood. (C.D.)
3. Madhumeha : Powder of jambu seeds is useful in Madhumeha. (N.R.)

Parts Used : Fruit, Leaves, Bark.

Preparations & Dosage : Juice 10-20 ml.; Powder 3-6 gm.

Specific Formulations : Jambwadi ghrita, Jambwadi taila, Panchapallava yoga.

फलेन्द्रा कथिता नन्दी राजजम्बूर्महाफला ।
तथा सुरभिपत्रा च महाजम्बूरपि स्मृता ।
राजजम्बूफलं स्वादु विष्टम्भि गुरु रोचनम् ॥
क्षुद्रजम्बु: सूक्ष्मपत्रा नादेयी जलजम्बुका ॥
जम्बू: संग्राहिणी रूक्षा कफं पित्तास्रदाहजित् ॥ भा०प्र०

Research Studies: Syzygium cumini seed kernel (aqueous suspension) was screened for its antidiabetic activity at the dose levels of 1g. 2g. 4g. and 6g./kg body weight 48 kg dose level was found to exhibit maximum hypoglycaemic effect in rabbits, 3 hrs. after medication. Like tolbutamide, the drug may also be promoting endogenous release of insulin. It also produced a promoting significant decrease in blood sugar level in alloxan diabetic rats (Ancient Science of Life, Vol VI, No 2; October,1986. pp.80-84)

46
DĀḌIMA

Punica granatum Linn. Family : Punicaceae

Chief Characters :

1. Big shrub grows upto 6 m. height.
2. Simple leaf, opposite phyllotaxy.
3. Red coloured flowers, Bisexual flowers.
4. Fruit - berry.

Synonyms : Dantabeeja, Lohitapushpa, Karaka, Kuchaphala, Vrittaphala.

Gana :

Charaka : Hridya, Chardinigrahana.

Sushruta : Parushakadi.

Properties : Rasa - Kashaya, Madhura, Amla; Guna - Laghu, Snigdha; Virya - Ushna and Vipaka - Madhura, Amla (Amla pradana phala).

Pharmacological Actions : Tridoshahara, Hridya, Deepaniya, Balya, Grahi, Shukrala, Tarpana, Medhya.

Indications : Trishna, Daha, Jwara, Raktapitta, Raktatisara, Raktarshas.

Therapeutic Uses :

1. Bleeding piles : Fruit rind of dadima is used as decoction. (C.S.)
2. Diarrhoea : Decoction of bark of dadima and kutaja mixed with honey checks severe diarrhoea with blood immediately. (B.P.)

Parts Used : Fruit, Epicarp of fruit, Root bark.

Preparations & Dosage : Fruit juice 20-50 ml.; Bark decoction 40-80 ml.

Specific Formulations : Dadimashtaka churna, Bhaskara lavana.

दाडिम: करको दन्तबीजो लोहितपुष्पक: ।
तत्फलं त्रिविधं स्वादु स्वाद्वम्लं केवलाम्लकम् ॥

तत्तु स्वादु त्रिदोषघ्नं तृड्दाहज्वरनाशनम् ।
हृत्कण्ठमुखगन्धघ्नं तर्पणं शुक्रलं लघु ॥
कषायानुरसं ग्राही स्निग्धं मेधाबलावहम् ॥
स्वाद्वम्लं दीपनं रुच्यं किञ्चित् पित्तकरं लघु ।
अम्लन्तु पित्तजनकमामं वातकफापहम् ॥ भा०प्र०

Research Studies: Punica granatum extract in a dose of 1.0 gm/kg orally increased pentobarbitone sleeping time by 27.0 % in rats. The extract (1&2 gm/kg. orally) provided protection against castor oil induced diarrhoea in rats. A relaxant effect was observed on isolated rabbit's ileum and rat's uterus. (Ref. Annual report CCRAS 1978-79)

47
DHĀTAKĪ

Woodfordia fruiticosa Linn. Family : Lythraceae

Chief Characters :

1. Big shrub grows upto 3 m. height.
2. Simple leaf, opposite phyllotaxy.
3. Red flowers, bisexual flowers.
4. Panicle inflorescence.
5. Fruit - capsule.

Synonyms : Vahnijwala, Tamrapushpi, Subhiksha, Madakara, Kunjara, Bahupushpi, Dhatupushpi.

Gana :

Charaka : Purisha sangrahaniya, Mutravirajaniya, Sandhaniya.

Sushruta : Priyangwadi, Ambashthadi.

Properties : Rasa - Kashaya, Katu; Guna - Laghu, Ruksha; Virya - Sheeta and Vipaka - Katu.

Pharmacological Actions : Kaphapittahara, Madakari.

Indications : Atisara, Raktapitta, Trishna, Visarpa, Vrana, Krimi.

Therapeutic Uses :

1. Dysentry : One should take the paste of dhataki and aragvadha. (C.D.)
2. Wound : The wound should be dusted with the powder of barks of dhataki and lodhra. (C.D.)
3. Leucorrhoea : Paste of dhataki should be taken with rice water in leucorrhoea. (G.N.)

Parts Used : Flower.

Preparations & Dosage : Powder 1-3 gm.

Specific Formulations : Dhatakyadi churna, Dhatakyadi taila.

धातकी धातुपुष्पी च ताम्रपुष्पी च कुञ्जरा ।
सुभिक्षा बहुपुष्पी च वह्निज्वाला च सा स्मृता ॥
धातकी कटुका शीता मृदुकृत्तुवरा लघुः ।
तृष्णातीसारपित्तास्रविषक्रिमिविसर्पजित् ॥ भा०प्र०

48
INDRAVĀRUṆĪ

Citrullus colocynthis Lamark. Family : Cucurbitaceae

Chief Characters :

1. Climber grows upto 3-4 m. length with hairs (Scabrid).
2. Simple leaf, alternate phyllotaxy.
3. Yellow coloured flowers.
4. Fruit - fleshy fruit, pepo.

Synonyms : Indravaruni : Indri, Chitra, Chitraphala, Gavakshi, Vishala, Gavadani. Maha indravaruni : Varuni, Vishala, Mahatphala, Shwetapushpa, Mrigakshi, Mrigairvaru, Mrigadani.

Gana :

Charaka : Rechana, Moolini.

Sushruta : Adhobhagahara, Shyamadi.

Properties : Rasa - Tikta; Guna - Laghu, Ruksha, Tikshna; Virya - Ushna and Vipaka - Katu.

Pharmacological Actions : Kaphapittahara, Rechana, Garbhapatana.

Indications : Kamala, Udara, Krimi, Kustha, Prameha, Pleehodara, Shwasa, Kasa, Vrana, Sandhivata, Mudhagarbha, Galaganda, Gandamala, Gulma, Granthi.

Therapeutic Uses :

1. Jaundice : Indravaruni mixed with jaggery is useful. (SS)
2. Arthritis : The root of indravaruni should be mixed with pippali and jaggery and taken in the dose of 10 gm. It alleviates arthritis. (B.P.)
3. Gandamala : The root of indravaruni taken with cow's urine alleviates even severe and chronic cervical adenitis. (C.D.)
4. Warts : The root of indravaruni pounded with bull's urine is pasted on affected part. (R.M.)

Parts Used : Fruit, Root.

Preparations & Dosage : Fruit powder $\frac{1}{8}$-$\frac{1}{2}$ gm.; Root powder 1-3 gm.

Specific Formulations : Indravarunyadi churna, Narayana churna.

ऐन्द्रीन्द्रवारुणी चित्रा गवाक्षी च गवादनी ।
वारुणी च पराऽप्युक्ता सा विशाला महाफला ॥
श्वेतपुष्पा मृगाक्षी च मृगैर्वारुर्मृगादनी ।
गवादनीद्वयं तिक्तं पाके कटु सरं लघु ॥
वीर्योष्णं कामलापित्तकफप्लीहोदरापहम् ॥
श्वासकासापहं कुष्ठगुल्मग्रन्थिव्रणप्रणुत् ।
प्रमेहमूढगर्भामगण्डामयविषापहम् ॥ भा०प्र०

<u>Research Studies:</u> The active principle is colocynthin and it acts as gastro intestinal irritant. It produces severe abdominal pain, yellow vomiting, watery stools often blood stained collapse, and ocassionally death. The fatal dose is 1-2 gms and fatal period is usually 24 hrs. Treatment consists of stomach wash with warm water and administration of demulcents and stimulants. In case of dehydration, intravenous glucose and saline should be administered.

49

KŪṢMĀṆḌA

Benincasa hispida Thumb. Family : Cucurbitaceae

Chief Characters :

1. Annual climber grows upto 10 m. height.
2. Covered with small hairs.
3. Simple leaf.
4. Yellow coloured flowers, unisexual flowers.
5. Fruit - big fruit with many seeds, Pepo.

Synonyms : Pushpa phala, Peetapushpa, Bruhat phala, Sthira phala.

Gana :

Shakavarga (B.P.)

Properties : Rasa - Madhura; Guna - Laghu, Snigdha, Guru (Pakwaphala); Virya - Sheeta and Vipaka - Madhura.

Pharmacological Actions : Pittavatahara, Brimhana, Vrishya, Deepana, Hridya, Vastishodhana.

Indications : Mutrakriccha, Mutraghata, Prameha, Ashmari, Trishna, Aruchi, Apasmara, Shwasa, Shoola, Manasika roga (Unmada, apasmara).

Therapeutic Uses :

1. Asthma and cough : Powder of kushmanda root taken with warm water alleviates asthma and cough immediately. (B.P.)
2. Retention of Urine : Kushmanda juice mixed with hingu and Yavaksara removes pain in pelvis, genitals and dysuria. (B.P.)
3. Epilepsy : Ghrita cooked in eighteen times kushmanda juice with the paste of madhuyashti alleviates epilepsy and promotes intellect, speech and voice. (A.H.)

Parts Used : Fruit, Seed, Seed oil.

Preparations & Dosage : Fruit 10-20 gm.; Seed powder-3-6 gm.; Seed oil 5-10 ml.

Specific Formulations : Kushmandavalehya, Kushmanda ghrita, Kushmanda khanda, Kushmanda guda kalyanaka.

कूष्माण्डं स्यात्पुष्पफलं पीतपुष्पं बृहत्फलम् ॥
कूष्माण्डं बृंहणं वृष्यं गुरु पित्तास्रवातनुत् ।
बालं पित्तापहं शीतं मध्यमं कफकारकम् ॥
वृद्धं नातिहिमं स्वादु सक्षारं दीपनं लघु ।
बस्तिशुद्धिकरं चेतोरोगहृत्सर्वदोषजित् ॥ भा०प्र०

Research Studies: Benincasa hispida (alcoholic extract) lowered fasting blood sugar level of 61.2mg/ml. to 41.6mg/ml. after 5 hrs of administration in rabbits. The blood sugar lowering effect persisted upto 24 hrs. The extract showed no effect on carraqeenin induced inflammation and open field performance in rats. (Annual report 1978-79, CCRAS). The alcoholic extract of Benincasa hispida in 10 and 30 mg/kg I.V. caused fail of mean arterial blood pressure. (Annual report 1977-78 CCRIMH)

50
MAṆḌŪKAPARṆĪ

Centella asiatica Linn. Family : Apiaceae

Chief Characters :

1. Perennial herb, procumbent with a weak stem.
2. Simple leaf.
3. Pale voilet coloured flowers.
4. Cyamose inflorescence.
5. Fruit - cremocarp.

Synonyms : Manduki, Divya, Twastri, Mahoushadhi.

Gana :

Charaka : Vayahsthapana, Tiktaskandha.

Sushruta : Tiktavarga.

Properties : Rasa - Tikta, Madhura; Guna - Laghu; Virya - Sheeta and Vipaka - Madhura.

Pharmacological Actions : Kaphapittahara, Vayahsthapana, Medhya, Smritiprada, Hridya, Sara, Rasayana, Swarya.

Indications : Kushta, Pandu, Prameha, Shotha, Raktapitta, Raktavikara, Jwara, Kasa.

Therapeutic Uses :

1. Boils : Local application of the juice of mandukaparni relieves boils. (G.N.)
2. Udara roga : One should take vegetable of trivrit and mandukaparni cooked in their own juice and water without sours salt and fat, steamed or slightly steamed for a month keeping on non-cereal diet. When thirsty one should take the fresh juice of the plant. (C.S.)
3. Intelligent promoting Rasayana : Juice of mandukaparni is life giving, disease destroyer, promotes strength, digestive power, complexion, voice and intellect promoting rasayana. (C.S.)

Parts Used : Panchanga.

Preparations & Dosage : Juice 10-20 ml.

Specific Formulations : Brahmi taila, Saraswatarishta, Saraswata ghrita, Brahmipanaka.

मण्डूकपर्णी माण्डूकी त्वाष्ट्री दिव्या महौषधी ।
× × ×
स्वर्या स्मृतिप्रदा कुष्ठपाण्डुमेहास्रकासजित् ।
विषशोथज्वरहरी तद्वन्मण्डूकपर्णिनी ॥ भा०प्र०

Research Studies: Studies have shown that the plant has a glycoside which dissolves the waxy coating of leprosy germs and make it easy for the body to destroy them. Experiments in which active glycoside has been purified have revealed that it is also active against T.B. bacilli.

Alcoholic extract of C. asiatica from the leaves of the plant was found to potantiate narcosis induced by phenobarbitone by 68.15%. (Annual report, CCRAS, 1979-80)

51

PAṬOLA

Trichosanthes dioica Roxb. Family : Cucurbitaceae

Chief Characters :

1. Climber grows upto 15 m. height.
2. Heart or rectangular shaped leaves.
3. Male and female flowers occurs on different branches consists of white coloured flowers.
4. Fruit - berry with many seeds.

Synonyms : Rajiphala, Beejagarbha, Kulaka, Karkasachada, Panduka, Amritaphala, Kasa bhanjanan, Kushtaha.

Gana :

Charaka : Truptighna, Trishnanigrahana.

Sushruta : Patoladi, Aragwadhadi.

Properties : Rasa - Tikta, Katu; Guna - Laghu, Snigdha; Virya - Ushna and Vipaka - Katu.

Pharmacological Actions : Kaphapittahara, Deepana, Vrishya, Rechana, Varnya.

Indications : Jwara, Daha, Amlapitta, Kushta, Kandu.

Therapeutic Uses :

1. Oedema : In oedema vegetable of patola is wholesome. (C.S.)
2. Masurika : One should take decoction of root of patola to alleviate pittaja masurika. (B.P.)

Parts Used : Fruit, Leaf.

Preparations & Dosage : Juice 10-20 ml.; Decoction 50-100 ml.

Specific Formulations : Patoladi kwatha, Patoladi chruna.

पटोलः कुलकस्तिक्तः पाण्डूकः कर्कशच्छदः ।
राजीफलः पाण्डुफलो राजेयश्चामृतफलः ॥
बीजगर्भः प्रतीकश्च कुष्ठहा कासभञ्जनः ।
पटोलं पाचनं हृद्यं वृष्यं लघ्वग्निदीपनम् ।
स्निग्धोष्णं हन्ति कासास्रज्वरदोषत्रयक्रिमीन् ॥
पटोलस्य भवेन्मूलं विरेचनकरं सुखात् ॥
नालं श्लेष्महरं पत्रं पित्तहारी फलं पुनः ।
दोषत्रयहरं प्रोक्तं तद्वत्तिक्ता पटोलिका ॥ भा०प्र०

52
HIṄGU

Ferula foetida Regal. Family : Apiaceae

Chief Characters :

1. Plant grows upto 2 m. height.
2. Simple leaf, alternate phyllotaxy.
3. Small yellow coloured flowers.
4. Compound or simple umbel inflorescence.
5. Fruit - cremocarp.

Synonyms : Jatuka, Bahlika, Ramatha, Sahasravedhi.

Gana :

Charaka : Deepaniya, Shwasahara, Sanjnasthapana, Katuka skandha.

Sushruta : Pippalyadi, Ushakadi.

Properties : Rasa - Katu; Guna - Laghu, Snigdha, Tikshna; Virya - Ushna and Vipaka - Katu.

Pharmacological Actions : Kaphavatahara, Pittavardhaka, Hridya, Pachana, Ruchya, Chakshusya, Artavajanana, Balya, Bhedaniya, Anulomana.

Indications : Shoola, Gulma, Krimi, Udara, Artavaroga, Apasmara, Murccha, Anaha.

Therapeutic Uses :

1. Caries : In dental caries slightly heated hingu should be kept on caries tooth. (V.M.)
2. Amenorrhoea : Intake of burnt hingu with jaggery induces menstruation. (Anubhuta)
3. Hricchula : Pills made of hingu and kumkuma should be given. (Anubhuta)

Parts Used : Gum Resin.

Preparations & Dosage : 125-500 mg.

Specific Formulations : Hingvashtaka churna, Hingu triguna taila, Hingu karpura vati, Rajah pravartini vati.

सहस्रवेधी जतुकं बाह्लीकं हिङ्गु रामठम् ॥
हिङ्गूष्णं पाचनं रुच्यं तीक्ष्णं वातबलासनुत् ।
शूलगुल्मोदरानाहकृमिघ्नं पित्तवर्धनम् ॥ भा०प्र०

53
ŚATAPUṢPĀ

Anethum sowa Roxb. Family : Apiaceae

Chief Characters :

1. Perennial herb.
2. Bifoliate or trifoliate compound leaves.
3. Yellow coloured flowers.
4. Compound umbel inflorescence.
5. Fruit - cremocarp.

Synonyms : Atilambi, Sitachatra, Madhura, Karavi, Misi, Satahwa, Samhita chatrika.

Properties : Rasa - Katu, Tikta; Guna - Laghu, Tikshna; Virya - Ushna and Vipaka - Katu.

Pharmacological Actions : Vatakaphahara, Deepana, Pittakrita.

Indications : Jwara, Shoola, Vrana, Netraroga, Ajeerna.

Therapeutic Uses :

1. Vatarakta : Shatapushpa pounded with milk should be applied externally to remove pain in vatarakta predominant in vata. (C.S.)
2. Bees sting : Paste of shatapushpa mixed with rocksalt and ghee should be applied. It counteracts the poison. (B.S.)
3. Piles : In dry piles the haemorrhoids should be fomented with lumps of vacha and satapushpa mixed with unctuous substances. (B.S.)

Parts Used : Seed, Oil, Arka (Volatile oil).

Preparations & Dosage : Powder 1-3 gm.; Oil 1-3 drops; Arka 20-40 ml.

Specific Formulations : Satapushpadi lepa, Satapushpadi kashaya, Arka soya.

शतपुष्पा शताह्वा च मधुरा कारवी मिसिः ।
अतिलम्बी सितच्छत्रा संहितच्छत्रिकाऽपि च ॥
शतपुष्पा लघुस्तीक्ष्णा पित्तकृद्दीपनी कटुः ।
उष्णा ज्वरानिलश्लेष्मव्रणशूलाक्षिरोगहृत् ॥ भा०प्र०

54

MIŚREYA

Foeniculum vulgare Mill. Family : Apiaceae

Chief Characters :

1. Perennial herb.
2. Paripinnate compound leaf, alternate phyllotaxy.
3. Yellow coloured flowers.
4. Compound umbel inflorescence.
5. Fruit - cremocarp.

Synonyms : Madhurika, Misri, Chatra, Madhura, Saleya, Saleena.

Properties : Rasa - Madhura, Katu, Tikta; Guna - Laghu, Ruksha; Virya - Sheeta (D.N., K.N.); Ushna (B.P.) and Vipaka - Madhura.

Pharmacological Actions : Vatapittahara (D.N.), Deepana, Pachana, Hridya, Shukrahara.

Indications : Jwara, Shoola, Krimi, Agnimandya, Vibandha, Chardi, Kasa, Yonishoola, Netraroga.

Therapeutic Uses :

1. Adhmana : Enema with decoction of mishreya should be given.
2. Headache : An ointment of seed paste of mishreya should be done.

Parts Used : Fruit, Oil, Root.

Preparations & Dosage : Fruit powder 3-6 gm.; Oil 5-10 drops; Arka 20-40 ml.

Specific Formulations : Misreya arka, Misreya churna.

छत्रा शालेयशालीनो मिश्रेया मधुरा मिसिः ।
मिश्रेया तद्गुणा प्रोक्ता विशेषाद्योनिशूलनुत् ॥
अग्निमान्द्यहरी हृद्या बद्धविट्कृमिशुक्रहृत् ।
रूक्षोष्णा पाचनी कासवमिश्लेष्मानिलान्हरेत् ॥ भा०प्र०

55
DHĀNYAKA

Coriandrum sativum Linn. Family : Apiaceae

Chief Characters :

1. Annual herb grows upto 40 cms. height.
2. Decompound leaf, alternate phyllotaxy.
3. White/light pink coloured flowers.
4. Compound umbel inflorescence.
5. Fruit - cremocarp.

Synonyms **:** Chatra, Kustumbaru, Vitunnaka, Dhanaka, Dhanya, Dhana, Dhanaeyaka, Kunati, Dhenuka.

Gana :

Charaka : Trishna prashamana, Sheeta prashamana.

Sushruta : Guduchyadi.

Properties : Rasa - Kashaya, Tikta, Madhura, Katu; Guna - Laghu, Snigdha; Virya - Ushna and Vipaka - Madhura (B.P.).

Pharmacological Actions : Tridoshahara, Grahi, Deepana, Pachana, Avrishya, Mutrala, Pittahara (Ardra).

Indications : Trishna, Daha, Jwara, Chardi, Krimi, Arshas, Kasa, Shwasa, Karshyatwa.

Therapeutic Uses :

1. Vatarakta : Intake of dhanyaka 10 gm. and jeeraka 20 gm. cooked with jaggery relieves vatarakta. (H.S.)
2. Cough and Asthma : Dhanyaka mixed with sugar should be given with rice water in treatment of cough of children. (V.S.)
3. Thirst : In thirst emerging as a complication in other diseases cold infusion of dhanyaka added with sugar and honey is useful. It relieves daha (burning sensation) also. (A.H.)

Parts Used : Fruit, Panchanga (Whole plant).

Preparations & Dosage : Powder-3-6 gm.; Cold infusion 20-30 ml.

Specific Formulations : Dhanyaka lehya, Dhanyaka panchaka kashaya, Dhanyakadi hima.

धान्यकं धानकं धान्यं धाना धानेयकं तथा ।
कुनटी धेनुका छत्रा कुस्तुम्बुरु वितुन्नकम् ॥
धान्यकं तुवरं स्निग्धमवृष्यं मूत्रलं लघु ।
तिक्तं कटूष्णवीर्यञ्च दीपनं पाचनं स्मृतम् ॥
ज्वरघ्नं रोचकं ग्राही स्वादुपाकित्रिदोषनुत् ।
तृष्णादाहवमिश्वासकासकार्श्यक्रिमिप्रणुत् ॥
आर्द्रन्तु तद्गुणं स्वादु विशेषात्पित्तनाशनम् ॥ भा०प्र०

56
AJAMODĀ

Apium graveolens Linn. Family : Umbelliferae

Chief Characters :

1. Biennial shrub, grows upto 2 m. height.
2. Compound leaf.
3. White flowers.
4. Umbel inflorescence.
5. Fruit - cremocarp.

Synonyms : Kharaswa, Deepya, Karavi, Mayura, Brahma kusha, Locamastaka.

Gana :

Charaka : Shoola prashamana, Deepaniya.

Sushruta : Pippalyadi.

Properties : Rasa - Katu, Tikta; Guna - Laghu, Ruksha, Tikshna; Virya - Ushna and Vipaka - Katu.

Pharmacological Actions : Kaphavatahara, Deepana, Vrishya, Balya, Hridya, Vidahi, Mutrala.

Indications : Shoola, Hikka, Adhmana, Krimi, Chardi, Agnimandya, Shotha, Udara, Vastiruja, Netraroga, Aruchi, Arshas.

Therapeutic Uses :

1. Shoola : Fruit powder should be given with hot water. (Anubhuta)
2. Oedema : Powder of root of ajamoda alleviates oedema of whole body. (Anubhuta)

Parts Used : Fruit, Root.

Preparations & Dosage : Powder 1-3 gm.; Arka 5-10 ml.

Specific Formulations : Ajamodadi chruna, Ajamodadi vataka, Ajamodarka.

अजमोदा खराश्वा च मयूरो दीप्यकस्तथा ।
तथा ब्रह्मकुशा प्रोक्ता कारवीलो च मस्तका ॥
अजमोदा कटुस्तीक्ष्णा दीपनी कफवातनुत् ।
उष्णा विदाहिनी हृद्या वृष्या बलकरी लघुः ॥
नेत्रामयकृमिच्छर्दिहिक्काबस्तिरुजो हरेत् । भा०प्र०

57

YAVĀNĪ

Carum copticum Benth. Family : Apiaceae

Chief Characters :

1. Annual herb grows upto 1 m. height.
2. Paripinnate compound leaf, alternate phyllotaxy.
3. Small white coloured flowers.
4. Compound umbel inflorescence.
5. Fruit - cremocarp.

Synonyms : Ajamodika, Deepyaka, Bhutika, Yavanaka, Yavanika, Ugra gandha, Brahmadarbha, Deepya.

Gana :

Chaturbeeja (B.P.)

Charaka : Shoola Prashamana.

Properties : Rasa - Katu, Tikta; Guna - Laghu, Ruksha, Tikshna; Virya - Ushna and Vipaka - Katu.

Pharmacological Actions : Kaphavatahara, Deepana, Pachana, Ruchya, Shukrahara.

Indications : Anaha, Gulma, Udara, Pleeha, Krimi, Shoola.

Therapeutic Uses :

1. Gulma : Buttermilk added with the powder of yavani and bida salt should be taken. It acts as appetiser and carminative.
2. Diseases of teeth : In the night yavani and vaca should be chewed. (H.S.)
3. Urticaria : One who takes yavani with jaggery keeping on wholesome diet becomes free from urticaria in a week. (V.M.)

Parts Used : Fruit.

Preparations & Dosage : Powder 1-3 gm.; Oil 1-3 drops; Arka 20-40 ml.

Specific Formulations : Yavanishadava, Yavanikadi ghrita.

यवानिकोग्रगन्धा च ब्रह्मदर्भाऽजमोदिका ॥
सैवोक्ता दीप्यका दीप्या तथा स्याद्यवसाह्वया ।

यवानी पाचनी रुच्या तीष्णोष्णा कटुका लघु: ॥
दीपनी च तथा तिक्ता पित्तला शुक्रशूलहृत् ।
वातश्लेष्मोदरानाहगुल्मप्लीहकृमिप्रणुत् ॥ भा०प्र०

Research Studies: When C. copticum seed powder was fed (1% mixed with powdered rabbit feed) for four weeks to normal albino rabbits, hypocholesterolemic hypotriglyceridemic and hypo-phospholi-pidemic effect were observed from the first week itself. The serum cholesterol binding reserve and high denisty lipoprotein levels, on the other hand, showed an increase in the corresponding periods.

58

JĪRAKA

Cuminum cyminum Linn. Family : Apiaceae

Chief Characters :

1. Annual herb.
2. Simple leaf dissected into 3 parts.
3. Small white coloured flowers.
4. Compound umbel inflorescence.
5. Fruit - cremocarp.

Synonyms : Shweta jiraka : Jarana, Ajaji, Kana, Dirgha jiraka, Krishna jiraka : Sugandha, Udgara shodhana, Brihat jiraka : Kalajaji, Sushavi, Upakalika, Karavi, Prithvika, Prithvi, Upakunchi, Kunchi.

Gana :

Charaka : Shoola prashamana.

Sushruta : Pippalyadi.

Properties : Rasa - Katu; Guna - Laghu, Ruksha; Virya - Ushna and Vipaka - Katu.

Pharmacological Actions : Kaphavatahara, Deepana, Pachana, Grahi, Medhya, Ruchya, Balya, Chakshusya, Garbhashaya shuddhikara, Vishahara, Vrishya.

Indications : Garbhashaya roga, Jwara, Arochaka, Atisara, Grahani, Krimi, Gulma, Chardi, Adhmana, Kushta, Vishama jwara.

Therapeutic Uses :

1. Vishama jwara : Jeeraka combined with jaggery alleviates irregular fever. It also improves digestion and destroys diseases caused by vata. (C.D.)
2. Amla pitta : Ghrita 640 gm. should be cooked with paste of jeeraka and dhanyaka. It removes kapha, pitta and anorexia, improves digestion and checks vomiting. (V.M.)
3. Scorpion bite : Paste of jeeraka mixed with ghee and rocksalt applied warm removes pain of scorpion sting. (C.D.)

Parts Used : Seed.

Preparations & Dosage : Powder 3-6 gm.

Specific Formulations : Jeerakadyarista, Jeeraka ghrita, Jeerakadi modaka.

जीरको जरणोऽजाजी कणा स्याद्दीर्घजीरकः ॥
जीरकत्रितयं रूक्षं कटूष्णं दीपनं लघु ।
संग्राही पित्तलं मेध्यं गर्भाशयविशुद्धिकृत् ॥
ज्वरघ्नं पाचनं वृष्यं बल्यं रुच्यं कफापहम् ।
चक्षुष्यं पवनाध्मानगुल्मच्छर्द्यतिसारहृत् ॥ भा०प्र०

59

KṚṢṆAJĪRAKA

Carum carvi Linn. Family : Umbellifereae

Chief Characters :

1. Perennial shrub grows upto 60 cms. height.
2. Alternate phyllotaxy, simple leaf.
3. White coloured flowers.
4. Umbel inflorescence.
5. Fruit - cremocarp.

Synonyms : Sugandha, Udgara shodhana, Krishnajeera, Jarana, Karavi, Kashmira jiraka.

Gana :

Haritakyadi varga (B.P.)

Properties : Rasa - Katu; Guna - Laghu, Ruksha; Virya - Ushna and Vipaka - Katu.

Pharmacological Actions : Kaphahara, Deepana, Pachana, Grahi, Vatahara, Pittala, Medhya, Chakshusya, Garbhasaya sodhana.

Indications : Jeerna jwara, Atisara, Gulma, Adhmana, Prasutivikara, Grahini, Shopha, Chardi, Agnimandya.

Therapeutic Uses :

1. Malaria fever : Intake of krishnajeeraka with equal quantity of jaggery and a bit of maricha checks quartidian fever immediately. (B.P.)
2. Pratishyaya : Inhalations of krishnajeeraka relieve cold. (V.S.)
3. Mukhapaka : The powder made up of krishnajiraka, kushta and kutajabeeja should be chewed and stomatitis relieves within three days.

Parts Used : Seed, Fruit.

Preparations & Dosage : Powder 1-3 gm.

कृष्णजीर: सुगन्धश्च तथैवोद्गारशोधन: ।। भा०प्र०

60
MAÑJIṢṬHĀ

Rubia cordifolia Linn. Family : Rubiaceae

Chief Characters :

1. Perennial herb grows upto 4 m. height.
2. Simple leaf.
3. Green coloured flowers.
4. Cyamose inflorescence.
5. Oval shaped fruit.

Synonyms : Yojanavalli, Vastraranjani, Vikasa, Samanga, Jingi, Bhanditaki, Kalameshika, Mandukaparni, Bhandiri, Bhandi, Rasayani, Aruna, Kala, Raktangi, Raktayashtika, Gandiri, Manjusha.

Gana :

Charaka : Jwarahara, Varnya, Vishaghna.

Sushruta : Priyangvadi, Pitta samshamana.

Properties : Rasa - Madhura, Tikta, Kashaya; Guna - Guru, Ruksha; Virya - Ushna and Vipaka - Katu.

Pharmacological Actions : Kaphapitta shamaka, Varnya, Swarya, Vishahara.

Indications : Jwara, Kushta, Visarpa, Prameha, Shotha, Yoniruja, Karnaruja, Vrana, Netraroga, Raktatisara, Mutrakriccha.

Therapeutic Uses :

1. Manjisthameha : One should take decoction of manjistha and chandana. (S.S.)
2. Vyanga : Manjistha powder should be taken with honey.

Parts Used : Root.

Preparations & Dosage : Decoction 50-100 ml.; Pwoder 1-3 gm.

Specific Formulations : Mahamanjisthadi kwatha, Pinda taila, Manjisthadyarka.

मञ्जिष्ठा विकसा जिङ्गी समङ्गा कालमेषिका ॥
मण्डूकपर्णी भण्डीरी भण्डी योजनवल्ल्यपि ।
रसायन्यरुणा काला रक्ताङ्गी रक्तयष्टिका ॥

भण्डीतकी च गण्डीरी मञ्जूषा वस्त्ररञ्जिनी ।
मञ्जिष्ठा मधुरा तिक्ता कषाया स्वरवर्णकृत् ॥
गुरुरुष्णा विषश्लेष्मशोथयोन्यक्षिकर्णरुक् ।
रक्तातीसारकुष्ठास्त्रवीसर्पव्रणमेहनुत् ॥ भा०प्र०

Research Studies: Rubidin anthraquinene, isolated from alcoholic extract of Rubia cordifolia, possesses potent antioxidant property. The antioxidant property of the preparation has been found to be better than that of EDTA, tris, mannitol,vitamin-E and P-benzoguinone. (Indian Journal of Biochemistry and Biophysics, Vol. 34, June 1997, pp. 302-306)

61
MADANAPHALA

Randia dumetorum Lamk. Family : Rubiaceae

Chief Characters :

1. Small tree grows upto 4 m. height.
2. Tree is covered with thorns.
3. Simple leaf, opposite phyllotaxy.
4. White coloured flowers.
5. Fruit - berry.

Synonyms : Chardana, Madana, Vishapushpaka, Pindi, Pinditaka, Pinda, Shalyaka, Marubaka.

Gana :

Charaka : Asthapanopaga, Anuvasanopaga.

Sushruta : Aragwadhadi, Mushkakadi.

Properties : Rasa - Madhura, Tikta; Guna - Laghu, Ruksha; Virya - Ushna and Vipaka - Katu.

Pharmacological Actions : Kaphavatahara, Lekhana, Vamanakara

Indications : Kushta, Shotha, Gulma, Vrana, Vidradhi, Pratishyaya, Anaha.

Therapeutic Uses :

1. Parshwa shoola : Madana pounded with sour gruel (kanjika) is applied as a paste on navel to relieve pain. (C.D.)
2. Raktapitta : Ksheerayavagu processed with seeds of mandana is useful in adhogata raktapitta. (C.D.)

Parts Used : Fruit.

Preparations & Dosage : Pwoder 1-2 gm.; For vamana 3-6 gm..

Specific Formulations : Madanaphaladivarti, Madanadi churna.

मदनश्छर्दनः पिण्डो नटः पिण्डीतकस्तथा ।
करहाटो मरुबकः शल्यको विषपुष्पकः ॥
मदनो मधुरस्तिक्तो वीर्योष्णो लेखनो लघुः ।
वान्तिकृद्विद्रधिहरः प्रतिश्यायव्रणान्तकः ॥
रूक्षः कुष्ठकफानाहशोथगुल्मव्रणापहः ॥ भा०प्र०

Research Studies: In anesthetized dogs RDG-I in doses of 2,4,8 mg./kg. produced hypotension and respiratory depression. It produced positive inotropic and chronotropic effects on prefused frog heart preparation. In isolated rabbit heart, it increased the heart rate and amplitude of contraction. It prolonged pentobarbitone induced hypnosis in mice significantly. (Annual report, CCRAS, 78-80)

62
GANDHAPRASĀRIṆĪ

Paederia foetida Linn. Family : Rubiaceae

Chief Characters :

1. Climbs covered with foul smelling hairs.
2. Simple leaf, opposite phyllotaxy.
3. Small white flowers.
4. Panicle inflorescence.
5. Fruit - pyrenes with broad wings.

Synonyms : Prasarini, Sarini, Gandhadya, Balya, Rajabala, Bhadraparni, Pratanini, Bhadra, Bala, Katambara.

Gana :

Guduchyadi. (B.P.)

Properties : Rasa - Tikta; Guna - Guru; Virya - Ushna and Vipaka - Katu.

Pharmacological Actions : Vatahara, Sara, Kaphahara, Balya, Vrishya, Sandhanakara.

Indications : Vatavyadhi, Amavata, Mutrakriccha, Arshas, Shotha, Vatarakta.

Therapeutic Uses :

1. Dysuria : Paste of prasarini when taken with coconut water regularly alleviates dysuria and gravels. (V.M.)
2. Vatavyadhi : Oil prepared with the paste, decoction of prasarini root along with addition of milk and oil should be used both externally (as abhyanga) and internally. (C.S.)

Parts Used : Root, Leaf.

Preparations & Dosage : Juice 10-20 ml.; Decoction 50-00 ml.

Specific Formulations : Prasarini taila, Prasarini lehya.

प्रसारणी राजबला भद्रपर्णी प्रतानिनी ।
सरणी सारणी भद्रा बला चापि कटम्भरा ॥
प्रसारणी गुरुर्वृष्या बलसन्धानकृत्सरा ।
वीर्योष्णा वातहृत्तिक्ता वातरक्तकफापहा ॥ भा०प्र०

63
JAṬĀMĀṀSĪ

Nardostachys jatamansi DC. Family : Velarianaceae

Chief Characters :

1. Perennial shrub having root-stock.
2. Radical and cauline leaves are present.
3. Rose coloured flowers.
4. Head inflorescence.
5. Fruit - white coloured long fruit covered with hairs.

Synonyms : Bhutajata, Tapaswini, Pisitha, Vilomasa, Nalada, Jatila.

Gana :

Charaka : Samjnasthapana, Kandughna, Tiktaskandha.

Properties : Rasa - Tikta, Kashaya, Madhura, ; Guna - Laghu, Snigdha; Virya - Sheeta and Vipaka - Katu.

Pharmacological Actions : Tridoshahara, Medhya, Balya.

Indications : Kushta, Visarpa, Daha, Jwara.

Therapeutic Uses :

1. Wound : Oil processed with mamsi is a good healing agent for accidental wounds. (S.S.)
2. Akshepaka vata : Intake of decoction prepared from jatamamsi (1 tola) ashwagandha ($\frac{1}{4}$ tola), powder of khurasani ajavayan (1 $\frac{1}{2}$ masha) and water (10 tola) alleviates akshepaka vata. (S.Y.S.)

Parts Used : Root.

Preparations & Dosage : Powder 2-4 gm.; Decoction 40-80 ml.

Specific Formulations : Mamsyadi kwatha, Rakshoghna ghrita.

जटामांसी भूतजटा जटिला च तपस्विनी ।
मांसी तिक्ता कषाया च मेध्या कान्तिबलप्रदा ॥
स्वाद्वी हिमा त्रिदोषास्त्रदाहवीसर्पकुष्ठनुत् ॥ भा०प्र०

Research Studies: In 1955 Gujral et al undertook a systematic study of 33 different plants selected from Ayurvedic literature for diuretic property. According to authors, N. jatamamsi, Sccharum officinarum (Ikshu), Oroxylum indicum (Shyonaka) and Viola odorata (Banapsha) showed good diuretic activity. (ARMI) RB Arora reported that N. jatamamsi is having hypotensive property. (ICMR, 1975, Serial No. 51)

64
BHṚṄGARĀJA

Eclipta alba Linn. Family : Asteraceae

Chief Characters :

1. Annual herb grows upto 50 cms. height.
2. Simple leaf, opposite phyllotaxy.
3. Small white flowers.
4. Head inflorescence (Heterogamous head).
5. Fruit - appears as triangular with small seeds.

Synonyms : Markava, Kesaraja, Kesaranjana, Bhringa, Angaraka, Bhringara.

Properties : Rasa - Tikta, Katu; Guna - Laghu, Snigdha, Tikshna; Virya - Ushna and Vipaka - Katu.

Pharmacological Actions : Kaphavatahara, Balya, Rasayana, Keshya, Dantya, Chakshusya, Twachya.

Indications : Kushta, Krimi, Shwasa, Kasa, Shotha, Pandu, Netraroga, Shiroruja, Hridroga.

Therapeutic Uses :

1. Gastritis : Powder of haritaki and bhringaraja mixed with old jaggery controls vomiting caused by hyperacidity. (C.D.)
2. Diarrhoea : Pill made of bhringaraja with water alleviates diarrhoea with mucous, blood and griping. (V.S.)
3. Cough and asthma : Oil prepared with juice of bhringaraja is useful in cough and asthma. (S.S.)

Parts Used : Panchanga (Whole plant).

Preparations & Dosage : Juice 5-10 ml.

Specific Formulations : Bhringarajasava, Shadbindu taila.

भृङ्गराजो भृङ्गरजो मार्कवो भृङ्ग एव च ।
अङ्गारकः केशराजो भृङ्गारः केशरञ्जनः ॥
भृङ्गारः कटुकस्तीक्ष्णो रूक्षोष्णः कफवातनुत् ।
केश्यस्त्वच्यः कृमिश्वासकासशोथामपाण्डुनुत् ।
दन्त्यो रसायनो बल्यः कुष्ठनेत्रशिरोऽर्त्तिनुत् ॥ भा०प्र०

65
PUṢKARAMŪLA

Inula racemosa Hook. F. Family : Asteraceae

Chief Characters :

1. Herb grows upto 3 m. height.
2. Consists of radical and cauline leaves.
3. Yellow coloured flowers.
4. Heterogamous head inflorescence.
5. Fruit - achene.

Synonyms : Pushkara, Poushkara, Padmapatra, Kashmeera, Kushtabheda.

Gana :

Charaka : Shwasahara, Hikkanigrahana.

Properties : Rasa - Tikta, Katu, ; Guna - Laghu, Tikshna; Virya - Ushna and Vipaka - Katu.

Pharmacological Actions : Kaphavatahara, Deepana.

Indications : Hikka, Shwasa, Kasa, Parshwa shoola, Vatakaphaja jwara, Shopha, Pandu, Aruchi.

Therapeutic Uses :

1. Cough and asthma : Pushkaramoola powder should be taken with honey. It alleviates cough, asthma and heart diseases.
2. Hridroga : One should take pushkaramoola root powder to alleviate hridroga. The powder consisting of haritaki, vacha, rasna, pippali, sunthi, sathi and pushkaramula is very useful in relieving hridroga. (B.P.)

Parts Used : Root.

Preparations & Dosage : Powder 1-3 gm.

Specific Formulations : Pushkaradi churna, Haritakyadi churna.

उक्तं पुष्करमूलं तु पौष्करं पुष्करं च तत् ।
पद्मपत्रं च काश्मीरं कुष्ठभेदमिमं जगु: ॥
पौष्करं कटुकं तिक्तमुक्तं वातकफज्वरान् ।
हन्ति शोथाऽरुचिश्वासान् विशेषात्पार्श्वशूलनुत् ॥ भा०प्र०

66
KUṢṬHA

Saussurea lappa C.B. Clarke   Family : Asteraceae

Chief Characters :

1. Annual shrub grows upto 2 m. height.
2. Consists of radical and cauline leaves.
3. Pale voilet flowers.
4. Homogamous head inflorescence.
5. Fruit - achene.

Synonyms : Vapya, Kashmeera, Utpala, Poushkara, Rogahwaya, Paribhavya.

Gana :

Charaka : Shukrashodhana, Lekhaniya, Asthapanopaga.
Sushruta : Eladi.

Properties : Rasa - Tikta, Katu, Madhura, ; Guna - Laghu, Ruksha, Tikshna; Virya - Sheeta and Vipaka - Katu.

Pharmacological Actions : Vatakaphahara, Shukrala, Lekhaniya.

Indications : Shwasa, Kasa, Hikka, Jwara, Vatarakta, Visarpa, Kustha, Apasmara.

Therapeutic Uses :

1. Apasmara and Unmada : Old ghee processed with brahmi juice, vaca, kushtha and shankhapushpi alleviates insanity and epilepsy. (C.S.)
2. Arumsika : Kushta is roasted on an earthenpan, powdered and mixed with oil. Its application on scalp destroys itching, discharge, burning sensation and pain. (A.H., C.D.)

Parts Used : Root.

Preparations & Dosage : Powder $\frac{1}{2}$-1 gm.

Specific Formulations : Kushtadi churna, Kushtadi taila.

कुष्ठं रोगाह्वयं वाप्यं पारिभव्यं तथोत्पलम् ॥
कुष्ठमुष्णं कटु स्वादु शुक्रलं तिक्तकं लघु ।
हन्ति वातास्रवीसर्पकासकुष्ठमरुत्कफान् ॥ भा०प्र०

Research Studies: The drug has remarkable effect in controlling bronchial asthma, especially those of the vago-tonic type. (IJMR, 1929, 351) Saussurine causes relaxation of bronchial muscles, partly by direct action on the muscle, and partly through the vagus. The essential oil acts as expectorant while excreted through the bronchial mucous membrane.

It is therefore largely used in the treatment of bronchial asthma. It is also used as carminative and diuretic. It is an antiseptic and is eliminated by the genito-urinary tract which it stimulates. It is possible that the aphrodisiac effect is due to local irritation. (PMMT)

67
CITRAKA

Plumbago zeylanica Linn. Family : Plumbaginaceae

Chief Characters :

1. Perennial shrub grows upto 1 m. height.
2. Simple leaf, alternate phyllotaxy.
3. White flowers.
4. Spike inflorescence.
5. Fruit - capsule.

Synonyms : Anala, Peeti, Dahana, Vahnisanganaka, Pati, Vyala, Ushna, Analanama.

Gana :

Charaka : Deepaniya, Shoola prashamana, Bhedaniya, Arshoghna, Lekhaniya.

Sushruta : Pippalyadi, Mustadi, Amalakyadi, Varunadi, Aragwadhadi.

Properties : Rasa - Katu; Guna - Laghu, Ruksha, Tikshna; Virya - Ushna and Vipaka - Katu.

Pharmacological Actions : Vatakaphahara, Deepana, Pachana, Grahi, Rasayana.

Indications : Grahani, Arshas, Shoola, Krimi, Kasa, Udara, Pandu, Kushta, Shotha.

Therapeutic Uses :

1. Diarrhoea : Intake of citraka root paste with buttermilk alleviates diarrhoea. (C.S.)
2. Medoroga : Intake of citraka root with honey keeping on wholesome diet is useful in reducing obesity. (B.S.)
3. Pandu roga : One should take roots of bala and citraka with warm water. (S.S.)

Parts Used : Root bark.

Preparations & Dosage : Powder 1-2 gm.

Specific Formulations : Chitrakadi vati, Chitrakadi ghrita, Chitraka haritaki.

चित्रकोऽनलनामा च पाठी व्यालस्तथोषणः ।
चित्रकः कटुकः पाके वह्निकृत्पाचनो लघुः ॥
रूक्षोष्णो ग्रहणीकुष्ठशोथार्शः कृमिकासनुत् ।
वातश्लेष्महरो ग्राही वातघ्नः श्लेष्मपित्तहृत् ॥ भा०प्र०

<u>Research Studies:</u> The plumbagin acetate when administered orally showed 80% anti-implantation effect while plumbagin benzoate derivatives in the same dose exhibited 83.3% anti-implantation effect. (Annual report 1976-77, CCRIMH)

It was observed that the root of Plumbago rosea in a dose of 600mg/day orally has a radio-sensitising effect on oral carcinoma as evidenced by the increased severity of mucosal reactions when given along with radiations. (Annual report 1979-80, CCRAS)

68
VIḌAṄGA

Embelia ribes Burm. F. Family : Myrsinaceae

Chief Characters :

1. Perennial shrub, climber.
2. Simple leaf, alternate phyllotaxy.
3. Light yellow coloured flowers.
4. Panicle inflorescence.
5. Fruit - round black coloured small fruits.

Synonyms : Tandula, Chitratandula, Krimighna, Vella, Amogha, Jantunashana.

Gana :

Charaka : Krimighna, Kushtaghna, Truptighna.

Sushruta : Surasadi, Pippalyadi.

Properties : Rasa - Katu, Kashaya; Guna - Laghu, Ruksha, Tikshan; Virya - Ushna and Vipaka - Katu.

Pharmacological Actions : Vatakaphahara, Deepana, Krimighna, Vishahara.

Indications : Krimi, Shoola, Udara, Adhamana, Kushta, Vibandha.

Therapeutic Uses :

1. Krimi kushta : Vidanga excels as anthelmintic and used in food and drinks, bath, fumigation and external applications. (C.S.)
2. Ardhavabhedaka : Vidanga and black tila in equal quantity are pounded together and taken as snuff to alleviate hemicrania. (B.S.)

Parts Used : Fruit.

Preparations & Dosage : Powder 5-10 gm.

Specific Formulations : Vidangarishta, Vidangadi loha, Vidanga taila.

पुंसि क्लीबे विडङ्गः स्यात्कृमिघ्नो जन्तुनाशनः ।
तण्डुलश्च तथा वेल्लममोघा चित्रतण्डुलः ॥
विडङ्गं कटु तीक्ष्णोष्णं रूक्षं वह्निकरं लघु ।
शूलाध्मानोदरश्लेष्मकृमिवातविबन्धनुत् ॥ भा०प्र०

69
LODHRA

Symplocos racemosa Roxb. Family : Styraceae

Chief Characters :

1. Small tree grows upto 6-7 m. height.
2. Simple leaf, alternate phyllotaxy.
3. White flowers.
4. Racemose inflorescence.
5. Fruit - drupe.

Synonyms : Sthulavalkala, Jeeranapatra, Brihatpatra, Kramuka patti, Lakshaprasadana.

Gana :

Charaka : Shonita sthapana, Sandhaniya, Purishasangrahani-ya, Kashayaskandha.

Sushruta : Lodhradi, Nyagrodhadi.

Properties : Rasa - Kashaya; Guna - Laghu, Ruksha; Virya - Sheeta and Vipaka - Katu.

Pharmacological Actions : Kaphapittahara, Grahi, Chakshusya.

Indications : Raktapitta, Atisara, Pravahika, Shotha, Jwara, Pradara.

Therapeutic Uses :

1. Shwetapradara : Paste of lodhra should be taken with decoction of nyagrodha bark. (C.S.)
2. Dysentry : Lodhra with curd is useful in dysentry. (B.P.)
3. Yuvana pidika : Paste of lodhra, dhanyaka and vaca is useful as an external application. (V.R.)

Parts Used : Bark.

Preparations & Dosage : Powder 1-2 gm.; Decoction 50-100 ml.

Specific Formulations : Lodhrasava, Lodhradi kwatha.

लोध्रस्तिल्वस्तिरीटश्च शावरो गालवस्तथा ।
द्वितीयः पट्टिकालोध्रः क्रमुकः स्थूलवल्कलः ॥
जीर्णपत्रो बृहत्पत्रः पट्टी लाक्षाप्रसादनः ।
लोध्रो ग्राही लघुः शीतश्चक्षुष्यः कफपित्तनुत् ॥
कषायो रक्तपित्तासृग्ज्वरातीसारशोथहृत् ॥ भा०प्र०

70
SAPTAPARṆA

Alstonia scholaris R. Br. Family : Apocyanaceae

Chief Characters :

1. Evergreen tree grows upto 20 m. height.
2. Whorled phyllotaxy.
3. Light green coloured flowers.
4. Cyamose inflorescence.
5. Fruit - follicle.

Synonyms : Vishala twak, Sharada, Shalmali patraka, Vishamacchada, Sharadi.

Gana :

Charaka : Kushtaghna, Udarda prashamana, Kashaya skandha, Tiktaskandha.

Sushruta : Aragwadhadi, Lakshadi.

Properties : Rasa - Tikta, Kashaya; Guna - Laghu, Snigdha; Virya - Ushna and Vipaka - Katu.

Pharmacological Actions : Tridoshahara, Hridya, Deepana.

Indications : Shoola, Gulma, Krimi, Shwasa, Vrana, Amavata, Kushta.

Therapeutic Uses :

1. Kushta : Decoction of saptaparna processed in oil and ghee is useful in kushta on internal as well as external administration.
2. For purification of breast milk : Decoction of guduchi and saptaparna's bark mixed with shunthi should be given for purification of breast milk. (C.S.)

Parts Used : Bark.

Preparations & Dosage : Decoction 40-80 ml.

Specific Formulations : Saptacchadadi taila, Saptacchadadi kwatha.

सप्तपर्णो विशालत्वक् शारदो विषमच्छदः ॥
सप्तपर्णो व्रणश्लेष्मवातकुष्ठास्रजन्तुजित् ।
दीपनः श्वासगुल्मघ्नः स्निग्धोष्णस्तुवरः सरः ॥ भा०प्र०

71
KUṬAJA

Holarrhena antidysentrica Linn. Family : Apocyanaceae

Chief Characters :

1. Small tree grows upto 4-5 m. height.
2. Simple leaf, alternate phyllotaxy.
3. White coloured flowers.
4. Cyamose inflorescence.
5. Fruit - follicle.

Synonyms : Sakrasakhi, Mallikapushpa, Pandura druma, Yavaphala, Girimallika, Vatsaka, Kalinga, Indravruksha. Seed names : Yava, Indrayava, Bhadrayava, Kalinga.

Gana :

Charaka : Arshoghna, Kandughna, Sthanyasodhana, Asthapanopaga.

Sushruta : Aragwadhadi, Pippalyadi, Haridradi, Lakshadi.

Properties : Rasa - Tikta, Kashaya, Katu; Guna - Laghu, Ruksha; Virya - Sheeta and Vipaka - Katu.

Pharmacological Actions : Kaphapittahara,Deepana, Grahi, Upashoshana, Aamahara.

Indications : Arshas, Atisara, Krimi, Kushta, Shoola, Trishna, Amavata, Raktapitta, Ashmari.

Therapeutic Uses :

1. Bleeding : Decoction of kutaja bark with shunthi checks mucous and blood. (C.S.)
2. Calculus and gravels : Kutaja bark taken with curd along with wholesome diet expels gravels through urethra. (B.P.)
3. Diarrhoea : Intake of decoction of indrayava along with meet soup diet checks diarrhoea caused by pitta. (C.S.)

Parts Used : Bark, Seed.

Preparations & Dosage : Powder 3-6 gm.; Decoction 50-100 ml.

Specific Formulations : Kutajarista, Kutajavalehya, Kutajasura.

कुटजः कूटजः कौटो वत्सको गिरिमल्लिका ॥
कालिङ्गः शक्रशाखी च मल्लिकापुष्प इत्यपि ।
इन्द्रो यवफलः प्रोक्तो वृक्षकः पाण्डुरद्रुमः ॥
कुटजः कटुको रूक्षो दीपनस्तुवरो हिमः ।
अर्शोतीसारपित्तास्रकफतृष्णाऽऽमकुष्ठनुत् ॥ भा०प्र०

72
SARPAGANDHĀ

Rauwolfia serpentina Linn. Family : Apocyanaceae

Chief Characters :

1. Perennial shrub grows upto 1 m. height.
2. Simple leaf, opposite phyllotaxy.
3. White and light pink coloured flowers.
4. Cyamose inflorescence.
5. Fruit - drupe.

Synonyms : Chandramara, Dhavalavitapa.

Properties : Rasa - Tikta; Guna - Ruksha; Virya - Ushna and Vipaka - Katu.

Pharmacological Actions : Kaphavata shamaka, Nidrajanaka.

Indications : Anidra, Bhrama, Unmada, Apasmara, Shoola, Jwara, Agnimandya, Krimi, Raktavata, Sirogatavata.

Therapeutic Uses :

1. Diarrhoea : One should take the powder of roots of sarpagandha and eshwari. (Chunekar)
2. Chonic fever : Paste of sarpagandha, maricha, ativisha, vidlavana alleveiates chronic fever. (Chunekar)
3. Psoriasis : The root powder mixed with triphala is useful in psoriasis. (Bhel)

Parts Used : Root.

Preparations & Dosage : Powder 3-6 gm.

Specific Formulations : Sarpagandhaghana vati, Sarpagandhadi churna.

नाकुली सुरसा नागसुगन्धा गन्धनाकुली ।
नकुलेष्टा भुजङ्गाक्षी सर्पाङ्गी विषनाशिनी ॥
नाकुली तुवरा तिक्ता कटुकोष्णा विनाशयेत् ।
भोगिलूतावृश्चिकाखुविषज्वरकृमिव्रणान् ॥ भा०प्र०

73
KARAVĪRA

Nerium indicum Mill. Family : Apocyanaceae

Chief Characters :

1. Shrub grows upto 4 m. height.
2. Whorled phyllotaxy.
3. White or rose coloured flowers.
4. Paniculate inflorescence.
5. Fruit - follicle.

Synonyms : Hayamaraka, Ashwamaraka, Chandata, Prathihasa.

Gana :

Charaka : Tiktaskandha, Kushtaghna.
Sushruta : Lakshadi, Shirovirechana.

Properties : Rasa - Katu, Tikta; Guna - Laghu, Ruksha, Tikshna; Virya - Ushna and Vipaka - Katu.

Pharmacological Actions : Kaphavatahara, Kushtaghna, Vranashodhana, Vranaropana, Chakshusya.

Indications : Kushta, Krimi, Kandu, Ashmari, Upadamsha, Palithya, Netrakopa, Indralupta, Dushtavrana.

Therapeutic Uses :

1. Kushta : Karavira (whole plant) decoction is used for both external and internal administration to alleviate kushta. (C.S.)
2. Upadamsha : The root of karavira pounded with water and applied as paste alleviates venereal diseases. (B.P.)

Parts Used : Root, Root-bark.

Preparations & Dosage : Powder 30-125 mg.

Specific Formulations : Karaveeradi taila, Karaveera yoga, Hayamaradi taila.

करवीरः श्वेतपुष्पः शतकुम्भोऽश्वमारकः ।
द्वितीयो रक्तपुष्पश्च चण्डातो लगुडस्तथा ॥
करवीरद्वयं तिक्तं कषायं कटुकञ्च तत् ।
व्रणलाघवकृन्नेत्रकोपकुष्ठव्रणापहम् ॥
वीर्योष्णं कृमिकण्डूघ्नं भक्षितं विषवन्मतम् ॥ भा०प्र०

Research Studies: The water soluble portion of alcoholic extract of leaves of Nerium indicum produced positive inotropic and negative chronotropic effects on frog heart and reversed heart failure produced in isolated rabbit heart with pento barbitone sodium or perfusion of half calcium Ringer Lock's solution. (Kohli et al 1967) Effect of this extract has been studied and compared with strophanthin on HLP of dog. It has negative chronotropic effect in both control and hypodynamic HLP. It has reversed the experimentally induced heart failure as judged by various parameters in HLP of dog. (JRIM, Vol. IV, No. 1)

Peruvoside, isolated from seeds of Thevetia nerifolia has been shown to be a very good cardiac glycoside by clinical pharmacological studies. Its speed of action is comparable to ouabian, by the intravenous route of adminstration. Its oral absorbability is comparable to that of digitoxin. Reports of clinical trials indicate that peruvoside has a very high degree of efficacy and very low toxicity. Thus in many ways, peruvoside is a novel and effective glycoside. (Arora R.B. & Rangaswami S., Peruviside and other Cardinotonic Glycosides of Thevetia nerifolia Juss; 1972)

74
ARKA

Calotropis gigantea Linn. Family : Asclepiadaceae

Chief Characters :

1. Perennial shrub grows upto 3-6 ft. height.
2. Simple leaf, opposite deccusate phyllotaxy.
3. Pale voilet flowers.
4. Umbellate inflorescence.
5. Fruit - follicle.

Synonyms : Shwetarka : Ganeruka, Shwetapushpa, Pratapara, Sadapushpa, Mandara, Alarka.
Raktarka : Arkaparna, Shuklaphala, Vikeerana, Asphota, Raktapushpa.

Gana :

Charaka : Bhedaniya, Vamanopaga, Swedopaga.

Sushruta : Adhobhagahara, Arkadi.

Properties : Rasa - Katu, Tikta; Guna - Laghu, Ruksha, Tikshna; Virya - Ushna and Vipaka - Katu.

Pharmacological Actions : Vatahara (R.N.), Deepana, Vishahara, Sara, Vrishya (flower), Pachana.

Indications : Kushta, Kandu, Purishaja krimi, Udara, Pleeha, Gulma, Pleehavriddhi, Arshas, Shwasa, Kasa, Shotha.

Therapeutic Uses :

1. Cough : In the morning sugar is soaked with 2-3 drops of latex and swallowed in the evening, the diet being sweet and unctuous. (S.B.)
2. Splenomegaly : Arka leaves mixed with salt are burn by closed heating. This alkali should be taken with curd water in severe splenomegaly. (V.M., B.P.)

Parts Used : Root-bark, Kshara, Flower, Leaf, Latex.

Preparations & Dosage : Root-bark powder $\frac{1}{2}$-1 gm.; Flower 1-3 gm.; Kshara $\frac{1}{2}$-1 gm.

Specific Formulations : Arka lavana, Arka taila.

अलर्ककुसुमं वृष्यं लघु दीपनपाचनम् ।
अरोचकप्रसेकार्शःकासश्वासनिवारणम् ॥
रक्तार्कपुष्पं मधुरं सतिक्तं कुष्ठकृमिघ्नं कफनाशनं च ।
अर्शो विषं हन्ति च रक्तपित्तं संग्राहि गुल्मे श्वयथौ हितं तत् ॥

भा०प्र०

Research Studies: The crude latex of C. procera and its protein fractions were found to possess high fibrinolytic and anticoagulant activity in rabbit and human plasma. Recently Prakash et al., (1978) reported that 50% ethanolic extract of the leaves of Calotropis procera and C. gigantea have 20%, 20.6% anti implantation activity when administered at the dose of 50, 200 mg/kg body weight respectively. (Probe 27 (4); 315-323)

75
SĀRIVĀ

Hemidesmus indicus Linn. Family : Periplocaceae

Chief Characters :

1. Perennial herb grows upto 6 m. height.
2. Simple leaf, opposite phyllotaxy.
3. Pale voilet flowers.
4. Cyamose inflorescence.
5. Fruit - follicle.

Synonyms : Krishna sariva : Gopi, Gopavadhu, Shyama, Ananta, Utpala sariva, Asphota.

Shweta sariva : Gopalata, Chandana, Krusodari, Shyama, Spota, Gopavalli, Gopakanya.

Gana :

Charaka : Jwarahara, Dahaprashamana, Stanyasodhana, Purishasangrahaniya, Madhuraskandha.

Sushruta : Sarivadi, Vidarigandhadi, Vallipanchamoola.

Properties : Rasa - Madhura, Tikta; Guna - Guru, Snigdha; Virya - Sheeta and Vipaka - Madhura.

Pharmacological Actions : Tridoshahara, Grahi, Amavishahara, Sukrakara.

Indications : Agnimandya, Aruchi, Atisara, Jwara, Kushta, Kandu, Prameha, Shwasa, Kasa, Pradara.

Therapeutic Uses :

1. Wound : Sariva root alone is capable of cleansing all types of wounds. (C.D.)
2. Bronchial asthma : Ghee cooked with the double quantity of the decoction of sariva is useful. (S.S.)

Parts Used : Root.

Preparations & Dosage : Hot infusion 50-100 ml.; Kalka 5-10 gm.

Specific Formulations : Sarivadyasava, Pinda taila.

सारिवायुगलं स्वादु स्निग्धं शुक्रकरं गुरु ।
अग्निमान्द्यारुचिश्वासकासामविषनाशनम् ॥

<u>Research Studies:</u> 2 hydroxy- 4 methoxy. benezaldehyde isolated from the root of the plant was screened for antiinflammatory activity against chronic inflammation in albino rats. Drug in 100 mg/kg. dose orally was found to possess significant action. The drug also revealed significant anti fungal activity in experiments and clinical studies. (CCRAS, Annual reports, 1977-78)

76
KUPĪLU

Strychnos nux-vomica Linn. Family : Loganiaceae

Chief Characters :

1. Tree grows upto 20 m. height.
2. Simple leaf.
3. Light green coloured flowers.
4. Cyamose inflorescence.
5. Fruit - round and pink coloured.

Synonyms : Vishatinduka, Karaskara, Kakatinduka, Vishatindu, Kulaka, Jalada, Deerghapatrala, Garadruma, Kakapiluka, Markata tinduka.

Gana :

Sushruta : Surasadi.
Amradi phala varga (B.P.)

Properties : Rasa - Katu, Tikta; Guna - Laghu; Virya - Ushna (R.N.), Sheeta (B.P.) and Vipaka - Katu.

Pharmacological Actions : Kaphavatahara (R.N.), Vishahara, Grahi.

Indications : Kushta, Kandu, Arshas, Vrana, Vataroga, Rakta-vikara.

Therapeutic Uses :

1. Visuchika : The root bark of kupilu should be pounded with neem juice and made into pills to alleviate visuchika.
2. Wound : Leaf paste should be used as anointment on dushta vrana.
3. Vajikarana : Vishatinduka, marica and loha bhasma are mixed together and used orally in impotence. This recipe is also useful to check the bedwetting.

Parts Used : Seed.

Preparations & Dosage : Powder 60-250 mg.

Specific Formulations : Agnitundi vati, Krimimudgara rasa, Vat-agajankusha, Vishatinduka taila.

तिन्दुको यस्तु कथितो जलदो दीर्घपत्रकः ॥
कुपीलुः कुलकः काकतिन्दुकः काकपीलुकः ।
काकेन्दुर्विषतिन्दुश्च तथा मर्कटतिन्दुकः ॥
कुपीलुः शीतलं तिक्तं वातलं मदकृल्लघु ।
परं व्यथाहरं ग्राहि कफपित्तास्रनाशनम् ॥ भा०प्र०

77
KIRĀTATIKTA

Swertia chirata Buch. Ham. Family : Gentianaceae

Chief Characters :

1. Annual shrub grows upto 2 m. height.
2. Simple leaf, opposite phyllotaxy.
3. Greenish white or pale voilet coloured flowers.
4. Panicle inflorescence.
5. Fruit - capsule.

Synonyms : Kairatha, Katutikta, Bhunimba, Ramasenaka, Kandatikta, Kirataka, Anaryatikta.

Gana :

Charaka : Stanyasodhana, Trishna nigrahana, Tiktaskandha.
Sushruta : Aragwadhadi.

Properties : Rasa - Tikta; Guna - Laghu, Ruksha; Virya - Sheeta and Vipaka - Katu.

Pharmacological Actions : Kaphapittahara, Sarakam (Sara), Stanyasodhana, Nidraharana (Nepala kiratatikta).

Indications : Arshas, Krimi, Kushta, Shotha, Vrana, Raktapitta.

Therapeutic Uses :

1. For purifying milk : One should administer decoction of kiratatikta. (C.S.)
2. Vomiting : Paste of kiratatikta mixed with equal quantity of sugar or honey checks vomiting and nausea. (A.S.)
3. Oedema : Paste of kiratatikta and shunthi destroys chronic oedema caused by tridoshas. (C.S.)
4. Malaria : Ayush-64 consisting of kiratatikta, saptaparni, kuberakgha and katu karohini relieves malaria caused by P. vivax and P. falciparum (CCRAS). Andrographis paniculata (kalamegha) is considered as kiratatikta in South India.

Parts Used : Panchanga (Whole plant).

Preparations & Dosage : Decoction 50-100 ml.; Powder 1-3 gm.

Specific Formulations : Sudarshana churna, Kiratadi kwatha.

किराततिक्तः कैरातः कटुतिक्तः किरातकः ।।
काण्डतिक्तोऽनार्यतिक्तो भूनिम्बो रामसेनकः ।
किरातकोऽन्यो नैपालः सोऽर्द्धतिक्तो ज्वरान्तकः ।।
किरातः सारको रूक्षः शीतलस्तिक्तको लघुः ।
सन्निपातज्वरश्वासकफपित्तास्रदाहनुत् ।
कासशोथतृषाकुष्ठज्वरव्रणकृमिप्रणुत् ।। भा०प्र०

<u>Research Studies:</u> The ether and petroleum ether extracts of Swertia chirata exhibited only 50% and 40% anthelminthic activity respectively. Chloroform extract exhibited neuromuscular blocking activity on dorsalis muscle preparation of ascarislumbricoides. (CCRAS, Annual report, 1978-79)

Swertia chirata, a source of an important Ayurvedic drug Chirata, is reputed for its better, anthelminthic, antimalarial and antidiarrhoeal properties. (Journal of Medicinal and Aromatic Plant Sciences V. 19 (4) : p. 955-963, 1997)

78
ŚAṄKHAPUṢPĪ

Convolvulus pluricaulis Chois. Family : Convolvulaceae

Chief Characters :

1. Perennial shrub consists of root stock.
2. Simple leaf, altenate phyllotaxy.
3. Light rose colour flowers, bisexual flowers.
4. Fruit - capsule.

Synonyms : Shankhahwa, Mangalya kusuma.

Properties : Rasa - Tikta, Kashaya; Guna - Snigdha, Picchila; Virya - Sheeta (R.N.), Ushna (D.N.) and Vipaka - Madhura.

Pharmacological Actions : Tridoshahara, Swarya, Medhya-rasayana.

Indications : Apasmara, Unmada, Bhrama, Anidra.

Therapeutic Uses :

1. Insanity and epilepsy : Old ghee cooked with brahmi juice, kushta and shankhapushpi alleviates insanity and epilepsy. (C.S.)
2. Intellect promoting rasayana : Shankhapushpi is consisdered as the most superior drug among medhya rasayana (intelligence promoting drugs). (C.S.)

Parts Used : Panchanga (whole plant).

Preparations & Dosage : Kalka 10-20 gm.

Specific Formulations : Shankhapushpi rasayana, Shankhapushpi taila.

शङ्खपुष्पी तु शङ्खाह्वा माङ्गल्यकुसुमाऽपि च ।
शङ्खपुष्पी सरा मेध्या वृष्या मानसरोगहृत् ॥
रसायनी कषायोष्णा स्मृतिकान्तिबलाग्निदा ।
दोषापस्मारभूताश्रीकुष्ठक्रिमिविषप्रणुत् ॥ भा०प्र०

Research Studies: In clinical study, C. pluricaulis provided significant relief in symptoms besides a quantitative reduction in axiety level and necroticism in the cases of anxiety neurosis. The treatment has also produced reduction in the level of plasma cortisol and catecholamines. In the experimental study, the drug showed slight sedation but no analgesic and anti convulsive activity. The drug decreased blood pressure in dogs. (JRIMYH 12:3, 1977)

79

TRIVṚT

Operculina turpethum Linn. Family : Convolvulaceae

Chief Characters :

1. Perennial climber grows upto 10 m. height.
2. Simple leaf, alternate phyllotaxy.
3. White flowers occur singly or in groups.
4. Fruit - capsule.

Synonyms : Sarvanubhuti, Sarala, Rechani, Tribhandi, Triputa, Nishotra, Palindi, Ardhachandra, Sushenika, Suvaha.

Gana :

Charaka : Bhedaniya.

Sushruta : Shyamadi.

Properties : Rasa - Tikta, Katu; Guna - Laghu, Ruksha, Tikshna; Virya - Ushna and Vipaka - Katu.

Pharmacological Actions : Kaphapittahara, Rechana, Vatala.

Indications : Jwara, Shotha, Udara, Pandu, Kamala, Arshas.

Therapeutic Uses :

1. Fever : One should take powder of trivrut with honey for alleviating acute fever. (S.S.)
2. Piles : Trivrut powder mixed in decoction of triphala should be given. (C.S.)

Parts Used : Root bark.

Preparations & Dosage : Powder 1-3 gm.

Specific Formulations : Avipattikara churna, Trivrtadi ghrita.

श्वेता त्रिवृत् त्रिभण्डी स्यात् त्रिवृता त्रिपुटाऽपि च ।
सर्वानुभूतिः सरला निशोता रेचनीति च ॥
श्वेता त्रिवृद्रेचनी स्यात्स्वादुरुष्णा समीरहृत् ।
रूक्षा पित्तज्वरश्लेष्मपित्तशोथोदरापहा ॥ भा०प्र०

80

KAṆṬAKĀRĪ

Solanum surattense Burm. F. Family : Solanaceae

Chief Characters :

1. Perennial herb, procumbent.
2. Pinnatifid leaves, opposite phyllotaxy.
3. Violet coloured flowers.
4. Umbellate cyme inflorescence.
5. Fruit - berry.

Synonyms : Vyaghri, Nidhigdika, Kshudra, Duhsparsha, Kantalika, Kantakini.

Gana :

Charaka : Kasahara, Hikkanigrahana, Sheetaprashamana, Shotha hara, Kanthya, Angamarda prashamana.
Sushruta : Brihatyadi, Laghu panchamoola, Varunadi.

Properties : Rasa - Katu, Tikta; Guna - Laghu, Ruksha, Tikshna; Virya - Ushna and Vipaka - Katu.

Pharmacological Actions : Kaphavatahara, Deepana, Pachana, Sara, Shukra rechana, Mutrala, Ashmari bhedana.

Indications : Krimi, Pratishyaya, Kasa, Shwasa, Hikka, Shotha, Hridroga, Parshwapida, Mutrakriccha, Ashmari, Peenasa, Jwara.

Therapeutic Uses :

1. Cough : Ghee processed with kantakari juice alleviates all types of coughs, asthma, hoarseness of voice and indigestion. (S.S.)
2. Asthma : Intake of kantakari and amalaki fruit (equal quantity) mixed with hingu (½ part) and honey alleviates asthma within three days. (S.S.)

Parts Used : Root, Panchanga (Whole plant).

Preparations & Dosage : Decoction 40-80 ml.

Specific Formulations : Vyagri haritaki, Kantakari ghrita.

कण्टकारी तु दुःस्पर्शा क्षुद्रव्याघ्री निदिग्धिका ।
कण्टालिका कण्टकिनी धावनी बृहती तथा ॥

श्वेतपुष्पी कण्टकारी—

श्वेता क्षुद्रा चन्द्रहासा लक्ष्मणा क्षेत्रदूतिका ।।
गर्भदा चन्द्रमा चन्द्री चन्द्रपुष्पा प्रियङ्करी ।।
कण्टकारी सरा तिक्ता कटुका दीपनी लघुः ।।
रूक्षोष्णा पाचनी कासश्वासज्वरकफानिलान् ।
निहन्ति पीनसं पार्श्वपीडाकृमिहृदामयान् ।।
तयोः फलं कटु रसे पाके च कटुकं भवेत् ।
शुक्रस्य रेचनं भेदि तिक्तं पित्ताग्निकृल्लघु ।
हन्यात्कफमरुत्कण्डूकासमेदःकृमिज्वरान् ।।
तद्वत् प्रोक्ता सिता क्षुद्रा विशेषात् गर्भकारिणी ।। भा०प्र०

Research Studies: Gluco-alkaloidal saponin fraction of S. xanthocarpum caused a marked increase in force of centraction of the hypodynamic heart and produced significant expectorant effect. (Annual report 1969-70 & 1970-71, CCRIMH)

81
BṚHATĪ

Solanum indicum Linn. Family : Solanaceae

Chief Characters :

1. Perennial herb grows upto 3 m. height.
2. Pinnatifid simple leaf, alternate phyllotaxy.
3. Light voilet coloured flowers.
4. Fruit - fleshy fruit.

Synonyms : Vartaki, Mahati, Hinguli, Simhi, Dushpraharshini, Kuli, Rashtrika, Mahoshtra.

Gana :

Charaka : Kanthya, Hikkanigrahana, Shotha hara, Angamarda prashamana.

Sushruta : Brihatyadi, Laghu panchamoola.

Properties : Rasa - Katu, Tikta; Guna - Laghu, Ruksha, Tikshna; Virya - Ushna and Vipaka - Katu.

Pharmacological Actions : Kaphavatahara, Pachana, Grahi, Hridya.

Indications : Agnimandhya, Shoola, Jwara, Shwasa, Kasa, Aruchi, Kushta, Asyavairasya.

Therapeutic Uses :

1. Alopecia : Juice of Brihati (fruit) mixed with honey by local application destroys alopecia. (G.N.)
2. Cough : Brihati fruit is slightly steamed in water, pounded and cooked in ghee. Then it is mixed with powdered rocksalt and taken internally for improving digestion and alleviating cough. (Kshemakutuhalam)

Parts Used : Root, Fruit.

Preparations & Dosage : Decoction 40-80 ml., Powder 3-6 gm.

Specific Formulations : Dashamoolarista, Brihatyadi kwatha.

वार्त्ताकी क्षुद्रभण्टाकी महती बृहती कुली ।
हिङ्गुली राष्ट्रिका सिंही महोष्ट्री दुष्प्रधर्षिणी ॥
बृहती ग्रहणी हृद्या पाचनी कफवातहृत् ॥
कटुतिक्ताऽऽस्यवैरस्यमलारोचकनाशिनी ।
उष्णा कुष्ठज्वरश्वासशूलकासाग्निमान्द्यजित् ॥ भा०प्र०

82
AŚWAGANDHĀ

Withania somnifera Linn. Family : Solanaceae

Chief Characters :

1. Perennial shrub grows upto 2 m. height.
2. Simple leaf, alternate phyllotaxy.
3. Green and yellow coloured flowers occur in fasicles.
4. Fruit - berry.

Synonyms : Varahakarni, Vajigandha, Vajee, Vajeekari, Balya, Kushtagandhini, Pivari, Gatrakari, Hayawaya, Balada.

Gana :

Charaka : Balya, Brimhaniya, Madhuraskandha, Virechanopaga.

Properties : Rasa - Katu, Tikta, Kashaya; Guna - Snigdha, Laghu; Virya - Ushna and Vipaka - Katu.

Pharmacological Actions : Vatakaphahara, Balya, Rasayana, Shukrala.

Indications : Kshaya, Kasa, Shwasa, Shopha, Granthi, Apachi, Vrana, Shwitra, Vandhyatva, Nidra nasha.

Therapeutic Uses :

1. Rasayana : One who takes powder of ashwangandha root in late winter mixed with honey and ghee alongwith milk regains youthfulness even in old age. (R.M.)
2. Infertility : Intake of ghee processed with ashwagandha decoction and milk cures infertility in woman. (C.D.)

Parts Used : Root, Leaf, Kshara.

Preparations & Dosage : Powder-3-6 gm., Kshara 1-2 gm.

Specific Formulations : Ashwagandharishta, Aswagandhadi churna.

गन्धान्ता वाजिनामादिरश्वगन्धा हयाह्वया ।
वराहकर्णी वरदा बलदा कुष्ठगन्धिनी ॥
अश्वगन्धाऽनिलश्लेष्मश्वित्रशोथक्षयापहा ।
बल्या रसायनी तिक्ता कषायोष्णाऽतिशुक्रला ॥ भा०प्र०

Research Studies: In a double blind study shade dried roots of the plant are powdered and made as tablets of 0.5 gm. each and administered in the dose of 2 tabs. 3 times a day with milk to healthy volunteers for a period of 1 year. Results have shown significant increase in haemoglobin, RBC, hair melanin, and in seated strature in the treated group as compared to control group. Serum cholesterol and calcium levels of nails have also been decreased in treated group. (Kuppurajan et al) On another study, this drug provided significant relief in symptoms of anxiety neurosis beside a quantitative reduction in anxiety level and neuroticism. (Singh R.H. et al)

In another study, drug Ashwagandha has been found to be useful in cases of acute rheumatoid arthritis and no substantial improvement was observed in cases of chronic rheumatoid arthritis, osteoarthritis and periarthritis of shoulder. (Bector N.P. et al) This drug is also possesing haematinic property.

The alcoholic extract on intraperitoneal administration showed a highly significant anti-pyretic activity as well as analgesic activity in albino rats. (Annual report 76-77, CCRIMH)

83

DHATTŪRĀ

Datura metel Linn. Family : Solanaceae

Chief Characters :

1. Annual shrub, grows upto 1 m. height.
2. Simple leaves, alternate phyllotaxy.
3. Voilet with white flowers, bisexual flowers.
4. Fruit - septifragal capsule.

Synonyms : Dhurta, Unmatta, Kanakakanakahwaya, Shivapriya, Drvata, Kitava, Matula, Matulaputraka, Turi, Madana, Mahamohi.

Gana :

Upavisha (R.R.S.)

Properties : Rasa - Tikta, Katu, Madhrua, Kashaya; Guna - Laghu, Ruksha; Virya - Ushna and Vipaka - Katu.

Pharmacological Actions : Vatahara, Vishaghna, Deepana, Pittala, Kaphahara (R.N.), Madakari.

Indications : Kushta, Kandu, Jwara, Vrana, Mutrakriccha, Yuka, Liksha, Krimi, Visha.

Therapeutic Uses :

1. Filariasis : Seeds of dhattura used in increasing dose like pippali vardhamana, with cold water relieves severe filariasis. (V.S.)
2. Alopecia : The nearly vein should be punctured and the surface is scarified deeply and pasted with juice of dhattura leaves. (A.H.)

Parts Used : Leaf, Flower, Seed.

Preparations & Dosage : Powder-50-100 mg.

Specific Formulations : Kankasava, Sutashekhara rasa, Unmatta rasa.

धत्तूरधूर्त्तधुत्तूरा उन्मत्तः कनकाह्वयः ।
देवता कितवस्तूरी महामोही शिवप्रियः ॥
मातुलो मदनश्चास्य फले मातुलपुत्रकः ।
धत्तूरो मदवर्णाग्निवातकृज्ज्वरकुष्ठनुत् ॥
कषायो मधुरस्तिक्तो यूकालिक्षाविनाशकः ।
उष्णो गुरुर्व्रणश्लेष्मकण्डूकृमिविषापहः ॥ भा०प्र०

84
PĀRASĪKA YAVĀNĪ

Hyoscyamus niger Linn. Family : Solanaceae

Chief Characters :

1. Annual herb covered with hairs.
2. Simple leaves, alternate phyllotaxy.
3. Greenish voilet coloured flowers.
4. Fruit - capsule.

Synonyms : Turushka, Madakarini, Yavani, Yaavani.

Properties : Rasa - Tikta, Katu; Guna - Guru, Ruksha; Virya - Ushna and Vipaka - Katu.

Pharmacological Actions : Kaphavatahara, Madakari, Grahi, Deepana, Pachana, Shukrahara, Ruchya.

Indications : Krimi, Shoola, Gulma, Anaha, Agnimandya, Pleeha, Atisara.

Therapeutic Uses :

1. Worms : Parasika yavani mixed with jaggery and taken with stale water expels the intestinal worms. (V.M.)
2. Nidranasha (Insomnia) : Parasika yavani is taken in the dosage of 575 mg for inducing good sleep. (Yadavaji)

Parts Used : Seed, Leaf, Flower.

Preparations & Dosage : Powder 250 mg-1 gm.

Specific Formulations : Parasiyadi churna, Mamsyadi kwatha.

पारसीकयवानी तु यवानीसदृशी गुणः ।
विशेषात्पाचनी रुच्या ग्रहणी मादिनी गुरुः ॥ भा०प्र०

85
KAṬUKĪ

Picrorhiza kurroa Royal. Family : Scrophulariaceae

Chief Characters :

1. Perennial shrub covered with hairs.
2. Simple leaves rounded and glabrous leaves.
3. White and blue coloured flowers.
4. Spike inflorescence.
5. Fruit - loculicidal capsule.

Synonyms : Matyasakala, Sakuladani, Chakragni, Katvi-katuka, Katurohini, Krishnabheda, Katambara, Ashoka, Tikta, Matsyapitta, Kandaruka, Rohini.

Gana :

Charaka : Bhedaniya, Lekhaniya, Stanyashodhana, Tiktaskandha.

Sushruta : Patoladi, Pippalyadi, Mustadi.

Properties : Rasa - Tikta; Guna - Laghu, Ruksha; Virya - Sheeta and Vipaka - Katu.

Pharmacological Actions : Kaphapittahara, Bhedana, Deepana, Lekhana, Hridya.

Indications : Vishamjwara, Kamala, Udara, Arochaka, Jwara, Krimi, Hridroga, Shotha, Shwasa, Kasa, Daha, Prameha, Kushta, Raktadosha.

Therapeutic Uses :

1. Hridroga : In heart disease caused by pitta, one should take paste of katuka and yashtimadhu with sugar-water. (C.S.)
2. Jaundice : Intake of katukarohini powder or paste alleviates jaundice. (Anubhuta)

Parts Used : Root, Rhizome.

Preparations & Dosage : Powder 1/2-1 gm.; 3-6 gm. for rechana.

Specific Formulations : Arogyavardhini rasa, Tiktadya ghrita, Tiktadi kwatha, Katukadya taila.

कट्वी तु कटुका तिक्ता कृष्णभेदा कटम्भरा ।
अशोका मत्स्यशकला चक्राङ्गी शकुलादनी ।
मत्स्यपित्ता काण्डरुहा रोहिणी कटुरोहिणी ।।
कट्वी तु कटुका पाके तिक्ता रूक्षा हिमा लघुः ।।
भेदिनी दीपनी हृद्या कफपित्तज्वरापहा ।
प्रमेहश्वासकासास्रदाहकुष्ठक्रिमिप्रणुत् ।। भा०प्र०

Research Studies: The alcoholic extract of the drug reduced markedly the S.G.O.T. and S.G.P.T. concentration in rabbits whose livers were damaged by carbon tetrachloride injection. Improvement in BSP clearance test was also noted in these rabbits. The total biliary output in the treated groups of animals have shown appreciable increase in comparision to the control group. (Pandey & Chaturvedi 1968, 1970) Total extracts of roots revealed marked hydrochloretic and anti bacterial activities suggesting its potential value in infective hepatitis and urinary tract infections. (Vohra et al 1972)

In order to establish its anti-allergic activity, its effect was studied an experimentally induced anaphylactic reaction (Schultz-Dalle phenomenon) and an Konzett-Roessler preparation Pieroliv showed a prominent anti-allergic activity and that activity could be due to inhibition of phenomenon of sensitization by immunomodulation.

Picroliv regulates lipid metabolism in plasmodium berghei induced liver damage in mice.

Protective effect of picroliv against alcohol induced hepatotoxicity in rat. (Indian Journal of Pharmacology, V. 29/1, Feb. 1997)

86
BRĀHMĪ

Bacopa monnieri Linn. Family : Scrophulariaceae

Chief Characters :

1. Annual shrub, grows upto 40 cms. height.
2. Simple leaf, opposite phyllotaxy.
3. Light blue coloured flowers, bisexual flowers.
4. Fruit - capsule.

Synonyms : Somavalli, Matsyakshi, Kapotavega, Kapotavanka, Saraswati.

Properties : Rasa - Tikta, Kashaya; Guna - Laghu; Virya - Sheeta and Vipaka - Madhura.

Pharmacological Actions : Kaphapittahara, Medhya, Rasayana, Swarya, Smritiprada, Ayushya, Vishahara.

Indications : Jwara, Shotha, Kushta, Prameha, Pandu, Kasa.

Therapeutic Uses :

1. Epilepsy : In epilepsy brahmi juice should be taken with milk. (C.S.)
2. Insanity : Brahmi juice when taken along with kushta powder and honey relieves insanity. (C.D.)
3. Calculi : One should take brahmi leaf, gokshuru and yashti to alleviate calculi. (S.S.)

Parts Used : Panchanga (Whole plant).

Preparations & Dosage : Juice 10-20 ml.

Specific Formulations : Saraswatarishta, Brahmi ghrita.

ब्राह्मी कपोतवङ्का च सोमवल्ली सरस्वती ।
ब्राह्मी हिमसरातिक्ता लघुर्मेध्या च शीतला ।।
कषायामधुरा स्वादु पाकाऽऽयुष्या रसायनी ।
स्वर्या स्मृतिप्रदा कुष्ठपाण्डुमेहास्रकासजित् ।।
विषशोथज्वरहरी तद्वन्मण्डूकपर्णिनी ।। भा०प्र०

Research Studies: Brahmi (Bacopa monnieri) has shown hypotensive action and reduced the clinical features of anxiety neurosis. It has also produced reduction in the level of plasma cortisol and urinary catecholamines in the cases of anxiety neurosis. When studied experimentally, for its psychotropic effect in rats, it has shown significant barbiturate hypnosis potentiation effect and caused a reduction in the level of acetylcholine and catecholamine in the whole brain tissue. (R.H. Singh et al 1977-78)

87

ŚYONĀKA

Oroxylum indicum Linn. Family : Bignoniaceae

Chief Characters :

1. Tree grows upto 12 m. height.
2. Bipinnate compound leaf, alternate phyllotaxy.
3. Voilet coloured flowers.
4. Racemose inflorescence.
5. Fruit - loculicidal capsule.

Synonyms : Tuntuka, Kutannata, Katvanga, Katambara, Mandukaparna, Nata, Soshana, Aralu, Sukanasa, Deergavrinta, Ashirimbhi, Prithusimba.

Gana :

Charaka : Shothahara, Sheeta prashamana, Anuvasanopaga.

Sushruta : Rodhradi, Veeratarvadi, Brihat panchamoola.

Properties : Rasa - Madhura, Tikta, Kashaya; Guna - Laghu, Ruksha ; Virya - Ushna (B.P., R.N.), Sheeta (D.N.) and Vipaka - Katu.

Pharmacological Actions : Kaphavata shamaka, Deepana, Grahi, Vatakara (Pakwaphala).

Indications : Atisara, Kasa, Shotha, Amavata, Gulma, Arshas, Krimi.

Therapeutic Uses :

1. Diarrhoea : The juice of shyonaka obtained by putapaka (closed heating) is useful in diarrhoea. (C.D.)
2. Amavata : Shyonaka decoction mixed with eranda taila relieves amavata, sandhivata and other vata disorders.

Parts Used : Root bark.

Preparations & Dosage : Powder-3-6 gm.; Decoction 40-80 ml.

Specific Formulations : Dashamoolarishta, Shyonaka putapaka, Brihat panchamuladi kwatha.

श्योनाकः शोषणश्च स्यान्नटकट्वङ्गटुण्टुकाः ।
मण्डूकपर्णपत्रोर्णशुकनासकुटन्नटाः ॥

दीर्घवृन्तोऽरलुश्चापि पृथुशिम्बः कटम्भरः ।
श्योनाको दीपनः पाके कटुकस्तुवरो हिमः ।
ग्राही तिक्तोऽनिलश्लेष्मपित्तकासप्रणाशनः ।
टुण्टुकस्य फलं बालं रूक्षं वातकफापहम् ।
हृद्यं कषायं मधुरं रोचनं लघु दीपनम् ।
गुल्मार्शःकृमिहृत् प्रौढं गुरुवातप्रकोपणम् ॥ भा०प्र०

88

PĀṬALĀ

Stereospermum suaveolens DC. Family : Bignoniaceae

Chief Characters :

1. Tree grows upto 20 m. height.
2. Imparipinnate compound leaf, opposite phyllotaxy.
3. Light yellow coloured flowers.
4. Panicle inflorescence.
5. Fruit - loculicidal capsule.

Synonyms : Madhuduti, Phaleruka, Patali, Amogha, Krishnavrinta, Tramapushpi, Kalasthali, Shitapatala, Gandhapatala, Kastapatala, Kuberakshi, Ativallabha, Mushkaka, Mokshaka, Patalasita.

Gana :

Charaka : Shothahara.

Sushruta : Aragwadhadi, Adhobhagahara.

Properties : Rasa - Tikta, Kashaya; Guna - Laghu, Ruksha; Virya - Ushna (R.N.), Anushna (B.P.), Sheeta (Pushpa, phala) and Vipaka - Madhura.

Pharmacological Actions : Tridoshahara, Hridya, Kanthya.

Indications : Shotha, Shwasa, Chardi, Trishna, Arshas, Aruchi, Amlapitta, Hikka.

Therapeutic Uses :

1. Gastritis : Decoction prepared with patala, patola, dhanyaka and shunthi should be given. (C.D.)
2. Calculi : Alkali of patala removes calculi. (S.S.)

Parts Used : Root bark, Flower, Seed, Leaf, Kshara.

Preparations & Dosage : Root bark decoction 50-100 ml., Kshara 1-1.5 gm..

Specific Formulations : Dashamoolarista, Brihat panchamuladi kwatha.

पाटलि: पाटलाऽमोघा मधुदूतो फलेरुहा ।
कृष्णवृन्ता कुबेराक्षी कालस्थाल्यलिवल्लभा ॥

ताम्रपुष्पी च कथिताऽपरा स्यात्पाटला सिता ।
मुष्कको मोक्षको घण्टापाटलिः काष्ठपाटला ॥
× × ×
पुष्पं कषायं मधुरं हिमं हृद्यं कफास्त्रनुत् ।
पित्तातिसारहृत्कण्ठ्यं फलं हिक्काऽस्त्रपित्तहृत् ॥ भा०प्र०

89
VĀSĀ

Adathoda vasica Linn. Family : Acanthaceae

Chief Characters :

1. Perennial shrub, grows upto 4 m. height.
2. Simple leaves, opposite phyllotaxy.
3. White flowers.
4. Spike inflorescence.
5. Fruit - capsule.

Synonyms : Vasika, Simhasya, Atarusha, Bhishakmatha, Vrisha, Simhi, Vasaka, Simhika, Vajidanta, Tamra, Simhaparna.

Gana :

Charaka : Tiktaskandha.

Sushruta : Durvadigana.

Properties : Rasa - Tikta, Kashaya; Guna - Laghu, Ruksha; Virya - Sheeta and Vipaka - Katu.

Pharmacological Actions : Kaphapittahara, Swarya, Hridya, Vatakara.

Indications : Shwasa, Kasa, Jwara, Rajayakshma, Chardi, Prameha, Kushta, Raktapitta.

Therapeutic Uses :

1. Intrinsic haemorrhage : Powder of vasa flowers dried in shade should be taken with honey. (S.B.)
2. Cough : Powder of haridra cooked with vasa juice and taken with fatty layer of milk checks dry cough. (S.B.)
3. Difficult labour : Paste of root of vasa should be applied on navel and vagina. It expels the confounded fetus. (C.D.)

Parts Used : Leaf, Root, Flowers.

Preparations & Dosage : Leaf juice 10-20 ml.; Flower juice 10-20 ml.; Root decoction 40-80 ml.

Specific Formulations : Vasavaleha, Vasarishta.

वासको वासिका वासा भिषङ्माता च सिंहिका ।

सिंहास्यो वाजिदन्ता स्यादाटरूषोऽटरूषकः ॥
अटरूषो वृषस्ताम्रः सिंहपर्णश्च स स्मृतः ।
वासको वासकृत्स्वर्यः कफपित्तास्रनाशनः ॥
तिक्तस्तुवरको हृद्यो लघुशीतस्तृषार्त्तिहृत् ।
श्वासकासज्वरश्छर्दिमेहकुष्ठक्षयापहः ॥ भा०प्र०

Research Studies: The roots, bark and leaves exibited bronchodilator activity both in vitro and in vivo studies, the roots were found to be less potent as compared to bark and leaves. (Annual reports, CCRAS 1979-80) It is concluded that vasicine possesses bronchodilatory activity which is potentiated in the presence of vasicinone. It was also observed that vasicine caused contraction as well as induced rhythmic contractile movements of uterus. This showed abortificient activity (100%) in most of the laboratory animals unassociated with undesirable effects. At a dose of 60 mg. and above, which will hardly cost 50 paise, it proved 100% effective for the termination of pregnancy of up to 5 months. Vasicine holds the promise of an ideal abortifacient particularly so because it act through the release of endogenous natural prostglandins. (C.K. Atal, Chemistry & Pharmacology of Vasicine-A new Oxytocin and Abortifacient, RRL Jammu)

90
NIRGUṆḌĪ

Vitex negundo Linn. Family : Verbenaceae

Chief Characters :

1. Branched shrub grows upto 3 m. height.
2. Compound leaf, opposite phyllotaxy.
3. Light blue coloured flowers.
4. Panicle inflorescence.
5. Fruit - drupe.

Synonyms : Sindhuvara, Shwetapushpa, Sindhuka, (White variety), Sephali, Neelapushpi, Suvaha (Blue variety).

Gana :

Charaka : Vishaghna, Krimighna.

Sushruta : Surasadi.

Properties : Rasa - Katu, Tikta, Kashaya; Guna - Laghu, Ruksha; Virya - Ushna and Vipaka - Katu.

Pharmacological Actions : Vatakaphahara, Keshya, Chakshusya.

Indications : Shotha, Amavata, Krimi, Shoola, Vrana, Kushta, Kasa, Pradara, Jwara, Aruchi.

Therapeutic Uses :

1. Osteoarthritis : Powder of nirgundi root should be taken with oil. It is useful in arthritis, lumbago and trembling. (R.R.S.)
2. Sciatica : The decoction of leaves prepared on simmering heat relieves sciatica. (G.N.)
3. Ringworm : The external application of leafy juice cures ringworm. (G.N.)

Parts Used : Leaf, Root, Seed.

Preparations & Dosage : Leaf juice 10-20 ml.; Root bark powder 3-6 gm.; Seed powder 3-6 gm.

Specific Formulations : Nirgundi taila, Nirgundi kalpa.

सिन्दुवारः श्वेतपुष्पः सिन्दूकः सिन्दुवारकः ।
नीलपुष्पी तु निर्गुण्डी शेफाली सुवहा च सा ॥

सिन्दुकः स्मृतिदस्तिक्तः कषायः कटुको लघुः ।
केश्यो नेत्रहितो हन्ति शूलशोथाममारुतान् ॥
कृमिकुष्ठारुचिश्लेष्मज्वरान्नीलापि तद्विधा ।
सिन्दुवारदलं जन्तुवातश्लेष्महरं लघु ॥ भा०प्र०

Research Studies: The ethyl acetate extract at a dose of 50 mg/kg. orally produced definite anti-inflammatory effect against carrageenine, 5 HT and Bradykinin. The extract was found to supress the primary as well as secondary phage of inflammation significantly. (Annual report, CCRIMH 1977-78)

91
AGNIMANTHA

Clerodendron phlomidis Linn. Family : Verbenaceae

Chief Characters :

1. Shrub grows upto 4 m. height.
2. Simple leaf, opposite phyllotaxy.
3. White flowers.
4. Panicle inflorescence.
5. Fruit - drupe.

Synonyms : Jaya, Shriparna, Ganakarika, Tarkari, Vataghni, Vaijayantika, Nadaeyi, Jayanti.

Gana :

Charaka : Shothahara, Sheeta prashamana, Anuvasanopaga.

Sushruta : Veeratarvadi, Varunadi, Vatasamshamana, Brihat panchmoola.

Properties : Rasa - Katu, Tikta, Kashaya, Madhura; Guna - Laghu, Ruksha; Virya - Ushna and Vipaka - Katu.

Pharmacological Actions : Kaphavatahara, Deepana, Pachana, Vibandhahara.

Indications : Shotha, Pandu, Agnimandya, Vibandha, Agnimantha particularly useful in Vatajashotha.

Therapeutic Uses :

1. Prameha : Vasameha—should take decoction of agnimantha. (S.S.)
2. Obesity : Charaka prescribes the decoction of agnimantha as a good remedy for obesity. (C.S.)
3. Sheetapitta : Intake of agnimantha root paste with ghee alleviates, sheetapitta, udarda, kotha within seven days. (C.D.)

Parts Used : Leaf, Root bark.

Preparations & Dosage : Powder 1-3 gm.; Juice 10-20 ml.; Decoction 50-100 ml.

Specific Formulations : Dashamoolarishta, Agnimantha kashaya, Chyavanaprasha.

अग्निमन्थो जयःसस्याच्छ्रीपर्णी गणिकारिका ।
जया जयन्ती तर्कारी नादेयी वैजयन्तिका ॥
अग्निमन्थः श्वयथुनुद्वीर्योष्णः कफवातहृत् ।
पाण्डुनुत्कटुकस्तिक्तस्तुवरो मधुरोऽग्निदः ॥ भा०प्र०

92
BHĀRṄGĪ

Clerodendrum serratum Linn. Family : Verbanaceae

Chief Characters :

1. Perennial shrub, grows upto 2 m. height.
2. Simple leaves, opposite phyllotaxy.
3. Voilet coloured flowers.
4. Panicle inflorescence.
5. Fruit - drupe.

Synonyms : Padma, Kharasaka, Brahmana yastika, Phanji, Manjika, Bhrugubhava, Brahmani, Angaravalli.

Gana :

Sushruta : Pippalyadi, Arkadi.

Properties : Rasa - Katu, Tikta, Kashaya; Guna - Laghu, Ruksha; Virya - Ushna and Vipaka - Katu.

Pharmacological Actions : Kaphavatahara, Deepana, Pachana.

Indications : Shwasa, Kasa, Jwara, Peenasa, Shotha, Krimi, Vrana, Gulma, Raktadosha.

Therapeutic Uses :

1. Goitre : Local application of paste of bharangi pounded with sour gruel alleviates goitre, cervical adenitis and scrotal enlargement. (C.D.)
2. Bronchial asthma : Paste of bharangi and shunthi should be taken. (C.S.)
3. Inguinal Hernia : Intake of paste made of root of bhargi alleviates inguinal hernia. (V.S.)

Parts Used : Root.

Preparations & Dosage : Powder 3-6 gm.

Specific Formulations : Bharangi guda, Bharangyadi kwatha.

Bharangi is often adulterated with roots of Pigmacopremna herbacea, Gardenia turgida, Picrama quassioides and Elaedendron glaucum.

भार्गी भृगुभवा पद्मा फञ्जी ब्राह्मणयष्टिका ।
ब्राह्मण्यङ्गारवल्ली च खटशाकश्च हञ्जिका ॥
भार्गी रूक्षा कटुस्तिक्ता रुच्योष्णा पाचनी लघुः ।
दीपनी तुवरा गुल्मरक्तनुन्नाशयेद् ध्रुवम् ।
शोथकासकफश्वासपीनसज्वरमारुतान् ॥ भा०प्र०

93
GAMBHĀRĪ

Gmelina arborea Roxb. Family ; Verbenaceae

Chief Characters :

1. Tree grows upto 4-8 m. height.
2. Simple leaf, opposite phyllotaxy.
3. Yellow coloured flowers.
4. Panicle inflorescence.
5. Fruit - drupe.

Synonyms : Kashmari, Madhuparnika, Sriparni, Peetarohini, Heera, Bhadraparni, Kashmiri, Kashmarya, Mahakusumika, Madhu-rasa, Krishnavritta.

Gana :

Charaka : Shothahara, Daha prashamana, Virechanopaga.

Sushruta : Sarivadi, Brihat panchamoola.

Properties : Rasa - Tikta, Kashaya, Madhura; Guna - Guru; Virya - Ushna and Vipaka - Katu.

Pharmacological Actions : Vatapittahara, Deepana, Pachana, Bhedana. Medhya fruit : Brimhana, Vrishya, Keshya, Rasayana.

Indications : Shotha, Shoola, Brama, Arshas, Jwara, Shosha, Trishna, Daha, Raktapitta, Raktatisara, Vatarakta.

Therapeutic Uses :

1. Sheetapitta (Urticaria) : The ripe fruits of kashmarya are dried and then cooked with cow's milk and taken with the same keeping on wholesome diet. It destroys urticaria. (Y.R.)
2. Whitlow : Wrapping with seven tender leaves of kashmarya destroys the disease. (Y.R.)
3. Greying of hairs : Oil of gambhari taken as snuff relieves the disease. (S.G.)

Parts Used : Root, Fruit.

Preparations & Dosage : Root bark decoction 50-100 ml.; Fruit powder 1-3 gm.

Specific Formulations : Sriparni taila, Dasamoolarishta.

गम्भारी भद्रपर्णी च श्रीपर्णी मधुपर्णिका ।
काश्मीरी काश्मरी हीरा काश्मर्य: पीतरोहिणी ॥
कृष्णवृन्ता मधुरसा महाकुसुमिकाऽपि च ।
काश्मरी तुवरा तिक्ता वीर्योष्णा मधुरा गुरु: ॥
दीपनी पाचनी मेध्या भेदिनी भ्रमशोषजित् ।
दोषतृष्णाऽऽमशूलार्शोविषदाहज्वरापहा ॥
तत्फलं बृंहणं वृष्यं गुरु केश्यं रसायनम् ।
वातपित्ततृषारक्तक्षयमूत्रविबन्धनुत् ॥
स्वादु पाके हिमं स्निग्धं तुवराम्लं विशुद्धिकृत् ।
हन्याद्दाहतृषावातरक्तपित्तक्षतक्षयान् ॥ भा०प्र०

94
TULASĪ

Ocimum sanctum Linn. Family : Lamiaceae

Chief Characters :

1. Perennial shrub, grows upto 1 m. height.
2. Simple leaves, opposite decussate phyllotaxy.
3. Purple coloured flowers.
4. Thyrsus inflorescence.
5. Fruit - carcerulus with nutlets.

Synonyms : Surasa, Sulabha, Vishnuvallabha, Apetharakshasi, Gouri, Shoolagni, Pavani, Bahumanjari.

Gana :

Charaka : Shwasahara.

Sushruta : Surasadi.

Properties : Rasa - Katu, Tikta; Guna - Laghu, Ruksha; Virya - Ushna and Vipaka - Katu.

Pharmacological Actions : Kaphavatahara, Pittavardhaka, Deepana, Hridya, Dahakara.

Indications : Hikka, Kasa, Shwasa, Parshwashoola, Kushta, Mutrakriccha.

Therapeutic Uses :

1. Cough : The juice of black tulasi mixed with honey is useful in cough caused by kapha. (C.S.)
2. Vishama jwara : Juice of tulasi and dronapushpi mixed with marica powder should be taken to check vishama jwara including malaria. (S.G.)

Parts Used : Leaf, Root, Seed, Flower.

Preparations & Dosage : Leaf juice 10-20 ml.; Root decoction 50-100 ml.; Seed powder 3-6 gm.

Specific Formulations : Surasadi kashaya.

तुलसी सुरसा ग्राम्या सुलभा बहुमञ्जरी ।
अपेतराक्षसी गौरी भूतघ्नी देवदुन्दुभिः ॥
तुलसी कटुका तिक्ता हृद्योष्णा दाहपित्तकृत् ।

दीपनी कुष्ठकृच्छ्रास्त्रपार्श्वरुक्कफवातजित् ।
शुक्ला कृष्णा च तुलसी गुणैस्तुल्या प्रकीर्त्तिता ।। भा०प्र०

Research Studies: Ocimum sanctum was found to possess marked adaptogenic properties. Treatment of mice with the plant extract increased their swimming capacity tremendously. The stress induced ulcers in rats were also prevented. (Annual report 1977-78, CCRIMH)

Moudulation of specific and nonspecific immune response by Ocimum sanctum. It was observed that oral administration of aqueous extract of O. sanctum enhanced the antibody production in stressed rats, when compared to contol. O. sanctum can cause the restoration of the humoral response in immuno-suppressive state thereby making them protective from infections. (Indian journal of Pharmacology, Vol. 29/1 Feb 1997)

Effect of Tulasi leaf powder supplimentation on blood sugar levels, serum lipids and tissue lipids in diabetic rats (Plant Foods for Human Nutrition V. 50 (1) : p. 9-16, 1997)

95
DROṆAPUṢPĪ

Leucas cephalotus Spring. Family : Lamiaceae

Chief Characters :

1. Annual shrub, grows upto 1 m. height.
2. Simple leaves, opposite deccusate phyllotaxy.
3. White flowers.
4. Verticillaster inflorescence.
5. Fruit - carcerulus with nutlets.

Synonyms : Phalepushpa, Kshavapatra, Chatrini, Drona.

Properties : Rasa - Katu; Guna - Guru, Ruksha; Virya - Ushna and Vipaka - Madhura.

Pharmacological Actions : Kaphavatahara, Deepana, Bhedana.

Indications : Agnimandya, Kamala, Vishamajwara, Tamaka shwasa, Arshas, Pakshaghata, Prameha, Shotha, Krimi.

Therapeutic Uses :

1. Jaundice : Juice of dronapushpi should be used as collyrium in Jaundice. (V.M.)
2. Malaria fever : Juice of dronapushpi is efficacious in malaria fever. (S.G.)
3. Eye disease : The juice of dronapushpi pounded with rice water destroys the disorders of patala in eyes. (G.N.)

Parts Used : Panchanga (Whole plant).

Preparations & Dosage : Juice 10-20 ml.

द्रोणा च द्रोणपुष्पी च फलेपुष्पा च कीर्त्तिता ।
द्रोणपुष्पी गुरुः स्वादू रूक्षोष्णा वातपित्तकृत् ॥
सतीक्ष्णलवणा स्वादु पाका कट्वी च भेदिनी ।
कफामकामलाशोथतमकश्वासजन्तुजित् ॥ भा०प्र०

96
PUNARNAVĀ

Boerhaavia diffusa Linn. Family : Nyctaginaceae

Chief Characters :

1. Shrub procumbent grows upto 3-4 m. length.
2. Simple leaf, opposite phyllotaxy.
3. Light pink coloured flowers.
4. Panicle inflorescence.
5. Fruit - small fruits.

Synonyms : Kshudra, Vasshabu, Raktapushpa, Varshaketu, Kattilaka, Rakta, Shilatika, Shothagni, Shwetamoola, Deerghapatrika (Shweta).

Gana :

Charaka : Vayahsthapana, Kasahara.

Sushruta : Vidarigandhadi.

Properties : Rasa - Madhura, Tikta, Kashaya; Guna - Laghu, Ruksha; Virya - Ushna (D.N.), Sheeta (B.P.) and Vipaka - Katu.

Pharmacological Actions : Shweta : Kaphavatahara, Deepana, Vayahsthapana; Rakta : Kaphapittahara, Grahi.

Indications : Shotha, Udara, Pandu, Hridroga, Kasa, Shoola, Raktavikara.

Therapeutic Uses :

1. Sotha : Ghrita processed with decoction and paste of punarnava alleviates oedema. (C.D.)
2. Amavata : Paste of shati and shunthi taken with decoction of punarnava for a week alleviates amavata. (B.P.)

Parts Used : Root, Leaf, Panchanga (Whole plant).

Preparations & Dosage : Juice 5-10 ml.; Powder 1-3 gm.

Specific Formulations : Punarnavadi mandoora, Punarnavarista.

पुनर्नवा श्वेतमूला शोथघ्नी दीर्घपत्रिका ।
कटु कषायानुरसा पाण्डुघ्नी दीपनी परा ।

शोफानिलगरश्लेष्महरी ब्रध्नोदरव्रणुत् ॥
पुनर्नवाऽपरा रक्ता रक्तपुष्पा शिलाटिका ।
शोथघ्नी क्षुद्रवर्षाभूर्वर्षकेतुः कठिल्लकः ॥
पुनर्नवाऽरुणा तिक्ता कटुपाका हिमा लघुः ।
वातला ग्राहिणी श्लेष्मपित्तरक्तविनाशिनी ॥ भा०प्र०

Research Studies: In experiments with Boerhaevia diffusa there has been diuresis accompanied by increased excretion of sodium. Anti-inflammatory activity incarrageenin induced oedema was observed in ethylacetate extraction of B. diffusa. (Ref.-Annual report, CCRIMH 1972-73)

Effect of stress on plasma and adreno cortisol levels and immune responsiveness in rats : Modulation by one fraction of Boerhaevia diffusa. (Fitoterapia, v-68(6) : p. 498-500, 1997)

Hepatoprotective activity of Boerhaevia diffusa roots-A popular Indian ethnomedicine (Journal of Ethnopharmacology; V. 56 (1) : p. 61-66, 1997)

97
APĀMĀRGA

Achyranthes aspera Linn. Family : Amaranthaceae

Chief Characters :

1. Perennial shrub grows upto 1-3 ft. height.
2. Simple leaf, opposite phyllotaxy.
3. Green flowers.
4. Spike inflorescence.
5. Fruit - utricle.

Synonyms : Pratyakpushpi, Mayuraka, Shikhari, Kapipippali, Adhashalya, Markati, Durgraha, Kinihi, Kharamanjari.

Gana :

Charaka : Sirovirechanopaga, Krimighna, Vamaopaga.
Sushruta : Arkadi.

Properties : Rasa - Katu, Tikta; Guna - Laghu, Ruksha, Tikshna; Virya - Ushna, Sheeta (Raktaapamarga) and Vipaka - Katu, Madhura (Fruit).

Pharmacological Actions : Kaphavatahara, Medohara, Deepana, Pachana, Shirovirechana, Shona, Rochana.

Indications : Chardi, Adhmana, Shoola, Arshas, Udara, Apachi, Visuchi, Krimi, Kandu, Hridruja, Mutrakriccha, Sidhmakushta, Sadyovrana.

Therapeutic Uses :

1. Piles : Apamarga root is pounded mixed with honey and taken with rice water only. (S.S.)
   The paste of the seeds of apamarga taken with rice water alleviates bleeding piles. (S.G.)
2. Dysuria : Apamarga root taken with milk relieves dysuria. (V.D.)

Parts Used : Leaf, Root, Seed, Panchanga (Whole plant).

Preparations & Dosage : Juice 10-20 ml.; Kshara ½ -1 gm.

Specific Formulations : Apamarga taila, Shikari ghrita, Apamarga kshara taila.

अपामार्गस्तु शिखरी ह्यधःशल्यो मयूरकः ।
मर्कटी दुर्ग्रहा चापि किणिही खरमञ्जरी ॥
अपामार्गः सरस्तीक्ष्णो दीपनस्तिक्तकः कटुः ।
पाचनो रोचनश्छर्दि कफमेदोऽनिलापहः ॥ भा०प्र०

98
MARICA

Piper nigrum Linn. Family : Piperaceae

Chief Characters :

1. Perennial twinner, grows upto 10 m. height.
2. Simple leaf, alternate phyllotaxy.
3. Green flowers, male and female flowers occur on different branches.
4. Spike inflorescence.
5. Fruit - berry.

Synonyms : Vellaja, Ushna, Krishna, Dharmapattana.

Gana :

Charaka : Deepaniya, Shoolaprashamana, Krimighna.

Sushruta : Pippalyadi, Tryushana (Trikatu).

Properties : Rasa - Katu; Guna - Laghu, Tikshna, Ruksha; Virya - Ushna and Vipaka - Katu, Madhura (Ardra).

Pharmacological Actions : Kaphavatahara, Deepana, Avrishya, Pittakara, Sleshmapraseki (Ardra).

Indications : Pravahika, Kasa, Peenasa, Hridroga, Shwasa, Shoola, Krimi.

Therapeutic Uses :

1. Chronic dysentry : Intake of fine powder of pippali or marica checks even chronic dysentry. (A.H.)
2. Cough : One should take marica powder with ghee, honey and sugar. (C.S.)

Parts Used : Fruit.

Preparations & Dosage : Powder ½ -1 gm.

Specific Formulations : Marichadi taila, Tekarajamaricha.

मरिचं वेल्लजं कृष्णमूषणं घर्मपत्तनम् ॥
मरिचं कटुकं तीक्ष्णं दीपनं कफवातजित् ।
उष्णं पित्तकरं रूक्षं श्वासशूलकृमीन् हरेत् ॥
तदार्द्रं मधुरं पाके नात्युष्णं कटुकं गुरु ॥
किञ्चित् तीक्ष्णगुणं श्लेष्मप्रसेकि स्यादपित्तलम् ॥ भा०प्र०

99
PIPPALĪ

Piper longum Linn. Family : Piperaceae

Chief Characters :

1. Perennial climber grows upto 1 m. height.
2. Simple leaf, alternate phyllotaxy.
3. Green flowers, male and female flowers occur on different branches.
4. Spike inflorescence.
5. Fruit - berry.

Synonyms **:** Magadhi, Krishna, Vaidehi, Chapala, Kana, Kola, Upakulya, Ushna, Tikshna tandula, Soundi.

Gana :

Charaka : Deepaniya, Shoola prashamana, Kasahara, Hikkanigrahana.

Sushruta : Pippalyadi, Urdhvabhagahara.

Properties : Rasa - Katu; Guna - Laghu, Snigdha, Tikshna, Guru; Virya - Ushna (Sushka), Sheeta (Ardra) and Vipaka - Madhura.

Pharmacological Actions : Vatakaphahara, Sleshmakara Pittaprashamana (Ardhara), Pittakara (Sushka) Deepana, Rasayana, Vrishya, Rechana, Medhya.

Indications : Jwara, Shoola, Udara, Hikka, Prameha, Arshas, Pleehodara, Kushta, Kasa, Shwasa, Jeernajwara, Gulma, Sthaulya.

Therapeutic Uses :

1. Dysentry : By using fine powder of pippali or maricha dysentry even if chronic is destroyed. (A.H.)
2. Acute grastritis : Pippali with profuse honey should be taken. (V.M.)

   For eradication of the disease patient should take in morning ghee cooked with pippali decoction and paste added with profuse honey. (V.M.)

Parts Used : Fruit, Root.

Preparations & Dosage : Powder ½ -1 gm.

Specific Formulations : Pippalyasava, Vyoshadi vati, Guda pippali.

पिप्पली मागधी कृष्णा वैदेही चपला कणा ।
उपकुल्योषणा शौण्डी कोला स्यात्तीक्ष्णतण्डुला ॥
पिप्पली दीपनी वृष्या स्वादुपाका रसायनी ।
अनुष्णा कटुका स्निग्धा वातश्लेष्महरी लघुः ॥
पिप्पली रेचनी हन्ति श्वासकासोदरज्वरान् ।
कुष्ठप्रमेहगुल्मार्शः प्लीहशूलाममारुतान् ॥
आर्द्रा कफप्रदा स्निग्धा शीतला मधुरा गुरुः ।
पित्तप्रशमनी सा तु शुष्का पित्तप्रकोपिणी ॥
पिप्पली मधुसंयुक्ता मेदःकफविनाशिनी ।
श्वासकासज्वरहरी वृष्या मेध्याग्निवर्द्धिनी ॥
जीर्णज्वरेऽग्निमान्द्ये च शस्यते गुडपिप्पली ।
कासाजीर्णारुचिश्वासहृत्पाण्डुकृमिरोगनुत् ।
द्विगुणः पिप्पला चूर्णाद् गुडोऽत्र भिषजां मतः ॥ भा०प्र०

Research Studies: The alkaloid from Piper longum, piperine has been found on comparision with nikethamide and metrazol to be better than both in its ability to counteract respiratory depression produced by morphine and phenobarbitone in a dog. The studies with petroleum ether extract of Piper longum revealed its analeptic potency. This also possesses potent central nervous stimulant action. (Annual report, CCRIMH 1972-73, 74-75)

100
JĀTIPHALA

Myristica fragrans Houtt. Family : Myristicaceae

Chief Characters :

1. Tree grows upto 10 m. height.
2. Simple leaf, alternate phyllotaxy.
3. Whie flowers.
4. Racemose inflorescence.
5. The seed of fruit consists of aril and mac.

Synonyms : Jatikosha, Malatiphala, Puta.

Properties : Rasa - Katu, Tikta; Guna - Laghu, Tikshna; Virya - Ushna and Vipaka - Katu.

Pharmacological Actions : Kaphavatahara, Deepana, Rochana, Grahi, Swarya, shukrastambana.

Indications : Mukhavairasya, Chardi, Atisara, Grahini, Krimi, Trishna, Kasa, Shwasa, Peenasa, Shosha, Hridruja, Kushta.

Therapeutic Uses :

1. Cracks in feet : Paste of jatiphala destroys the cracks in feet. (B.S.)
2. Freckles : Application of paste of aril of Jatiphala removes freckles. (R.M.)
3. Thirst : In case of thirst and slight nausea water boiled with jatiphala and cooled should be given. (C.D.)

Parts Used : Seed, Mac (Japatri), Oil (Aril).

Preparations & Dosage : Powder ½ -1 gm.; Oil 1-3 drops.

Specific Formulations : Jathipaladi churna, Jathipaladi vati.

जातीफलं जातिकोशं मालतीफलमित्यपि ।
जातीफलं रसे तिक्तं तीक्ष्णोष्णं रोचनं लघु ।
कटुकं दीपनं ग्राही स्वर्यं श्लेष्मानिलापहम् ॥
निहन्ति मुखवैरस्यं मलदौर्गन्ध्यकृष्णताः ।
कृमिकासवमिश्वासशोषपीनसहृद्रुजः ॥

Research Studies: Nutmeg in combination with ginger, jaggery and ghee is an ageold indian household remedy against diarrhoea. Recent work confirms that nutmeg often works where other drugs have failed. P.G. inhibition is suspected to be the mechanism of this anti diarrhoeal effect. (PPT 1983)

(Hypolipidaemic effect of Myristica fragrans fruit extract in rabbits is also reported. Journal of Ethnopharmacology V. 55 (1) : 49-53, 1996)

101

TWAK

Cinnamonum zeylanicum Blume. Family : Lauraceae

Chief Characters :

1. Evergreen tree grows upto 6-8 m. height.
2. Simple leaf, opposite phyllotaxy.
3. Light green flowers.
4. Panicle inflorescence.
5. Fruit - berry.

Synonyms : Darusita, Varanga, Swadvi, Janutwak, Utkata.

Gana :

Vagbhata : Trijata.

Sushruta : Eladi.

Properties : Rasa - Katu, Tikta, Madhura; Guna - Laghu, Ruksha, Tikshna; Virya - Ushna and Vipaka - Katu.

Pharmacological Actions : Vatapittahara (B.P.), Shukrala, Varnya, Grahi.

Indications : Agnimandya, Aruchi, Hrillasa, Adhmana, Akshepaka vata, Kandu, Arshas, Peenasa, Kasa, Krimi, Hridroga, Danta shoola, Trishna, Mukha shosha, Chardi, Rajorodha (oil).

Therapeutic Uses :

1. Dysentry : Intake of one masha of twak powder cures dysentry. (T.N. Ghosh)
2. Rakta pradara : Twak powder should be given with rice water. Decoction of twak cures dysmennorhoea. (Anubhuta)

Parts Used : Bark, Oil, Leaf.

Preparations & Dosage : Bark powder 1-3 gm.; Oil 2-5 drops.

Specific Formulations : Sitopaladi churna, Eladi rasayana, Trijatakadi vati.

त्वक् स्वाद्वी तु तनुत्वक्स्यात्तथा दारुसिता मता ॥
उक्ता दारुसिता स्वाद्वी तिक्ता चानिलपित्तहृत् ।
सुरभिः शुक्रला बल्या मुखशोषतृषापहा ॥ भा०प्र०

102
KARPŪRA

Cinnamomum camphora Nees & Eberm. Family : Lauraceae

Chief Characters :

1. Tree grows upto 30 m. height.
2. Simple leaf, alternate phyllotaxy.
3. Light green coloured flowers.
4. Panicle inflorescence.
5. Fruit - pea shaped green coloured when unripen. Ripened fruits are black in colour.

Synonyms : Sheetabhra, Himavaluka, Ghanasara, Hima.

Gana :

Karpuradi. (B.P.)

Properties : Rasa - Tikta, Katu, Madhura; Guna - Laghu, Tikshna; Virya - Sheeta and Vipaka - Katu.

Pharmacological Actions : Kaphahara, Pachana, Vrishya, Chakshusya, Lekahana, Hridya, Medhya, Vishaghna, Madakara.

Indications : Kustha, Kandu, Krimi, Daha, Trishna, Vrana, Mukhavairasya, Netraroga.

Therapeutic Uses :

1. Accidental injury : Wound caused by accidental injury is filled with camphor mixed with ghee and bandaged. By this it heals free of infection and pus. (R.M.)
2. Corneal opacity : Fine powder of camphor should be used as collyrium in case of corneal opacity. (V.S.)

Parts Used : Exudate (Extract).

Preparations & Dosage : 125-175 mg.

Specific Formulations : Karpuradi rasa, Hingu karpura vati.

पुंसि क्लीबे च कर्पूरः सिताभ्रो हिमवालुकः ।
घनसारश्चन्द्रसंज्ञो हिमनामाऽपि स स्मृतः ॥
कर्पूरः शीतलो वृष्यश्चक्षुष्यो लेखनो लघुः ।
सुरभिर्मधुरस्तिक्तः कफपित्तविषापहः ॥
दाहतृष्णाऽस्यवैरस्यमेदोदौर्गन्ध्यनाशनः ।
कर्पूरो द्विविधः प्रोक्तः पक्वापक्वप्रभेदतः ।
पक्वात्कर्पूरतः प्राहुरपक्वं गुणवत्तरम् ॥ भा०प्र०

103
AGURU

Aquilaria agallocha Roxb. Family : Thymeliaceae

Chief Characters :

1. Big tree grows upto 60-70 ft. height.
2. Simple leaf, alternate phyllotaxy.
3. White flowers, umbel inflorescence.
4. Fruit - capsule.

Synonyms : Loha, Rajasa, Krimija, Anaryaja, Pravara, Yogaja, Vamshika, Krimijagdha, Anardraka.

Gana :

Charaka : Sheetaprashamana, Shwasahara, Shirovirechana, Tikta skandha.

Sushruta : Salasaradi, Eladi, Sleshma samshamana.

Properties : Rasa - Katu, Tikta; Guna - Laghu, Tikshna; Virya - Ushna and Vipaka - Katu.

Pharmacological Actions : Vatakaphahara, Pittala, Twachya, Rasayana.

Indications : Hikka, Shwasa, Kasa, Kushta, Prameha, Shotha, Dushtavrana, Karnaroga, Akshiroga, Dadru kushta.

Therapeutic Uses :

1. Hiccough : The powder of aguru mixed with honey is taken to check Hikka. (C.S.)
2. Skin disease : The aguru oil is efficacious in skin diseases such as ringworm etc. (S.S.)
3. Rasayana : Aguru is also recommended as rasayana. (A.H.)

Parts Used : Oil, Aromatic resinous wood.

Preparations & Dosage : Powder 1-3 gm.; Oil 1-5 drops.

Specific Formulation : Aguruvadi taila.

अगुरु प्रवरं लोहं राजार्हं योगजं तथा ।
वंशिकं कृमिजं वाऽपि कृमिजग्धमनार्यकम् ॥
अगुरूष्णं कटु त्वच्यं तिक्तं तीक्ष्णञ्च पित्तलम् ।
लघु कर्णाक्षिरोगघ्नं शीतवातकफप्रणुत् ॥
कृष्णं गुणाधिकं तत्तु लोहवद्वारि मज्जति ॥
अगुरुप्रभवः स्नेहः कृष्णागुरुसमः स्मृतः ॥ भा०प्र०

104
CANDANA

Santalum album Linn. Family : Santalaceae

Chief Characters :

1. Evergreen tree grows upto 8 m. height.
2. Simple leaf, opposite phyllotaxy.
3. Voilet coloured flowers, bisexual flowers.
4. Fruit - drupe.

Synonyms : Gandhasara, Malayaja, Srikanda, Chandana, Bhadrasi, Tailaparnika, Chandradyuti.

Gana :

Charaka : Daha prashamana, Trishnanigrahana, Kandughna, Angamardaprashamana.

Sushruta : Salasaradi, Sarivadi, Patoladi, Priyangvadi.

Properties : Rasa - Tikta, Madhura; Guna - Laghu, Ruksha; Virya - Sheeta and Vipaka - Katu.

Pharmacological Actions : Kaphapittahara, Daha prashamana, Varnya, Vishahara.

Indications : Daha, Trishna, Jwara, Shosha, Raktapitta, Prameha, Raktarshas, Raktatisara, Raktapradara, Pittaja roga.

Therapeutic Uses :

1. Prameha : Shukrameha : Decoction of arjuna and candaran is useful. (S.S.)
   Manjishthameha : Decoction of manjishtha and candana is useful. (S.S.)
2. Pradara : Should adminsiter candana mixed with milk, ghee, sugar and honey. (G.N.)
3. Shitapitta : Candana pounded with guduchi should be taken. (V.D.)

Parts Used : Oil, Heartwood.

Preparations & Dosage : Powder 3-6 gm.; Oil 5-10 drops.

Specific Formulations : Chandanasava, Chandanadi vati, Chandanadi taila.

श्रीखण्डं चन्दनं न स्त्री भद्रश्रीस्तैलपर्णिकः ।
गन्धसारो मलयजस्तथा चन्द्रद्युतिश्च सः ॥

उत्तमचन्दनस्य लक्षणम्—

स्वादे तिक्तं कषे पीतं छेदे रक्तं तनौ सितम् ।
ग्रन्थिकोटरसंयुक्तं चन्दनं श्रेष्ठमुच्यते ॥
चन्दनं शीतलं रूक्षं तिक्तमाह्लादनं लघु ।
श्रमशोषविषश्लेष्मतृष्णापित्तास्रदाहनुत् ॥ भा०प्र०

105
ERAṆḌA

Ricinus communis Linn. Family : Euphorbiaceae

Chief Characters :

1. Annual or perennial shrub grows upto 2-6 m. height.
2. Simple leaf, alternate phyllotaxy.
3. Green coloured flowers.
4. Panicle inflorescence.
5. Fruit - capsule.

Synonyms : Gandharvahasta, Panchangula, Amanda, Chitra, Deerghadouta, Vardhamana, Vyadambaka, Urubhuka, Taruna, Ru-trika (Shweta eranda); Urupuka, Rutrika, Rubu, Vyagrapuchcha (Rakta eranda).

Gana :

Charaka : Bhedaniya, Angamardaprashamana, Swedopaga.
Sushruta : Vidarigandhadi, Adhobhagahara, Vata samshamana.

Properties : Rasa - Madhura, Katu, Kashaya; Guna - Snigdha, Tikshna, Sukshma, Guru; Virya - Ushna and Vipaka - Madhura.

Pharmacological Actions : Kaphavatahara, Rechana, Twachya, Vrishya.

Indications : Gulma, Anaha, Shoola, Jwara, Vatakaphodara, Yakritpleehodara, Arshas, Krimi, Pravahika, Amavata, Katishoola, Sotha, Shwasa, Sirashoola,Anaha, Kasa, Bastishoola, Vriddhi, Mutrakriccha, Bradhna, Kushta.

Therapeutic Uses :

1. Amavata : Paste of shunthi mixed with decoction of eranda root should be cooked in closed heating. The juice there of mixed with honey alleviates severe pain caused by Amavata. (S.G.)
2. Obesity : In order to remove obesity one should take alkali of eranda leaves mixed with hingu. The diet should be rice with scum. (B.P.)

Parts Used : Root, Leaf, Oil, Seed.

Preparations & Dosage : Root paste 10-20 gm.; Oil 5-15 ml.

Specific Formulations : Erandapaka, Erandasaptaka kwatha, Erandamuladi kwatha.

शुक्ल एरण्ड आमण्डश्चित्रो गन्धर्वहस्तक: ।
पञ्चाङ्गुलो वर्द्धमानो दीर्घदण्डो व्यडम्बक: ॥
वातारिस्तरुणश्चापि बूकश्च निगद्यते ।
रक्तोऽपरो रुबूक: स्यादुरुबूको रुबुस्तथा ॥
व्याघ्रपुच्छश्च वातारिश्चक्षुरुत्तानपत्रक: ।
एरण्डयुग्मं मधुरमुष्णं गुरु विनाशयेत् ॥
शूलशोथकटीबस्तिशिर:पीडोदयज्वरान् ।
ब्रध्नश्वासकफानाहकासकुष्ठाममारुतान् ॥
एरण्डपत्रं वातघ्नं कफक्रिमिविनाशनम् ।
मूत्रकृच्छ्रहरं चापि पित्तरक्तप्रकोपणम् ।
वातार्यग्रदलं गुल्मबस्तिशूलहरं परम् ॥
कफवातकृमीन्हन्ति वृद्धिं सप्तविधामपि ।
एरण्डफलमत्युष्णं गुल्मशूलानिलापहम् ॥
यकृत्प्लीहोदरार्शोघ्नं कटुकं दीपनं परम् ।
तद्वन्मज्जा च विड्भेदी वातश्लेष्मोदरापहा: ॥ भा०प्र०

<u>Research Studies:</u> The aqueous extract of Ricinus communis Linn. (root bark) in the dose of 500 mg/100gm. did not inhibit the carrageenin induced oedema in rats. But the crude alcohol extract in the dose 100mg/100gm showed 72.2% inhibition of the oedema. The fraction II of the crude alcohol extract in the dose 10 mg/100 gm produced 65.12% inhibition. Acetyl salycilic acid showed 62.1% inhibition. when used in the doses of 30 mg/100 gm. (Sharma V. N. et al JRIM 4,1, 1969 pp. 47.51)

106
DANTĪ

Baliospermum axillare Blume. Family : Euphorbiaceae

Chief Characters :

1. Small shrub grows upto 2 m. height.
2. Simple leaf, alternate phyllotaxy.
3. Racemose inflorescence, monoecious plant.
4. Consists of green coloured flowers.
5. Fruit - capsule.

Synonyms : Nikumbha, Udumbaraparni, Erandaphala, Laghudanti, Vishalya, Shighra, Ghunapriya, Makulaka, Varahangi.

Gana :

Charaka : Rechana, Mulini.

Sushruta : Shyamadi, Adhobhagahara.

Properties : Rasa - Katu; Guna - Laghu, Tikshna; Virya - Ushna and Vipaka - Katu.

Pharmacological Actions : Kaphavatahara, Deepana, Rechana.

Indications : Arshas, Shoola, Kushta, Kandu, Ashmari, Shotha, Udara, Krimi, Vidaha.

Therapeutic Uses :

1. Piles : Leaves of danti fried in oil and ghee and added with fatty layer of curd should be given as vegetable. (C.S.)
2. Udara roga : Oil of danti and dravanti seeds should be given with curd water, soup, meat-soup etc. (C.S.)

Parts Used : Root, Seed, Leaf.

Preparations & Dosage : Bark powder 1-3 gm.; Seed powder 125-250 mg.; Leaf decoction 40-80 ml.

Specific Formulations : Dantyarishta, Dantiharitaki, Abhayadimodaka.

लघुदन्ती विशल्या च स्यादुदुम्बरपर्ण्यपि ।
तथैरण्डफला शीघ्रा श्येनघण्टा घुणप्रिया ॥
वाराहाङ्गी च कथिता निकुम्भश्च मकूलकः ।
द्रवन्ती शम्बरी चित्रा प्रत्यक्पर्ण्याखुपर्ण्यपि ॥

उपचित्रा श्रुतश्रोणी न्यग्रोधी च तथा वृषा ।
दन्तीद्वयं सरं पाकं रसे च कटु दीपनम् ॥
गुदाङ्कुराश्मशूलास्त्रकण्डूकुष्ठविदाहनुत् ।
तीक्ष्णोष्णं हन्ति पित्तास्त्रकफशोथोदरक्रिमीन् ॥ भा०प्र०

Research Studies: An investigation of the constituents responsible for the antitumour activity observed for extracts of B. montanum roots have afforded five new phorbol ester derivatives exhibiting anti-cancer activity. (Ogura M. Planta Med. 33 (2), 128 & 133, 1978)

107
ARJUNA

Terminalia arjuna Roxb. Family : Combretaceae

Chief Characters :

1. Big tree grows upto 20-40 m. height.
2. Simple leaf, opposite phyllotaxy.
3. Light green coloured flowers.
4. Spike inflorescence.
5. Fruit - consists of truncate wings.

Synonyms : Kakubha, Veerataru, Nadisarjaha, Indradaru, Veera, Dhavala, Veeravriksha.

Gana :

Charaka : Kashayaskandha, Udardaprashamana.
Sushruta : Nyagrodhadi, Salasaradi.

Properties : Rasa - Kashaya; Guna - Laghu, Ruksha; Virya - Sheeta, Ushna (Raja Nighantu) and Vipaka - Katu.

Pharmacological Actions : Kaphapittahara, Hridya, Udardaprashamana, Vrana shodhana, Rasayana.

Indications : Hridroga, Kshatakshaya, Raktapitta, Medoroga, Prameha, Raktatisara, Grahani, Arshas, Vrana, Mutraghata, Kandabhagna.

Therapeutic Uses :

1. Heart disease : Those who take arjuna bark with ghee, milk or jaggery-water are relieved of heart disease. (V.M.)
2. Prameha : Shukrameha—Decoction of arjuna and candana is useful. (S.S.). Puyameha—Decoction of dhava and arjuna is beneficial. (H.S.)
3. Kshayaja kasa : The bark powder to be pounded with vasas-warasa several times on internal administration with honey and sugar relieves kshayaja raktaja kasa. (B.P.)

Parts Used : Bark.

Preparations & Dosage : Powder 3-6 gm.; Decoction 50-100 ml.

Specific Formulations : Arjunarista, Arjuna ghrita, Nagarjunabhraka rasa, Arjuna ksheerapaka.

ककुभोऽर्जुननामाख्यो नदीसर्जश्च कीर्त्तितः ।
इन्द्रद्रुर्वीरवृक्षश्च वीरश्च धवलः स्मृतः ॥
ककुभः शीतलो हृद्यः क्षतक्षयविषास्त्रजित् ।
मेदोमेहव्रणान् हन्ति तुवरः कफपित्तहृत् ॥ भा०प्र०

Research Studies: The bark possesses a reputation of being a valuable cardiac tonic and is extensively used in this country for all sorts of cardiac troubles and complications.

The reputation of the drug and the fact that is extensively used and advertised as cardiac tonic led us to make a careful investigation of its action on animals. Experiments made with liquid extracts obtained from reputed manufacturers and prepared in the laboratory show that it causes a fall of blood pressure in intact animals even in very small doses. While larger doses cause death of the animal from stoppage of heart. On isolated hearts, the beats are rendered weaker and eventually the heart stops from direct action on the cardiac muscle. These findings are directly opposite to the general belief. Future work is in progress to sustantiate or controvent these observations. (B.N. Ghosh PMMT)

The bark of Terminalia arjuna has shown cardiac stimulant and diuretic activity. (Bose et al IJMS 10, 701-704, 1956) Hypocholesterolaemic effects of Terminelia arjuna tree bark (Journal of Ethnopharmacology V. 55(3) : p. 165-169, 1997)

An aqueous extract of Terminalia arjuna stem bark produced a transient decrease in blood pressure accompained by a slight decrease in heart rate. The hypotensive effect was observed with a fraction containing tannin related compounds (F_2) seperated from the aqueous extract.

108
UDUMBARA

Ficus racemosa Linn. Family : Moraceae

Chief Characters :

1. Tree grows upto 10 m. height.
2. Simple leaf, oval shaped leaves with acute tip.
3. Hypanthodium inflorescence.
4. Fruit - achene.

Synonyms : Jantuphala, Yajnanga, Shwetavalkala, Hemadugdhaka, Sadaphala, Apushpaka.

Gana :

Charaka : Mutra sangrahaniya, Kashayaskandha.
Sushruta : Nyagrodhadi.
Bhava Prakasha : Panchavalkala, Ksheerivriksha.

Properties : Rasa - Kashaya, Madhura; Guna - Guru, Ruksha; Virya - Sheeta and Vipaka - Katu.

Pharmacological Actions : Kaphapittahara, Varnya, Vranashotha ropana, Vrana ropana.

Indications : Raktapitta, Daha, Murccha, Trishna, Bhasmakagni, Atisara, Raktapradara.

Therapeutic Uses :

1. Raktapitta : The juice of the pounded fruit should be taken in raktapitta. (S.S.)
2. Excessive digestion : One should take udumbara bark mixed with woman's breast milk or payasa prepared with udumbara. (C.S.)

Parts Used : Bark, Root, Latex.

Preparations & Dosage : Powder 3-6 gm.; Decoction 50-100 ml.; Latex 6-10 drops.

Specific Formulations : Udumbara taila, Udumbara sara.

उदुम्बरो जन्तुफलो यज्ञाङ्गो हेमदुग्धक: ।।
उदुम्बरो हिमो रूक्षो गुरु: पित्तकफास्रजित् ।
मधुरस्तुवरो वर्ण्यो व्रणशोधनरोपण: ।। भा०प्र०

109
BHAṄGĀ

Cannabis sativa Linn. Family : Cannabinaceae

Chief Characters :

1. Annual shrub grows upto 1m. height covered with hairs.
2. Trifoliate compound leaf, alternate phyllotaxy.
3. Panicle inflorescence, male and female flower occur on different branches.
4. Consists of greenish white flowers.
5. Fruit - achene.

Synonyms : Vijaya, Jaya, Matulani, Madani, Ganja.

Gana :

Upavisha (R.R.S.)

Properties : Rasa - Tikta; Guna - Laghu, Tikshna, Vyavayi; Virya - Ushna and Vipaka - Katu.

Pharmacological Actions : Kaphavatahara, Grahi, Pachana, Deepana, Pittala, Madakari.

Indications : Amlapitta, Atisara, Grahani, Visuchi, Shoola, Dhanusthamba, Nidranasha, Madatyaya, Jalatrasa, Raktapradara, Pratishyaya.

Therapeutic Uses :

1. Diarrhoea : Bhanga and jatiphala in equal part mixed with indrayava in double quantity is made into a linctus. It checks all types of diarrhoea. (B.P.)
2. Coryza : Bhanga leaf juice processed through putapakwa process added with rocksalt, oil should be given to the patient. (Y.R.)

Parts Used : Leaf, Resin.

Preparations & Dosage : Bhanga 125-250 mg.; Ganja 60-125 mg., Charasa 30 mg.

Specific Formulations : Jatiphaladi churna, Madananda modaka.

भङ्गा गञ्जा मातुलानि मादिनी विजया जया ।

भङ्गा कफहरी तिक्ता ग्राहिणी पाचनी लघुः ।

तीक्ष्णोष्णा पित्तला मोहमदवाग्वह्निवर्द्धिनी ॥ भा०प्र०

Research Studies: Subsequent experience has confirmed the value of the drug as a remedy in tetanus and cholera. In the former disease we have obtained most satisfactory results, large doses are required and patient must be kept under the influence of the drug for some days. In cholera, its action may be compared with that of opium. It is most likely to be sucessfull when resorted too early in the disease. (Dymock)

110
DEVADĀRU

Cedrus deodara Roxb. Family : Pinaceae

Chief Characters :

1. Big tree grows upto 80 m. height.
2. Leaves-needle like 2-3 cms. long.
3. Monoecious plant, female and male cones on the same plant.
4. Seeds consists of a wing.
5. Seeds 1 cm. in length.

Synonyms **:** Indradaru, Drukilamala, Bhadradaru, Darubhadra, Mastadaru, Kilimam, Surabhuruha.

Gana :

Charaka : Stanya shodhana, Anuvasanopaga.
Sushruta : Vatasamshamana.

Properties : Rasa - Tikta, Kashaya; Guna - Laghu, Snigdha; Virya - Ushna and Vipaka - Katu.

Pharmacological Actions : Kaphavatahara, Deepana, Vibandhahara.

Indications : Adhmana, Jwara, Hikka, Prameha, Peenasa, Vibandha, Shosha, Kandu, Kushta, Krimi, Dushtavrana, Shopha, Vyanga, Tandra, Kasa, Raktadosha.

Therapeutic Uses :

1. Hiccough and asthma : To quench thirst, the patient should take decoction of devadaru. (C.S.)
2. Cough : Should take initially the oil extracted from the burnt wood of devadaru added with trikatu and yavaksara. (A.H.)

Parts Used : Oil, Wood.

Preparations & Dosage : Powder 3-6 gm.; Oil 20-40 drops.

Specific Formulations : Devadarvadi churna, Devadarvadi taila.

देवदारु स्मृतं दारुभद्रं दार्विन्द्रदारु च ।
मस्तदारु द्रुकिलिमं किलिमं सुरभूरुहः ॥
देवदारु लघु स्निग्धं तिक्तोष्णं कटुपाकि च ।

विबन्धाध्मानशोथामतन्द्राहिक्काज्वरास्रजित् ।
प्रमेहपीनसश्लेष्मकासकण्डूसमीरनुत् ॥ भा०प्र०

Research Studies: The oil was found to possess significant anti inflammatory activity in carrageenin induced odema in rats. It was divoid of analgesic, sedative and motor incoordinating, activities in mice. However it caused a significant increase in pheno-barbitone induced hypnosis which may be due to inhibition of drug metabolising enzymes (Ind. Jr. of Phar. Sci; pp. 20-23). Anti allergic activity of C. deodara (Journal of Medicinal and Aromatic plants Sciences V. 19 (4) : p. 1007-1008, 1997)

111
TĀLĪŚAPATRA

Abbies webbiana Lindle. Family : Pinaceae

Chief Characters :

1. Big and evergreen tree grows upto 30 m. height.
2. Glabrous leaves with acute tip.
3. Male and female cones are present on the same plant.

Synonyms : Patradya, Dhatripatra, Shukodara, Hridya, Mukha-rogahara.

Gana :

Sushruta : Sirovirechana.

Properties : Rasa - Tikta, Madhura; Guna - Laghu, Tikshna; Virya - Ushna and Vipaka - Katu.

Pharmacological Actions : Kaphavatahara, Deepana, Hridya, Swarya.

Indications : Aruchi, Agnimandya, Gulma, Shwasa, Kasa, Kshaya, Hikka, Chardi, Raktapitta.

Therapeutic Uses :

1. Anorexia : Big pills made of talisha churna mixed with comphor and sugarcandy promote relish. (A.H.)
2. Tamaka shwasa : Powder of talisha mixed with vasa leaf juice should be used. (H.S.)

Parts Used : Leaf.

Preparations & Dosage : Powder 2-5 gm.

Specific Formulations : Talisadi churna, Talisadi vati.

Taxus baccata is also considered as one of the source plants of talispatri.

तालीसमुक्तं पत्राढ्यं धात्रीपत्रञ्च तत्स्मृतम् ॥
तालीसं लघु तीक्ष्णोष्णं श्वासकासकफानिलान् ।
निहन्त्यारुचिगुल्मामवह्निमान्द्यक्षयामयान् ॥ भा०प्र०

112
HARIDRĀ

Curcuma longa Linn. Family : Zingiberaceae

Chief Characters :

1. Perennial herb grows upto 1½ m. height.
2. Consists of root stock.
3. Long leaves with a long petiole.
4. Yellow coloured flowers.
5. Spike inflorescence.
6. Fruit - capsule.

Synonyms : Peeta, Yoshipriya, Nisha, Varavarnini, Haladi, Kanchani, Krimighna, Hattavilasini, Nisakhya.

Gana :

Charaka : Kushtaghna, Kandughna, Lekhaniya, Vishaghna.
Sushruta : Haridradi, Mustadi, Sleshma samshamana.

Properties : Rasa - Katu, Tikta; Guna - Ruksha, Laghu; Virya - Ushna and Vipaka - Katu.

Pharmacological Actions : Kaphavatahara, Varnya, Lekhana, Vishaghna.

Indications : Kushta, Kandu, Krimi, Prameha, Peenasa, Aruchi, Vrana, Kamala, Pandu, Shotha.

Therapeutic Uses :

1. Prameha : Haridra powder mixed with honey should be taken with the juice of amalaka. (C.S., S.S., A.S., A.H.)
2. Scabies and eczema : Cow's urine 80 ml. mixed with paste of haridra should be taken. (V.M.)

Parts Used : Tuberous root.

Preparations & Dosage : Juice 10-20 ml.; Powder 1-3 gm.

Specific Formulations : Haridra khanda, Vranasodhana taila.

हरिद्रा काञ्चनी पीता निशाऽऽख्या वरवर्णिनी ।
कृमिघ्नी हलदी योषित्प्रिया हट्टविलासिनी ॥
हरिद्रा कटुका तिक्ता रूक्षोष्णा कफपित्तनुत् ।
वर्ण्या त्वग्दोषमेहास्रशोथपाण्डुव्रणापहा ॥ भा०प्र०

Research Studies: A volatile oil isolated from the fresh rhizomes of C. longa was found to possess marked anti-inflammatory activity against histamine, eggalbumin, carrageenin induced hind paw oedema in rats. It also manifested anti-arthritic activity against formaline as well as freund's adjuvant induced arthritis in rats. (Annual report CCRIMH 1969-71)

113
ĀRDRAKA

Zingiber officinale Rose. Family : Zingiberaceae

Chief Characters :

1. Perennial herb grows upto 1 m. height.
2. Simple leaf occur on leafy stem.
3. Greenish yellow and one petal is red colour.

Synonyms : Ardrika, Shrungavera, Katubhadra.

Gana :

Charaka : Triptighna, Arshoghna, Deepaniya, Shoolaprashamana, Trishna nigrahana.
Sushruta : Pippalyadi, Trikatu.

Properties : Rasa - Katu; Guna - Guru, Ruksha, Tikshna; Virya - Ushna and Vipaka - Madhura.

Pharmacological Actions : Vatakaphahara, Deepana, Bhedana.

Indications : Anaha, Shoola, Udara, Chardi, Arshas, Kasa, Shosha, Sleepada, Hridroga, Shwasa.

Therapeutic Uses :

1. Udara roga : Intake of juice of ardraka mixed with equal quantity of milk is wholesome or oil cooked with ten times the same juice is useful. (C.S.)
2. Bronchial asthma and cough : Ardraka juice mixed with honey should be taken in case of cough, bronchial asthma, coryza and fever caused by kapha. (H.S.)

Parts Used : Rhizome.

Preparations & Dosage : Juice 5-10 ml.; Shunthi powder 1-2 gm.

Specific Formulations : Ardrakhandavalehya, Ardraka rasayana, Soubhagya shunthi, Nagaradi kwatha, Shunthyadi churna.

आर्द्रकं शृङ्गवेरं स्यात्कटुभद्रं तथाऽऽर्द्रिका ।
आर्द्रिका भेदिनी गुर्वी तीक्ष्णोष्णा दीपनी मता ॥
कटुका मधुरा पाके रूक्षा वातकफापहा ।
ये गुणाः कथिताः शुण्ठ्यास्तेऽपि सन्त्यार्द्रकेऽखिलाः ॥
भोजनाग्रे सदा पथ्यं लवणार्द्रकभक्षणम् ।

अग्निसन्दीपनं रुच्यं जिह्वाकण्ठविशोधनम् ।।
कुष्ठपाण्ड्वामये कृच्छ्रे रक्तपित्ते व्रणे ज्वरे ।
दाहे निदाघशरदोर्नैव पूजितमार्द्रकम् ।। भा०प्र०

Research Studies: Recently a preliminary study of the hypoglycaemic action of ginger juice conducted in diabetic and non-diabetic rats and rabbits showed a significant hypoglycaemic response in diabetic animals. (Sharma and Shukla 1977, JRIMYH 12(2) : 127)

Traditional uses, chemical constituents, anti emetics, antinauseatic, antiulcer, antiplatelet, antiinflammatory, anti-pyretic, cardiovascular, antiinfective, antioxidant and other activities of ginger have been reviewed. (British journal of phytotherapy V 4 (3) : p. 110-120, 1997)

114
ELĀ

Elattaria cardamomum Maton. Family : Zingiberaceae

Chief Characters :

1. Perennial shrub grows upto 3 m. height.
2. Long leaves with acute tip.
3. Pale voilet coloured flowers.
4. Panicle inflorescence.
5. Fruit - capsule.

Synonyms : Sukshma—Upakunchika, Dravidi, Korangi, Thutha, Truti. Brihat—Sthula, Bahula, Prithvika, Bhadrasha, Chandrabala, Nishkuti, Triputa.

Gana :

Charaka : Shwasahara, Angamarda prashamana, Katuka skandha.

Sushruta : Eladi, Pippalyadi.

Vagbhata : Trijataka, Chaturjataka

Properties : Rasa - Katu, Madhura; Guna - Laghu, Ruksha; Virya - Sheeta (Sukshma), Ushna (Brihat) and Vipaka - Katu.

Pharmacological Actions : Kaphavatahara, Hridya, Deepana, Rochana, Shukranashaka.

Indications : Mutrakriccha, Vastishoola, Shwasa, Kasa, Trishna, Kandu, Arshas, Chardi, Hridroga, Sirashoola.

Therapeutic Uses :

1. Dysuria : One should take only cardamom with juice of amalaka fruits. (S.S.)
2. Hridroga : Ela and pippalimula taken with ghee alleviates heart diseases and gulma. (B.S.)
3. Timira : Powdered ela should be dipped in goat's urine for three days and then used as powder-colyrium. It is useful in krimi, timira and pitta. (C.S.)

Parts Used : Seed.

Preparations & Dosage : Powder ½ -1 gm.

Specific Formulations : Eladi chruna, Eladyarishta, Eladi kwatha, Eladi gutika, Eladi modaka.

Amomum subulatum Roxb. is considered as the source plant of brihat ela.

सूक्ष्मोपकुञ्चिका तुत्था कोरङ्गी द्राविडी त्रुटिः ।
एला सूक्ष्मा कफश्वासकासार्शोमूत्रकृच्छ्रहृत् ।
रसे तु कटुका शीता लघ्वी वातहरी मता ॥
एला स्थूला च बहुला पृथ्वीका त्रिपुटाऽपि च ॥
भद्रैला बृहदेला च चन्द्रबाला च निष्कुटिः ।
स्थूलैला कटुका पाके रसे चानलकृल्लघुः ॥
रूक्षोष्णा श्लेष्मपित्तास्रकण्डूश्वासतृषाऽपहा ।
हृल्लासविषवस्त्यास्यशिरोरुग्वमिकासनुत् ॥ भा०प्र०

115
RASONA

Allium sativum Linn. Family : Liliaceae

Chief Characters :

1. Annual shrub.
2. Adventitious roots arise from the lower part of the stem.
3. Consists of fleshy leaf bases (cloves).
4. White coloured flowers.
5. Umbel inflorescence.
6. Fruit - capsule.

Synonyms : Ugragandha, Yavaneshta, Mahoushadha, Lashuna, Arishta, Mlechchakanda, Rasonaka.

Properties : Rasa - Madhura, Lavana, Katu, Tikta, Kashaya; Guna - Snigdha, Guru, Tikshna, Sara; Virya - Ushna and Vipaka - Katu.

Pharmacological Actions : Vatakaphahara, Vrishya, Brimhana, Balya, Varnya, Kanthya, Medhya, Netrya, Hridya, Rasayana.

Indications : Ajeerna, Gulma, Shoola, Vibhandha, Shwasa, Agnimandhya, Bhagna, Kasa, Krimi, Shopha, Rajayakshma, Hridroga, Aruchi, Kushta, Asthibhagna, Kukshishoola, Arshas.

Therapeutic Uses :

1. Vishamajwara : Rasona mixed with ghee should be taken every morning. (S.S.)
2. Wasting : One should use rasona with milk. (S.S.)
3. Wound : Paste of rasona applied to wound kills organism. (V.M.)

Parts Used : Oil, Tuber.

Preparations & Dosage : Paste 3-6 gm., Oil 1-2 drops.

Specific Formulations : Lashunadi vati, Rasonapinda, Hingu triguna taila.

लशुनस्तु रसोनः स्यादुग्रगन्धो महौषधम् ।
अरिष्टो म्लेच्छकन्दश्च यवनेष्टो रसोनकः ॥
यदाऽमृतं वैनतेयो जहार सुरसत्तमान् ।

तदा ततोऽपतद् बिन्दुः स रसोनोऽभवद् भुवि ॥
पञ्चभिश्च रसैर्युक्तो रसेनाम्लेन वर्जितः ।
तस्माद्रसोन इत्युक्तो द्रव्याणां गुणवेदिभिः ॥
कटुकश्चापि मूलेषु तिक्तः पत्रेषु संस्थितः ।
नाले कषाय उद्दिष्टो नालाग्रे लवणः स्मृतः ।
बीजे तु मधुरः प्रोक्तो रसस्तद्गुणवेदिभिः ॥
रसोनो बृंहणो वृष्यः स्निग्धोष्णः पाचनः सरः ।
रसे पाके च कटुकस्तीक्ष्णो मधुरको मतः ॥
भग्नसन्धानकृत्कण्ठ्यो गुरुः पित्तास्रवृद्धिदः ।
बलवर्णकरो मेधाहितो नेत्र्यो रसायनः ॥
हृद्रोगजीर्णज्वरकुक्षिशूलविबन्धगुल्मारुचिकासशोफान् ।
दुर्नामकुष्ठानलसादजन्तुसमीरणश्वासकफांश्च हन्ति ॥
मद्यं मांसं तथाऽम्लञ्च हितं लशुनसेविनाम् ।
व्यायाममातपं रोषमतिनीरं पयो गुडम् ।
रसोनमश्नन् पुरुषस्त्यजेदेतान् निरन्तरम् ॥ भा०प्र०

Research Studies: Allium sativum and A. ascalonicum have shown significant anti-coagulant and fibrinolytic activities by virtue of increasing whole blood coagulation time, prothrombine time and fibrinolytic activity. In addition to it, allium ascalonicum also possess significant hypocholestrolemic property. (JRIM Vol. IX, No. 4)

116
KUMĀRĪ

Aloe barbadensis Mill. Family : Agavaceae

Chief Characters :

1. Perennial shrub.
2. Ensiform leaves, leaves are fleshy with a ghee like mucous substance.
3. Yellowish pink flowers.
4. Fruit - loculicidal capsule.

Synonyms : Ghritakumari, Sthuladala, Vipulasrava, Gruhakanya, Kanya.

Gana :

Guduchyadi. (B.P.)

Properties : Rasa - Tikta, Madhura; Guna - Guru, Snigdha, Picchila; Virya - Sheeta and Vipaka - Katu.

Pharmacological Actions : Kaphavatahara, Bhedana, Rasayana, Brimhana, Balya, Vrishya, Chakshusya.

Indications : Yakrita vriddhi, Pleeha vriddhi, Gulma, Shoola, Vibandha, Kushta, Granthi, Agnidagdha vrana.

Therapeutic Uses :

1. Spleenomegaly : The juice of kumari mixed with haridra powder alleviates splenomegaly and scrofula. (S.G.)
2. Dysuria : If there is dysuria during fever, one should take the juice of kumari. (V.D.)
3. Mastitis : Kumari root mixed with haridra is applied as paste on breast to relieve pain. (B.P.)

Parts Used : Leaf, Root.

Preparations & Dosage : Juice 10-20 ml.

Specific Formulations : Kumaryasava, Rajah pravartini vati, Kumarika vati, Kumari paka.

कुमारी गृहकन्या च कन्या घृतकुमारिका ।
कुमारी भेदिनी शीता तिक्ता नेत्र्या रसायनी ॥
मधुरा बृंहणी बल्या वृष्या वातविषप्रणुत् ।

गुल्मप्लीहयकृद्वृद्धिकफज्वरहरी हरेत् ।
ग्रन्थ्यग्निदग्धविस्फोटपित्तरक्तत्वगामयान् ॥ भा०प्र०

Research Studies: Petroleum ether extract of Aloe vera is found to be effective against gastric ulceration in laboratory animals. Methanol extract of the same plant showed local anasthetic activity. (Annual report, 1972-73, CCRIM & H) Gastric acid secretion inhibitory and gastric lesion protective effects of Aloe preparation. (Thai Journal of Phyto Pharmacy V. 4 (1) ; p. 1-11, 1997)

117
ŚATĀVARĪ

Asparagus racemosus Willd. Family : Asparagaceae

Chief Characters :

1. Perennial shrub consisting of thorns.
2. Consists of groups of adventitious. roots.
3. Leaves are modified into cladodes.
4. White coloured flowers.
5. Racemose inflorescence.
6. Fruit - berry.

Synonyms : Indeevari, Sukshmapatra, Bahusuta, Shatamooli, Sheeta narayani, Bhiru, Virya, Madabhanjani, Peevari, Shatavirya, Shatpadi.

Gana :

Charaka : Balya, Vayah-sthapana, Madhura skandha.
Sushruta : Vidarigandhadi, Pitta prashamana, Kantaka panchamoola.

Properties : Rasa - Madhura, Tikta; Guna - Guru, Snigdha; Virya - Sheeta and Vipaka - Madhura.

Pharmacological Actions : Vatapittahara, Vrishya, Rasayana, Hridya, Shukrala, Netrya, Balya.

Indications : Atisara, Arshas, Grahini, Gulma, Kshaya, Prameha, Raktapitta, Shotha.

Therapeutic Uses :

1. Raktapitta : Milk processed with shatavari and gokshura checks haemorrhage particularly of urinary tract. (C.S.)
2. Dysuria : Powder of shatavari should be taken with cold water. (H.S.)
3. Shoola : Shatavari juice mixed with honey should be taken in morning. It alleviates burning, pain and all disorders of pitta. (V.M., S.G., B.S.)

Parts Used : Root (Tuber).

Preparations & Dosage : Juice 10-20 ml.; Decoction 50-100 ml.; Powder 3-6 gm.

Specific Formulations : Shatavari mandoora, Narayana taila.

शतावरी बहुसुता भीरुरिन्दीवरी वरी ।
नारायणी शतपदी शतवीर्या च पीवरी ॥
महाशतावरी चान्या शतमूल्यूर्ध्वकण्ठिका ।
सहस्रवीर्या हेतुश्च ऋष्यप्रोक्ता महोदरी ॥
शतावरी गुरुः शीता तिक्ता स्वाद्वी रसायनी ।
मेधाग्निपुष्टिदा स्निग्धा नेत्र्या गुल्मातिसारजित् ॥
शुक्रस्तन्यकरी बल्या वातपित्तास्रशोथजित् ।
महाशतावरी मेध्या हृद्या वृष्या रसायनी ॥
शीतवीर्या निहन्त्यर्शोग्रहणा नयनामयान् ।
तदङ्कुरस्त्रिदोषघ्नी लघुरर्शःक्षयापहा ॥ भा०प्र०

Research Studies: Alcoholic extract of Asparagus racemosus and A_2 fraction of this extract showed significant anti-oxytoxic activity. (Annual report, CCRIMH 1974-75)

The crude alcoholic and water-alcoholic (1:1) extracts of the root of Asparagus racemosus were studied for pharmacological effect. The drug caused hypotension both in normal as well as spinal cat under different conditions. Action was antagonized by atropine sulphate indicating cholinergic like effect. Inhibitory effect on the growth of E.histolytica in vitro and encouraging result in intestinal amoebiosis in rats was also noticed. Light hypoglycaemic effect in rabbit was also noticed when given orally and intravenously. (JRIM. Vol. VI, No.2, 1971)

118
VACĀ

Acorus calamus Linn. Family : Araceae

Chief Characters :

1. Perennial shrub.
2. Ensiform leaves.
3. Green coloured flowers.
4. Spadix inflorescence.
5. Fruit - berry.

Synonyms : Shadgrantha, Golomi, Ugragandha, Satparvika, Mangalya, Kshudrapatri, Jatila, Ugra, Lonasha.

Gana :

Charaka : Lekhaniya, Arshoghna, Truptighna, Samjnasthapana, Sheetaprashamana.
Sushruta : Pippalyadi, Vachadi, Mustadi.

Properties : Rasa - Katu, Tikta; Guna - Laghu, Tikshna; Virya - Ushna and Vipaka - Katu.

Pharmacological Actions : Kaphavatahara, Medhya, Lekhaniya, Sakrut-mutra vishdhana, Vamaka, Deepana.

Indications : Apasmara, Unmada, Jwara, Shoola, Krimi, Vibandha, Adhmana.

Therapeutic Uses :

1. Epilepsy : By using vacha powder with honey keeping on diet of milk and rice overcomes epilepsy, even if chronic and severe. (S.B., V.M., B.S.)
2. Amlapitta : One should take vacha mixed with honey and jaggery. (G.N.)

Parts Used : Root, Rhizome.

Preparations & Dosage : Powder 125-500 mg.

Specific Formulations : Vachadi ghrita, Vachadi churna, Saraswata churna, Medhya rasayana.

वचोग्रगन्धा षड्ग्रन्था गोलोमी शतपर्विका ।
क्षुद्रपत्री च मङ्गल्या जटिलोग्रा च लोमशा ॥
वचोग्रगन्धा कटुका तिक्तोष्णा वान्तिवह्निकृत्

विबन्धाध्मानशूलघ्नी शकृन्मूत्रविशोधिनी ।
अपस्मारकफोन्मादभूतजन्त्वनिलान् हरेत् ॥ भा०प्र०

Research Studies: The chloroform extract factor was studied for its effect on behavioural changes in conscious rats, rabbits, mice and monkeys. It was observed that the compound possessed dose dependant calming effect on all these animal species. It also offered protection against terecan, escamine, harmine, amphetamine and cardiozol induced restlessness, increased locomotory activity and convulsions (Annual report CCRIMH, 1975-76)

The extract was found to supress the primary as well as secondary phase of inflammation significantly. It was also found as potent analgesic at a dose of 5mg/1kg. (Annual report CCRIMH, 1977-78)

119
MUSTĀ

Cyperus rotundus Linn. Family : Cyperaceae

Chief Characters :

1. Perennial shrub.
2. Consists of stolons which store food material.
3. Leaves - narrow with acute tip.
4. Red coloured spikelets.
5. Fruit - nutlets.

Synonyms : Varida, Kodsesta, Hima, Sugandhi, Mushtaka, Kuruvinda (Musta)
Nagaramustaka-krodakaseruka, Bhadramusta, Gundra.

Gana :

Charaka : Lekhaniya, Trishnanigrahana, Kandughna, Stanyasodhana.
Sushruta : Mustadi, Vachadi.

Properties : Rasa - Tikta, Katu, Kashaya; Guṇa - Laghu, Ruksha; Virya - Sheeta and Vipaka - Katu.

Pharmacological Actions : Kaphapittahara, Deepana, Pachana, Grahi, Lekhana, Stanyasodhana.

Indications : Jwara, Trishna, Atisara, Krimi, Aruchi.

Therapeutic Uses :

1. Diarrhoea : Musta rhizomes twenty should be boiled in milk with three times water reduced to milk. Its intake checks mucous and pain. (S.S.)
2. Cough : Sharkaradi formulation should be given mixed with musta and marica in cough caused by pitta associated with kapha. (C.S.)

Parts Used : Rhizome.

Preparations & Dosage : Powder 3-6 gm.; Decoction 50-100 ml.

Specific Formulations : Shadanga paneeya, Gangadhara churna, Mustakadi churna, Mustakarishta.

मुस्तकं न स्त्रियां मुस्तं त्रिषु वारिदनामकम् ।
कुरुविन्दश्च संख्यातोऽपरः क्रोडकसेरुकः ॥

भद्रमुस्तञ्च गुन्द्रा च तथा नागरमुस्तकः ।
मुस्तं कटु हिमं ग्राहि तिक्तं दीपनपाचनम् ॥
कषायं कफपित्तास्रतृड्ज्वरारुचिजन्तुहृत् ।
अनूपदेशे यज्जातं मुस्तकं तत्प्रशस्यते ।
तत्रापि मुनिभिः प्रोक्तं वरं नागरमुस्तकम् ॥ भा०प्र०

Research Studies: Alcoholic extract of Cyperus rotundus was tested in doses of 0.5, 1.0 and 1.5 gm/kg orally for diuretic effect in rats and it was observed that the extract showed biphasic effect on urine flow. In doses of 0.5 and 1.0 gm/kg. of the urine flow was increased but with a dose of 1.5 gm/kg, it was reduced. Against castor oil induced diarrhoea, the alcoholic extract in doses of 0.5 & 1.0 gm/kg given orally showed protective effect at one hour after drug administration. (Annual report CCRAS, 1978-79)

120
UŚĪRA

Vetiveria zizanioides Linn. Family : Poaceae

Chief Characters :

1. Perennial herb grows upto 2 m. height.
2. Cauline leaves 1-2 ft. length occur in two rows.
3. Each flower is a spike, panicle inflorescence.
4. Consists of yellowish red coloured flowers.

Synonyms : Sevya, Nalada, Mrunala, Veerana, Abhaya, Jalavasa, Amrinala, Samagandhika.

Gana :

Charaka : Daha prashamana, Stanyajanana, Chardi nigrahana, Shukra shodhana.

Sushruta : Eladi, Sarivadi, Pitta samshamana.

Properties : Rasa - Tikta, Madhura; Guna - Ruksha, Laghu; Virya - Sheeta and Vipaka - Katu.

Pharmacological Actions : Kaphapittahara, Pachana, Stambhana.

Indications : Jwara, Trishna, Daha, Raktapitta, Chardi, Visarpa, Shosha, Vrana, Mutrakriccha.

Therapeutic Uses :

1. Raktapitta : Ushira and candana mixed in equal quantity along with sugar and rice water alleviates intrinsic haemorrhage. (C.S.)
2. Boils : External application of ushira relieves boils caused by excessive perspiration. (V.M.)

Parts Used : Root.

Preparations & Dosage : Powder 3-6 gm.; Hot infusion 50-100 ml.; Cold infusion 25-50 ml.

Specific Formulations : Usheerasava, Usheeradi churna, Usheeradi kwatha, Shadanga paneeya, Usheeradi taila.

वीरणस्य तु मूलं स्यादुशीरं नलदञ्च तत् ।
अमृणालञ्च सेव्यञ्च समगन्धिकमित्यपि ॥
उशीरं पाचनं शीतं स्तम्भनं लघु तिक्तकम् ॥
मधुरं ज्वरहृद्वान्तिमदनुत्कफपित्तहृत् ।
तृष्णाऽस्रविषवीसर्पदाहकृच्छ्रव्रणापहम् ॥ भा०प्र०

121
PIPPALĪMŪLA

Piper longum Linn. Family : Piperaceae

Chief Characters :

1. Perinneal herb growing upto 1 mt.
2. The leaves are alternate, spreading and without stipules.
3. The flowers are in solitary spikes.
4. Green coloured flowers on different branches.
5. Fruit - berry.

Synonyms : Pippali Magadhi, Krishna, Vaidehi, Chapala, Upakulya, Kana, Shyama, Kola, Shoundi etc.

Gana :

Charaka : Deepaniya.
Sushruta : Pippalyadi.

Properties : Rasa - Katu; Guna - Laghu, Snigdha; Virya - Ushna and Vipaka - Madhura.

Pharmacological Actions : Vatakaphahara.

Indications : Arshas, Kasa, Shwasa, Jirna jwara, Gulma, Udara, Amavata.

Therapeutic Uses :

1. The powder of pippalimoola given with honey after delivary to sootika prevents deposition of fat in the abdominal area. (B.P.)
2. Insomnia : The powder taken with honey relieves insomnia. (B.R.)

Parts Used : Root.

Preparations & Dosage : Powder 1-3 gm.

Specific Formulation : Panchakola churna.

ग्रन्थिकं पिप्पलीमूलमूषणं चटकाशिर: ।
दीपनं पिप्पलीमूलं कटूष्णं पाचनं लघु ॥
रूक्षं पित्तकरं भेदि कफवातोदरापहम् ।
आनाहप्लीहगुल्मघ्नं कृमिश्वासक्षयापहम् ॥ भा०प्र०

122
PALĀṆḌU

Allium cepa Linn. Family : Liliaceae

Chief Characters :

1. Annual bulb globular.
2. Leaves in two rows.
3. Inflorescence - umbel globular, many flowered.
4. Flowers white/lilac in colour.
5. Fruit capsule and contains black coloured seeds.

Synonyms : Yavaneshta, Mukhadushaka.

Properties : Rasa - Madhura, Katu; Guna - Guru, Snigdha; Virya - Anushna and Vipaka - Madhura.

Pharmacological Actions : Vatahara, Kaphakara, Balya, Vrishya.

Indications : Prameha, Raktarshas, Raktapitta.

Parts Used : Bulb, Seed.

Preparations & Dosage : Fresh juice 10-20 ml.

पलाण्डुर्यवनेष्टश्च दुर्गन्धो मुखदूषकः ।
पलाण्डुस्तु बुधैर्ज्ञेयो रसोनसदृशो गुणैः ॥
स्वादःपाके रसेऽनुष्णः कफकृन्नातिपित्तला ।
हरते केवलं वातं बलवीर्यकरो गुरुः ॥ भा०प्र०

SECOND PAPER

Part - A

General Introduction of 246 Dravyas

1
MAMĪRĀ

Thalictrum foliolosum D.C. Family : Ranunculaceae

Chief Characters :

1. Perinneal herb.
2. Compound leaf.
3. Green or violet coloured flowers, panicle inflorescence.
5. Fruit is achene.

Synonyms : Tiktamoola.

Properties : Rasa - Tikta; Guna - Ruksha; Virya - Ushna and Vipaka - Katu.

Pharmacological Actions : Kaphapittahara, Deepana, Pachana, Chakshushya. (B.P.)

Indications : Yakrit roga, Vishama jwara, Netraroga, Kushta, Prameha, Mutrakriccha, Kasa, Shwasa.

Therapeutic Uses :

1. Conjunctivitis : Collyrium prepared from it should be applied or eyedrops prepared from it can be used.
2. Leucoderma : Its paste can be used as anointment in leucoderma and kshudra rogas.

Parts Used : Root.

Preparations & Dosage : Powder 1-3 gm.

Coptis teeta wall. (Ranunculaceae) is considered as china Mamira and rhizome of this plant is being prescribed in the condition like Madhumeha, Vishama jwara and netra roga.

Thalietrum foliolosum is considered as one of the sources of trayamana.

ममीरा तिक्तमूला स्यात् कामरूपसमुद्भवा ।
स्निग्धखण्डितपत्रा च सितपुष्पाऽतितिक्तका ॥
तिक्तमूला कटुस्तिक्ता रूक्षोष्णा दीपनी सरा ।
चक्षुष्या पाचनी रुच्या कफपित्तहरा मता ॥
यकृदुत्तेजनी चैव विषमज्वरनाशिनी ।
नेत्रामये यकृद्रोगे कुष्ठे शोथे कफामये ॥
कासे श्वासे तथा मूत्रकृच्छ्रे मेहे च पूयजे ।
ज्वरौत्तरिकदौर्बल्ये ज्वरे चापि प्रशस्यते ॥ द्र०गु०वि०

2
NIRVIṢĀ

Delphinium denudatum **Wall.** Family : Ranunculaceae

Chief Characters :

1. It is an annual plant.
2. Radical and cauline leaves.
3. Blue coloured flowers, racemose inflorescence.
4. Fruit - follicle.

Properties : Rasa - Katu, Tikta; Guna - Laghu, Ruksha; Virya - Ushna and Vipaka - Katu.

Pharmacological Actions : Kaphavatahara, Vranaropana, Vishaghna.

Indications : Agnimandya, Pakshagata, Kushta, Kasa, Shwasa, Pratishyaya, Udara.

Therapeutic Uses :

Used as antidote for snake and acotine poisoning.

Parts Used : Root.

Preparations & Dosage : Powder ½ - 1 gm.

निर्विषा कटुका सोष्णा कफवातास्रदोषनुत् ।
अनेकविषदोषघ्नी व्रणसंरोपणी च सा ॥ रा०नि०

3
UPAKUÑCIKĀ

Nigella sativa Linn. Family : Ranunculaceae

Chief Characters :

1. Herb grows upto 60 cm.
2. Leaves are disected at the tip into 3 parts.
3. Light blue coloured flowers, bisexual flowers.
4. Fruit - follicle.

Synonyms : Kunchika, Upakunchi, Kalika, Prithu, Prithvika, Sthulajeeraka, Kalajaji.

Properties : Rasa - Katu, Tikta; Guna - Laghu, Ruksha; Virya - Ushna and Vipaka - Katu.

Pharmacological Actions : Kaphavata shamaka, Deepana, Pachana, Grahi, Chakshushya, Atisara, Adhmana, Gulma, Chardi, Agnimandya.

Indications : Vishamajwara, Adhmana, Gulma, Chardi, Atisara, Udgara.

Therapeutic Uses :

1. Dhumagandhi udgara : The powdered seed (3gm.) mixed with sugar relieves belching (Vrinda).
2. Irregular fever : Kalajaji taken with jaggery controls irregular fever. (B.P.)
3. Coryza : The powder of upakunchika should be inhaled. (C.S.)
4. For expelling placenta : The paste of ela, devadaru etc. containing upakunchika is administered for expulsion of placenta. (C.S.)

Parts Used : Seed.

Preparations & Dosage : Powder 1-3 gm.

जीरकत्रितयं रूक्षं कटूष्णं दीपनं लघु ।
सङ्ग्राहि पित्तलं मेध्यं गर्भाशयविशुद्धिकृत् ॥
ज्वरघ्नं पाचनं वृष्यं बल्यं रुच्यं कफापहम् ।
चक्षुष्यं पवनाध्मानगुल्मच्छर्द्यतिसारहृत् ॥ भा०प्र०

4
KĀNDĪRA

Ranunculus sceleratus Linn. Family : Ranunculaceae

Chief Characters :

1. Annual herb grows upto 1 m. height.
2. Simple leaf.
3. White coloured flowers, panicle inflorescence.
4. Fruit - achene.

Synonyms : Nasa samvedhana, Toyavalli, Kandekatuka, Sukandaka.

Properties : Rasa - Katu, Tikta; Guna - Tikshna, Ruksha; Virya - Ushna and Vipaka - Katu.

Pharmacological Actions : Kaphavatahara, Deepana, Pachana, Sara, Bhedana.

Indications : Gulma, Udara, Shoola, Agnimandya, Dushtavrana.

Therapeutic Uses :

1. Plague : Pills made of kandeera should be given.
2. Impotence : It is used as anointment.

Parts Used : Whole plant.

Preparations & Dosage : Powder 1-3 gm.

काण्डीरः काण्डकटुको नासासंवेदनः पटुः ।
उग्रकाण्डस्तोयवल्ली कारवल्लीसुकाण्डकः ॥
काण्डीरः कटुतिक्तोष्णः सरो दुष्टव्रणार्त्तिजित् ।
लतागुल्मोदरप्लीहशूलमन्दाग्निनाशनः ॥ ध०नि०

5
CAVYA

Piper chaba Linn. Family : Piperaceae

Chief Characters :

1. A climber with aerial roots.
2. Stem consists of approximately 20 ridges.
3. Simple leaf, round or elliptical in shape with acute tip.
4. Green coloured flowers.
5. Fruit - 1 to 2 inches in length, with red in colour.

Synonyms : Chavika, Ushana.

Gana :

Charaka : Triptighna, Deepaniya, Arshoghna.
Sushruta : Pippalyadi.

Properties : Rasa - Katu; Guna - Laghu, Ruksha; Virya - Ushna and Vipaka - Madhura.

Pharmacological Actions : Kaphavatahara, Pittakara, Bhedi, Pachana.

Indications : Udara, Anaha, Gulma, Krimi, Pleeha, Shwasa, Kshaya, Arsas.

Therapeutic Uses :

1. Diarrhoea : Tender leaves of cavika, shwetamula and kshirivriksha should be pounded and given with oil. (V.D.)
2. Udararoga : The paste of cavya and shunthi with milk should be administered internally. (S.S.)

Parts Used : Root, Fruit.

Preparations & Dosage : Powder 1-2 gm.

Specific Formulations : Panchakola phanta, Pranada gutika, Kankayan modaka, Chavyadi ghrita.

भवेच्चव्यं तु चविका कथिता सा तथोषणा ।
कणामूलगुणं चव्यं विशेषाद् गुदजापहम् ॥ भा०प्र०

6

CAMPAKA

Michelia champaka Family : Magnoliaceae

Chief Characters :

1. Tree.
2. Simple leaf.
3. Light yellow coloured flowers.
5. Fruit - silique.

Synonyms : Champeya, Hemapushpa, Gandhaphali.

Properties : Rasa - Katu, Tikta, Kashaya, Madhura; Guna - Laghu, Ruksha; Virya - Sheeta and Vipaka - Katu.

Pharmacological Actions : Kaphavatahara, Vishahara, Dahaprashamana.

Indications : Krimi, Mutrakricchra, Raktapitta, Kandu, Kushta, Visha.

Therapeutic Uses :

1. Incontinence of urine : Decoction of the root of champaka checks incontinence of urine. (V.D.)
2. Foul smell in vagina : Ghee mixed with tender leaves of campaka, flowers of jati and madhuka and heated in the sun is applied into the vagina. It removes foul smell. (G.N.)

Parts Used : Bark, Flower.

Preparations & Dosage : Bark decoction 50-100 ml., Powder 3-6 gm.

चम्पकः कटुकस्तिक्तः कषायो मधुरो हिमः ।
विषक्रिमिहरः कृच्छ्रकफवातास्रा पित्तजित् ॥ भा०प्र०

7
SĪTĀPHALA

Annona squamosa Family : Annonaceae

Chief Characters :

1. Tree.
2. Simple leaves, alternate phyllotaxy.
3. Green coloured flowers.
4. Fruit - Compound

Synonyms : Gandhagatra, Krishnabheeja.

Properties : Rasa - Madhura; Guna - Guru; Virya - Sheeta and Vipaka - Madhura.

Pharmacological Actions : Vatapittahara, Balya, Brimhana, Rechana (Root), Garbhapataka (Seed).

Indications : Daha, Raktapitta, Vidradhi, Krimi (Uka - LIksha).

Therapeutic Uses :

1. Seed and leaf of sitaphala is used as an external application to kill the lice.
2. Fever with rigor : Intake of 3½ leaves of sitaphala with salt checks fever with rigor. (S.B.)
3. Diabetes : In recent researches the leaf decoction exhibited hypoglycaemic action.

Parts Used : Root, Leaf, Seed, Fruit.

Preparations & Dosage : Decoction 40-60 ml.; Powder 1-3 gm.

The alcoholic extract of the aerial part of A. squamosa was found to have anti-cancer activity against human epidermal carcinoma of the nasopharynx in tissue culture (Bhakuni et al. 1969).

बलासवीर्यपात्राणि दात्राणि दवसम्पदाम् ।
प्रायशः स्वादुमात्राणि गण्डमात्राणि मन्महे ।। सि०भे०म०

8

KĀṢṬHADĀRU

Polyalthia longifolia Benth. Family : Anonaceae

Chief Characters :

1. Tree grows upto 20 m. height.
2. Simple leaf.
3. Light yellow coloured flowers.
4. Umbel inflorescence.
5. Fruit - Berries are fused to form fruit.

Synonyms : Devadari.

Properties : Rasa - Tikta, Katu; Guna - Laghu, Ruksha; Virya - Ushna and Vipaka - Katu.

Pharmacological Actions : Kaphapittahara, Deepana.

Indications : Jwara, Krimi, Kushta, Prameha.

Therapeutic Uses :

The decoction of the bark is used as a substitute for ashoka to checks menorrhagia and metrorrhagia.

Parts Used : Bark.

Preparations & Dosage : 50-100 ml.

काष्ठदारुः लघु रूक्षस्तिक्तः सकटुकोऽहिमः ।
दीपनः कृमिहृन् मेहे ज्वरे कुष्ठे च शस्यते ॥ द्र०गु०वि०

9
PĀTĀLAGARUḌĪ

Cocculus hirsutus Linn. Family : Menispermaceae

Chief Characters :

1. It is a perennial climber.
2. Panicle inflorescence.
3. Simple leaf, alternate phyllotaxy.
4. Consists of green coloured flowers.

Synonyms : Mahamoola, Chilahinta.

Properties : Rasa - Tikta; Guna - Laghu, Picchila; Virya - Ushna and Vipaka - Katu.

Pharmacological Actions : Kaphavatahara, Vrishya.

Indications : Agnimandya, Kustha, Mutrakricchra, Shukra dourbalya.

Therapeutic Uses :

1. Snake poisoning : The root of garudi is rubbed and applied as snuff, collyrium, paste and administered internally. It counteracts the snake poison if cyanosis has not developed. (R.M., G.N.)
2. Guinea worm : It is also useful in guinea worm. (Y.R.)

Parts Used : Root, Leaf.

Preparations & Dosage : Juice 10-20 ml.

छिलहिण्टो महामूल: पातालगरुडाह्वय: ।
छिलहिण्ट: परं वृष्य: कफघ्न: पवनापह: ॥ भा०प्र०

10
GIRI PARPAṬA

Podophyllum hexandrum Family : Berberidaceae

Chief Characters :

1. Simple leaves, alternate phyllotaxy.
2. White flowers arranged in racemose inflorescence.
3. Fruit - berry, red in colour.

Synonyms : Vanavrintaka.

Properties : Rasa - Katu, Tikta; Guna - Laghu, Tikshna; Virya - Ushna and Vipaka - Katu.

Pharmacological Actions : Pittahara, Rechana.

Indications : Vibandha, Anaha, Kushta, Udara, Kamala.

Parts Used : Root, Gum.

Preparations & Dosage : Powder 125-250 mg.

11
KAMALA
(Sacred Lotus)

Nelumbo nucifera Gaertn. Family : Nelumbonaceae

Chief Characters :

1. Perennial herb, aquatic plant.
2. Simple leaf, floats on water. Petiole is attached to the centre of the leaf.
3. Rose coloured large flowers.
4. Dry dehiscent fruit. Seeds - ½ inch in length and blackish in colour.

Synonyms : Padma, Nalinda, Aravinda, Mahotpala, Sahasrapatra, Shatapatra, Kusheshaya, Rajeeva, Pushkara, Pankeruha, Sarasa, Ambhoruha, Sarasiruha, Bisaprasuna.

Gana :

Charaka : Mutravirajaneeya.
Sushruta : Utpaladigana, Pittasamshamana.

Properties : Rasa - Kashaya, Tikta, Madhura; Guna - Laghu, Snigdha, Picchila; Virya - Sheeta and Vipaka - Madhura.

Pharmacological Actions : Kaphapittahara, Varnya, Grahi, Garbha- sthapana, Mutra virajaneeya.

Indications : Daha, Trishna, Mutrakriccha, Arshas, Raktapitta, Vi-spota, Visarpa.

Therapeutic Uses :

1. Gudabhramsa : The intake of tender leaves pounded and mixed with sugar arrests the prolapse of rectum. (C.D.)
2. Garbhapata : The powder of tuber of blue variety kamala admnistered with sugar and honey prevents abortion. (Sodhala)
3. Krimidanta : The root of kamala chewed relieves krimidanta. (Rajmartanda)

Parts Used : Flower, Seed, Root.

Preparations & Dosage : Seed powder 3-6 gm.; Root juice 10-20 ml.

Specific Formulations : Aravindasava.

Acharya Chunekar opines that :

Pundarika	:	White variety kamalam
Kokanada	:	Red variety kamalam
Indivara	:	Blue variety kamalam
Kamala	:	Suryavikasi
Kumuda	:	Chandravikasi

कमलं शीतलं वर्ण्यं मधुरं कफपित्तजित् ।
तृष्णादाहास्रविस्फोटविषवीसर्पनाशनम् ॥
पद्मबीजं हिमं स्वादु कषायं तिक्तकं गुरु ।
विष्टम्भि वृष्यं रूक्षं च गर्भस्थापकं परम् ।
कफवातहरं बल्यं ग्राहि पित्तास्रदाहनुत् ॥ भा०प्र०

12

KUMUDA

(Water Lily)

Nymphaea stellata Willd. Family : Nymphaeaceae

Chief Characters :

1. Perennial acquatic plant.
2. Round simple leaves, float on water.
3. Blue, pink, white coloured flowers.
4. Fruit - berry.
5. Seeds mustard in shape and whitish or blackish in colour.

Synonyms : Shweta kuvalaya, Kairava, Utpala.

Gana :

Charaka : Purishavirajaneeya, Mutravirajaneeya, Dahaprashamana.
Sushruta : Utpaladi.

Properties : Rasa - Madhura, Kashaya, Tikta; Guna - Laghu, Snigdha, Picchila; Virya - Sheeta and Vipaka - Madhura.

Pharmacological Actions : Kaphapittahara, Grahi, Varnya, Vishahara, Medhya, Dahaprashamana, Mutravirajaneeya.

Indications : Trishna, Jwara, Raktapitta, Prameha, Daha, Visarpa, Vispota, Arshas.

Therapeutic Uses :

1. Raktapitta : Utpala kshara mixed with honey and ghee checks Raktapitta associated with kapha. (C.S.)
2. Palita : The milk mixed with flowers is kept underground for one month and applied to gray hair for blackness. (Vrinda)
3. Chaladanta : The intake of milk boiled with utpala nala makes the loose teeth strong. (S.S.)

Parts Used : Root, Flower, Seed.

Preparations & Dosage : Juice 10-20 ml.; Powder 3-6 gm.

Specific Formulations : Neelotpaladi hima, Sarbhat neelufusa.

श्वेतं कुवलयं प्रोक्तं कुमुदं कैरवं तथा ।
कुमुदं पिच्छिलं स्निग्धं मधुरं ह्लादि शीतलम् ॥ भा०प्र०

13
SATYĀNĀŚĪ

Argemone mexicana Family : Papaveraceae

Chief Characters :

1. Thorny annual shrub.
2. Leaves - simple with serrated margins.
3. Yellow coloured flowers.
4. Fruit - capsule.

Synonyms : Katuparni, Hemavati, Hemaksheeri, Hemahwa, Peeta-dugdha, Choka (name of the root), Swarnaksheeri.

Properties : Rasa - Tikta, Katu; Guna - Laghu, Ruksha; Virya - Sheeta and Vipaka - Katu.

Pharmacological Actions : Kaphapittahara, Rechana, Bhedana, Vishahara.

Indications : Krimi, Kandu, Kushta, Anaha.

Therapeutic Uses :

1. Skin disorders & wound : The juice (latex) or seed oil is used as anointment in the inflammation of eye and wounds.
2. The seed oil or root powder is useful in constipation and abdominal pain.
3. Worms : The root powder should be given in the dosage of 3-4 gm.

Parts Used : Root, Seed, Latex, oil.

Preparations & Dosage : Powder 1-3 gm.; Latex 5-10 drops; Oil 10-30 drops; Juice 5-10 ml.

हेमाह्वा रेचनी तिक्ता मेदन्युत्क्लेशकारिणी ।
कृमिकण्डूविषानाहकफपित्तास्रकुष्ठनुत् ॥ भा०प्र०

14
MAKHĀNNA

Euryale ferox Family : Nymphaeceae

Chief Characters :

1. Annual herb, aquatic.
2. Leaves - floating round shaped.
3. Flowers are greenish from outside and red coloured inside.
4. Fruit - berry.

Synonyms : Padmabeejabha, Paneeyaphala, Ankalodya.

Properties : Rasa - Madhura, Kashaya, Tikta; Guna - Guru, Ruksha (B.P.), Snigdha, Picchila (D.N., R.N.); Virya - Sheeta and Vipaka - Madhura.

Pharmacological Actions : Pittahara (D.N.), Kaphavatakara (B.P.), Vrishya, Garbhasthapaka, Grahi, Balya, Kaphavatahara (R.N.).

Indications : Daha, Raktapitta, Shukrameha, Raktavikara.

Parts Used : Fruit.

Preparations & Dosage : Powder 5-10 gm.

Specific Formulations : Paushtika churna.

मखान्नं स्निग्धवृष्यं च गर्भसंस्थापकं परम् ।
वातपित्तहरं बल्यं शीतं पित्तास्रदाहनुत् ॥ द्र०गु०वि०

15
PARPAṬAKA

Fumaria parviflora Lam. Family : Fumariaceae

Chief Characters :

1. It is perennial plant.
2. Leaf blade either linear or quadrangular.
3. White coloured flowers, racemose inflorescence.

Synonyms : Varatikta, Parpata, Pamshuparyaya, Kavachanamaka, Rehu, Sukshmapatra.

Gana :

Charak : Trishna nigrahana.

Properties : Rasa - Tikta; Guna - Laghu; Virya - Sheeta and Vipaka - Katu.

Pharmacological Actions : Pittakaphahara, Vatala, Grahi, Trishna nigrahana.

Indications : Jwara, Trishna, Bhrama, Daha, Raktapitta.

Therapeutic Uses :

1. The fine powder of musta and parpataka with honey is used in atisara. (C.S.)
2. Decoction of parpataka with honey relieves vomiting. (Vrinda)
3. Parpata alone or combined with guduchi and amalaki alleviates fever caused by pitta. (A.S., V.M., B.P.)

Parts Used : Whole plant.

Preparations & Dosage : Powder 3-6 gm.; Decoction 50-100 ml.

Specific Formulations : Parpatadyarista, Shadangapaneeya.

पर्पटो वरतिक्तश्च स्मृतः पर्पटकश्च सः ।
कथितः पांशुपर्यायस्तथा कवचनामकः ॥
पर्पटो हन्ति पित्तास्रभ्रमतृष्णाकफज्वरान् ।
संग्राही शीतलस्तिक्तो दाहनुद्वातलो लघुः ॥ भा०प्र०

16
SARṢAPA

Brassica campestris Family : Cruciferae

Chief Characters :

1. Annual plant.
2. Simple leaves, alternate phyllotaxy.
3. Yellow coloured flowers, recemose inflorescence.
4. Fruit - black or reddish black in colour.

Synonyms : Katuka, Sneha, Tantubha, Kadambaka, Siddhartha (White variety), Katusneha.

Gana :

Charaka : Kandughna, Asthapanopaga, Sirovirechaneeya.
Sushruta : Pippalyadi.

Properties : Rasa - Katu, Tikta; Guna - Laghu, Snigdha; Virya - Ushna and Vipaka - Katu.

Pharmacological Actions : Kaphavatahara, Deepana.

Indications : Kandu, Kushta, Krimi.

Therapeutic Uses :

1. Oedema : Local application of the paste of mustard is useful. (C.S.)
2. Filariasis : Paste of sarsapa pounded with brihati leaves should be applied locally. (G.N.)
   - One should take mustard oil to alleviate filaria. (S.S.)
3. Disease of teeth : In case of spongy gums, sarsapa mixed with salt should be rubbed thereon. (H.S.)

Parts Used : Seed, Oil.

Preparations & Dosage : Seed powder 2-4 gm.

Specific Formulations : Sarshapadi pralepa.

सर्षपः कटुकस्नेहस्तन्तुभश्च कदम्बकः ।
गौरस्तु सर्षपः प्राज्ञैः सिद्धार्थ इति कथ्यते ॥
सर्षपस्तु रसे पाके कटुः स्निग्धः सतिक्तकः ।
तीक्ष्णोष्णः कफवातघ्नो रक्तपित्ताभिवर्धनः ॥
रक्षोहरो जयेत् कण्डूकुष्ठकोष्ठक्रिमिग्रहान् ।
यथा रक्तस्तथा गौरः किन्तु गौरो वरो मतः ॥ भा०प्र०

17

RĀJIKĀ

Brassica juncea Family : Cruciferae

Chief Characters :

1. Annual shrub.
2. Yellow coloured flowers, corymb inflorescence.
3. Fruit - silique.

Synonyms : Aasuri, Kshujjanika, Raji, Tikshnagandha, Kshutabhijanaka.

Properties : Rasa - Katu; Guna - Laghu, Tikshna, Ruksha; Virya - Ushna and Vipaka - Katu.

Pharmacological Actions : Kaphapittahara, Deepana, Raktapittakrit, Keshya.

Indications : Kushta, Kandu, Krimi.

Therapeutic Uses :

Enlargement of liver and spleen : Rajika mixed with equal quantity of salt and cow's urine should be taken in the dose of about 8 gm. . It alleviates the disorder. (G.N.)

Parts Used : Seed, Oil.

Preparations & Dosage : Seed powder 1-3 gm.

राजी तु राजिका तीक्ष्णगन्धा क्षुज्जनिकाऽऽसुरी ।
क्षवः क्षुत्ताभिजनकः कृष्णीका कृष्णसर्षपः ॥
राजिका कफपित्तघ्नी तीक्ष्णोष्णा रक्तपित्तकृत् ।
किञ्चिद्रूक्षाऽग्निदा कण्डूकुष्ठकोष्ठक्रिमीन्हरेत् ॥ भा०प्र०

18
CANDRAŚŪRA

Lepidium sativum Family : Cruciferae

Chief Characters :

1. Annual herb.
2. Simple leaf.
3. White coloured flowers, racemose inflorescence.
4. Fruit - silique.

Synonyms : Chandrika, Charmahantri, Pasumehanakarika, Nandini, Karvi, Bhadra, Uasapushpa.

Properties : Rasa - Katu, Tikta; Guna - Laghu, Ruksha, Tikshna; Virya - Ushna and Vipaka - Katu.

Pharmacological Actions : Kaphavatahara, Balya.

Indications : Atisara, Hikka, Shoola, Adhamana, Katishoola, Vataroga.

Therapeutic Uses :

1. Its paste is useful for external application in lumbago, arthritis and skin diseases.
2. Its powder or ksheerapaka alleviates vatavyadhi.

Parts Used : Seed.

Preparations & Dosage : Powder 1-3 mg.

Specific Formulations : Chaturbeeja churna (methika, chandrashura, kalajaji, yavani)

चन्द्रशूरं हितं हिक्कावातश्लेष्मातिसारिणाम् ।
असृग्वातगदद्वेषि बलपुष्टिविवर्धनम् ॥ भा०प्र०

19
KHŪBAKALĀ

Sisymbrium irio Family : Cruciferae

Chief Characters :

1. Annual plant, growing upto 1 mt. height.
2. Simple leaf.
3. Racemose inflorescence, yellow coloured.
4. Fruit - long and straight.

Properties : Rasa - Katu; Guna - Snigdha, Picchila; Virya - Ushna and Vipaka - Katu.

Pharmacological Actions : Vatasleshmahara, Balya, Swedani.

Indications : Jwara, Kasa, Shwasa, Swarabheda.

Therapeutic Uses :

1. Its arka is useful in visuchika. It alleviates thirst and vomiting.
2. Its avaleha being an expectorant is useful in chronic cough, asthma and laryngitis.
3. Its paste is useful for external application on inflammation of eyes, breasts etc.

Parts Used : Seed.

Preparations & Dosage : Powder 3-6 gm.

खाकसी सर्षपाभासा कटूष्णा पिच्छिला सरा ।
वातश्लेष्महरा बल्या स्वेदनी ज्वरकासनुत् ॥ द्र०गु०वि०

20
TODARĪ

Lepidium iberis Family : Cruciferae

Chief Characters :

1. It is a herb of 36 cm. height.
2. Radical leaves and cauline leaves present.
3. Small flowers, racemose inflorescence.
4. Fruit - legume.

Properties : Rasa - Katu, Tikta; Guna - Guru, Picchila; Virya - Ushna and Vipaka - Katu.

Pharmacological Actions : Vatasleshmahara, Mutrala, Vrishya, Rasayana.

Indications : Kasa, Shwasa, Daurbalya, Mutrakriccha, Prameha.

Therapeutic Uses :

1. Oedema : Paste made from its seeds is used as an external application.
2. Cough and asthma : Its avaleha alleviates cough and asthma.
3. Aphrodisiac : Its seed powder should be taken along with milk. It also acts as galactogoue.
4. Sandhivata : Its seed oil is useful for massaging on the painful joint for alleviating pain.

Parts Used : Seed.

Preparations & Dosage : Powder 3-6 gm.

तोदरी त्रिविधा श्वेता पीता रक्ता च वर्णतः ।
कटूष्णा पिच्छिला गुर्वी वातश्लेष्महरा सरा ॥
कासे श्वासे च दौर्बल्ये मूत्रकृच्छ्रे प्रशस्यते ॥ द्र०गु०वि०

21
MŪLAKA

Raphanus sativus Family : Cruciferae

Chief Characters :

1. Annual shrub.
2. Storage roots.
3. Small leaves covered with hairs.
4. Violet coloured flowers, racemose inflorescence.
5. Indehiscent legume.

Synonyms : Chanakyamulaka, Marusambhava.

Properties : Rasa - Katu, Tikta; Guna - Laghu; Virya - Ushna and Vipaka - Katu.

Pharmacological Actions : Tridoshahara, Pacahana, Swarya, Deepana, Grahi.

Indications : Jwara, Shwasa, Nasika, Kanthya, Netravyadhi, Kasa, Arsas, Gulma, Shoola.

Therapeutic Uses :

1. Mulaka and tila cures shopha. (G.N.)
2. Mulaka decoction and pippali churna relieves visuchika. (B.P.)
3. Fomentation with the pounded and heated dried radish externally on pile mass relieves the pain. (C.S.)
4. Juice of tender radish 40 ml. added with sugar alleviates anaemia and jaundice. (S.B.)

Parts Used : Root, Seed, Leaf.

लघूमूलं कटूष्णं स्याद्रुच्यं लघु च पाचनम् ।
दोषत्रयहरं स्वर्यं ज्वरश्वासविनाशनम् ।
नासिकाकण्ठरोगघ्नं नयनामयनाशनम् ॥
महत्तदेव रूक्षोष्णं गुरु दोषत्रयप्रदम् ।
स्नेहसिद्धं तदेव स्याद् दोषत्रयविनाशनम् ॥ भा०प्र०

22

TILAPARṆĪ

Cleome gynandra Linn. Family : Cleomaceae

Chief Characters :

1. Annual herb with pentafoliate leaves.
2. White coloured flowers arranged in corymb inflorescence.
3. Fruit - silique.

Synonyms : Suvarchala, Suryabhakta, Varada, Badara, Ravipreeta, Suryavasta, Brahma, Sudurlabha, Ajagandha, Putigandha, Barbaraka, Ugragandha.

Properties : Rasa - Katu; Guna - Ruksha; Virya - Sheeta (B.P.), Ushna (R.N.) and Vipaka - Madhura (B.P.), Katu (R.N.).

Pharmacological Actions : Kaphavatahara, Apittala, Shoolaprashamana.

Indications : Shwasa, Kasa, Kushta, Krimi, Prameha, Yonishoola, Pandushoola, Gulma, Jwara, Karnashoola.

Therapeutic Uses :

1. Fresh extract of tilaparni, tila taila, tankana, lemon juice relieve karnashoola. (S.S.)
2. Poultice of suryavarta and rasona should be applied on the goitre. By this blisters appear and fluid is discharged and thus growth subsides. (V.M.)
3. Ears should be filled up with juice of suryavarta or sinduvara or langali added with trikatu. It destroys organism in the ear. (V.M.)

Parts Used : Seed, Leaf, Root.

Preparations & Dosage : Seed powder 1-3 gm.; Leaf juice 5-10 ml.; Root powder 1-3 gm.

तिलपर्णी पूतिगन्धाऽत्युग्रगन्धा च रोमशा ।
तिलपर्णी कटूष्णा स्यात्तीक्ष्णा विस्फोटकारिणी ॥
विदाहिकृमिशूलघ्नी स्वेदला कफवातनुत् । द्र०गु०वि०

23
HIṀSRĀ

Capparis sepiaria Family : Capparidaceae

Chief Characters :

1. Perennial shrub.
2. Simple leaf.
3. White coloured flowers, umbel inflorescence.
4. Pea sized fruit.

Synonyms : Kanthari, Gridranakhi.

Properties : Rasa - Katu, Tikta; Guna - Laghu, Ruksha; Virya - Ushna and Vipaka - Katu.

Pharmacological Actions : Kaphavatahara, Deepana, Ruchya.

Indications : Raktagranthi, Shopha, Vatavyadhi.

Therapeutic Uses :

1. In swelling caused by vata, paste of himsra and rasna is useful. (V.M.)
2. The paste of himsra should be applied intravaginally to relieve itching. (C.S.)

Parts Used : Root, Leaf.

Preparations & Dosage : Decoction 50-100 ml.

कन्थारी कटुतिक्तोष्णा कफवातनिकृन्तनी ।
शोफघ्नी दीपनी रुच्या रक्तग्रन्थिरुजापहा ॥ भा०प्र०

24
VYĀGHRANAKHĪ

Capparis zeylanica Family : Capparidaceae

Chief Characters :

1. Perennial herb.
2. Simple leaf.
3. White coloured flowers.
4. Fruit - round, 4 cm. in length.

Synonyms : Ahimsra, Alpahimsra.

Gana :

Sushruta : Eladi.

Properties : Rasa - Katu, Tikta; Guna - Laghu, Ruksha; Virya - Ushna and Vipaka - Katu.

Pharmacological Actions : Kaphavatahara.

Indications : Agnimandhya, Shotha, Granthi.

Parts Used : Root, Leaf.

Preparations & Dosage : Decoction 50-100 ml.

नखद्वयं ग्रहश्लेष्मवातास्रज्वरकुष्ठहृत् ॥
लघूष्णं शुक्रलं वर्ण्यं स्वादु व्रणविषापहम् ।
अलक्ष्मीमुखदौर्गन्ध्यहृत्पाकरसयोः कटुः ॥ भा०प्र०

25

KARĪRA

Capparis decidua Edgew. Family : Capparidaceae

Chief Characters :

1. Perennial shrub.
2. Small leaves are seen on the tender branches.
3. Orange coloured thorns.
4. Red coloured flowers, corymb imflorescence.
5. Fruit - berry.

Synonyms : Apatra, Marubhuruha, Nigudapatra.

Gana :

Charaka : Tiktaskandha.

Properties : Rasa - Katu, Tikta; Guna - Laghu, Ruksha; Virya - Ushna and Vipaka - Katu.

Pharmacological Actions : Kaphavatahara, Bhedana, Vishaghna.

Indications : Krimi, Shotha, Vrana, Arshas.

Therapeutic Uses :

1. Arshas : The tender fruits washed and dried in the sun on internal administration with the cream of the curd relieves arshas. (S.B.M.)
2. Shotha : The intake of powder of the flower relieves shotha. The powdered fruit also cures the condtion. (S.B.M.)

Parts Used : Root bark.

Preparations & Dosage : Powder 1-3 gm.; Decoction 50-100 ml.

करीरः कटुकस्तिक्तः स्वेद्युष्णो भेदनः स्मृतः ।
दुर्नामकफवातामगरशोथव्रणप्रणुत् ॥ भा०प्र०

26

BANAPHŚĀ

Viola odorata Family : Violaceae

Chief Characters :

1. Perennial herb.
2. Simple leaf, alternate phyllotaxy.
3. Consists of bluish violet coloured flowers with aromatic odour.
4. Fruit—loculicidal capsule.

Properties : Rasa - Katu, Tikta; Guna - Laghu, Snigdha; Virya - Ushna and Vipaka - Katu.

Pharmacological Actions : Vatapittahara, Kaphahara.

Indications : Kasa, Shwasa, Jwara, Shotha.

Parts Used : Flower, Whole plant.

Preparations & Dosage : Powder 3-6 gm.

Specific Formulations : Banapshadi kwatha.

बनफ्सा कटुतिक्तोष्णा शीतज्वरनिवारणी ।
कासश्वासहरा त्वच्या सरा वातकफापहा ॥ द्र०गु०वि०

27
VIKAṄKATA

Flacourtia ramontchi Family : Flacourtiaceae

Chief Characters :

1. Perennial herb.
2. Simple leaf.
3. Racemose inflorescence.
4. Consists of yellow or green coloured flowers.
5. Indehiscent capsule.

Synonyms : Swadukantaka, Granthila, Kantaki, Sruvavriksha, Yajnavriksha, Vyaghrapada.

Properties : Rasa - Amla, Madhura; Guna - Laghu; Virya - Sheeta and Vipaka - Madhura.

Pharmacological Actions : Tridoshahara, Deepana, Pacahana, Mutrala.

Indications : Kamala, Pleeha vriddhi.

Therapeutic Uses :

1. Prameha : Arista, asava, leha and ayaskriti should be prepared of vikankita which is useful in prameha. (S.S.)
2. Cyst : In cyst caused by kapha, paste of vikankata, aragva-dha etc. should be applied. (S.S.)
3. Spider poisoning : Vikankata is used as intake collyrium, snuff, paste and bath in spider poisoning predoninant in all the three doshas. (A.H.)

Parts Used : Bark, Fruit, Leaf.

Preparations & Dosage : Decoction 50-100 ml.; Juice 10-20 ml.

विकङ्कतः स्रुवावृक्षो ग्रन्थिलः स्वादुकण्टकः ।
स एव यज्ञवृक्षश्च कण्टकी व्याघ्रपादपि ॥
विकङ्कतफलं पक्वं मधुरं सर्वदोषजित् ॥ भा०प्र०

28
PUNNĀGA

Caplophyllum inophyllum Linn. Family : Guttiferae

Chief Characters :

1. Tree.
2. Simple leaf, opposite phyllotaxy.
3. Panicle inflorescence, white flowers.
4. Fruit - yellow coloured drupe.

Synonyms : Tunga.

Properties : Rasa - Madhura, Kashaya; Guna - Laghu, Ruksha; Virya - Sheeta and Vipaka - Madhura.

Pharmacological Actions : Kaphapittashamaka.

Indications : Raktatisara, Raktapitta, Mutrakricchra, Amavata.

Therapeutic Uses :

Sprinkling with infusion of punnaga leaves or decoction of priyangu destroys corneal opacity. (V.M.)

Parts Used : Bark, Seed oil, Flowers, Leaves.

Preparations & Dosage : Bark decoction 50-100 ml.; Oil 2-5 drops.

पुन्नागो मधुरः शीतः सुगन्धिः पित्तनाशकृत् ॥ रा०नि०

29
SURAPUNNĀGA

Ochrocarpus longifolius Family : Guttiferae

Chief Characters :

1. Tree.
2. Simple leaves - glabrous.
3. White coloured polygamous flowers.
4. Fruit - berry.

Synonyms : Nameru, Suraparnika.

Gana :

Sushruta : Eladi.

Properties : Rasa - Madhura, Kashaya; Guna - Laghu, Ruksha; Virya - Sheeta and Vipaka - Madhura.

Pharmacological Actions : Kaphapittahara.

Indications : Raktapitta, Raktatisara, Pravahika, Amavata, Sandhivata.

Parts Used : Bark, Seed oil.

Preparations & Dosage : Decoction 50-100 ml.; Oil 2-5 drops.

सुरतुङ्गश्च पञ्चाह्वः पुंनागगुणसंयुतः ।। रा०नि०

30
TAMĀLA

Garcinia morella Family : Guttiferae.

Chief Characters :

1. A tree growing upto 15 m. height, monoecious.
2. Oval/elliptical shaped simple leaf, alternate phyllotaxy.
3. Fruit - cherry shaped berry.

Synonyms : Tapiccha, Kalaskandha, Amitadruma, Lokaskandha, Neeladhwaja, Neelatala.

Properties : Rasa - Katu, Tikta, Kashaya; Guna - Laghu, Ruksha; Virya - Ushna and Vipaka - Katu.

Pharmacological Actions : Kaphapittahara.

Indications : Gulma, Udavarta, Shoola, Udara, Shotha, Daha, Vispota.

Parts Used : Gum.

Preparations & Dosage : Powder 50-125 mg.

कङ्कुष्ठं तिक्तकटुकं वीर्ये चोष्णं प्रकीर्तितम् ।
गुल्मोदावर्तशूलघ्नं रसरञ्जं व्रणापहम् ॥ ध०नि०

31
SARJA

Vateria indica Linn. Family : Dipterocarpaceae

Chief Characters :

1. Tree.
2. Hairy shoot.
3. Simple leaf.
4. White flowers in panicle inflorescence.
5. Fruit - capsule.

Synonyms : Ajakarna, Marichapatraka, Sala.

Properties : Rasa - Katu, Tikta, Kashaya; Guna - Snigdha; Virya - Sheeta/Ushna and Vipaka - Katu.

Pharmacological Actions : Kaphahara, Vishahara, Vatapittahara.

Indications : Pandu, Kushta, Vrana, Prameha, Karnaroga.

Therapeutic Uses :

1. Grahaniroga : Sarjarasa mixed with less quantity of jaggery should be taken to controls grahani roga. (B.P.)
2. Whitlow : After fomenting with hot water the powder of sarjarasa should be applied to the wound and bandaged. (V.M.)
3. Cracks in feet : Powder of sarjarasa and rocksalt mixed with honey and mustard oil should be churned and applied locally. (V.M.)

Parts Used : Bark, Gum.

Preparations & Dosage : Bark decoction 50-100 ml.; Gum powder 1-3 gm.

सर्जस्तु तुवरस्तिक्तः हिमः स्निग्धोऽतिसारजित् ।
पित्तास्रदोषकुष्ठघ्नः कण्डूविस्फोटवातजित् ॥ रा०नि०

32
VṚKṢĀMLA

Garcinia indica Family : Guttiferae

Chief Characters :

1. Tree.
2. Simple leaf.
3. Monoecious flower.
4. Fruit - violet colour, in size of an orange Berry.

Synonyms : Tintidika, Chukra, Amlavrikshaka.

Properties : Rasa - Madhura, Amla; Guna - Guru, Ruksha; Virya - Ushna and Vipaka - Amla.

Pharmacological Actions : Vatahara, Kaphapittakara, Grahi, Deepana.

Indications : Trishna, Arshas, Grahani, Gulma, Shotha, Hridroga, Krimi.

Therapeutic Uses :

1. Gulma : Juice of Vrikshamla mixed with rocksalt should be given. (V.D.)
2. Thirst : Gargle of Vrikshamla and matulunga removes dryness of palate. (C.S.)

Parts Used : Oil, Fruit, Root bark.

Preparations & Dosage : Oil 3-5 gm.; Fruit sharbat 10-20 ml.; Root bark decoction 40-80 ml.

वृक्षाम्लमाममम्लोष्णं वातघ्नं कफपित्तलम् ।
पक्वं तु गुरु संग्राहि मधुराम्लरसं तथा ॥
अल्पोष्णं रोचनं रूक्षं दीपनं वातनाशनम् ।
तृष्णार्शोग्रहणीगुल्मशूलहृद्रोगजन्तुजित् ॥ भा०प्र०

33
AŚWAKARṆA

Dipterocarpus turbinatus Gaertn.   Family : Dipterocarpaceae

Chief Characters :

1. Big tree.
2. Simple leaf, oval shaped.
3. Light pink coloured flowers.
4. Racemose inflorescence.
5. Fruit - drupe.

Synonyms : Jaranadruma, Deerghapama, Kusikataru, Kaushika, Sasya, Samvarana, Sala, Marichapatra.

Properties : Rasa - Katu, Tikta; Guna - Snigdha, Laghu; Virya - Ushna and Vipaka - Katu.

Pharmacological Actions : Pittaraktahara, Kaphavatashamaka, Puyanashaka.

Indications : Jwara, Visarpa, Kandu, Sirashoola, Kushta, Visphota, Vrana, Dushtavrana.

Parts Used : Oil.

Preparations & Dosage : 5-10 drops.

अश्वकर्णः कटुस्तिक्तः स्निग्धः पूयास्रनाशनः ।
ज्वरविस्फोटकण्डुघ्नः शिरोदोषार्त्तिकृन्तनः ॥ रा०नि०

34
LATĀKASTŪRĪ

Hibiscus abelmoschus Family : Malvaceae

Chief Characters :

1. Annual shrub.
2. Simple leaf.
3. Yellow coloured inflorescence.
4. Loculicidal capsule.

Synonyms : Latakasturika.

Properties : Rasa - Tikta, Madhura, Katu; Guna - Laghu, Ruksha, Tikshna; Virya - Sheeta and Vipaka - Katu.

Pharmacological Actions : Kaphapitta shamaka, Deepana, Vrishya, Chakshushya.

Indications : Triśhna, Mutrakricchra, Mukharoga.

Therapeutic Uses :

1. Dysuria : The juice of root and leaves is useful to relieve dysuria.
2. Eye disorders : The fine powder made from it is applied to the eyes.

Parts Used : Seed.

Preparations & Dosage : Powder 1-3 gm.

लता कस्तूरिका तिक्ता स्वाद्वी वृष्या हिमा लघुः ।
चक्षुष्या दीपिनी श्लेष्मतृष्णाबस्त्यास्यरोगहृत् ॥ भा०प्र०

35
PĀRĪṢA

Thespesia populnea Linn. Family : Malvaceae

Chief Characters :

1. It is a tree, grows upto 20 m. in height.
2. Simple leaves, alternate phyllotaxy.
3. Yellow coloured flowers.
4. Fruit - capsule.

Synonyms : Kapichuta, Gardabhanda, Kamanada, Palasha, Kapitana, Suparshwaka, Parshvapippala.

Properties : Rasa - Amla, Madhura, Kashaya; Guna - Laghu, Ruksha/Snigdha (B.P.); Virya - Sheeta and Vipaka - Katu.

Pharmacological Actions : Kaphakara, Mutra sangrahaneeya, Shukrala, Grahi.

Indications : Prameha, Kushta, Yoniroga.

Therapeutic Uses :

1. Pumsavana : The woman who takes parsh vapippala mixed with jiraka and sarapunkha delivers male child. (B.P.)
2. Skin disorder: It is useful for external application in vrana, pama, kandu and other skin disorders.

Parts Used : Bark.

Preparations & Dosage : Decoction 50-100 ml.

कपीतनस्तु पारीषः सुपार्श्वः पार्श्वपिप्पलः ।
गर्दभाण्डश्च विज्ञेयः समुद्रतटशोभनः ॥
कपीतनो लघू रूक्षः कषायः शिशिरो हरेत् ।
कफपित्तप्रमेहास्रकुष्ठयोनिगदव्रणान् ॥ द्र०गु०वि०

36
KHATMĪ

Althoea officinalis Linn. Family : Malvaceae.

Chief Characters :

1. Perennial shrub.
2. Simple leaf, alternate phyllotaxy.
3. Consists of pink coloured flowers.
4. Fruit - capsule.

Properties : Rasa - Madhura; Guna - Snigdha, Guru, Picchila; Virya - Sheeta and Vipaka - Madhura.

Pharmacological Actions : Vatapittahara, Mutrala, Sara.

Indications : Pratishyaya, Kasa, Mutrakricchra.

Therapeutic Uses :

1. Paste prepared from its seeds and leaves is useful for external application in accidental wounds, mastitis etc.
2. Decoction made from its root or seeds is useful in dysentry and enteritis

Parts Used : Flower, Seed, Root.

Preparations & Dosage : Powder 3-6 gm.

खत्मी तु मधुरा स्निग्धा पिच्छिला शीतला गुरुः ।
वातपित्तहरा श्लेष्मसारणी मूत्रला सरा ।
प्रतिश्याये तथा कासे मूत्रकृच्छ्रे च शस्यते ॥ द्र०गु०वि०

37
KĀRPĀSA

Gossypium herbaceum Linn. Family : Malvaceae

Chief Characters :

1. It is annual or perennial shrub.
2. Heart shaped simple leaf.
3. Alternate phyllotaxy.
4. Yellow coloured flowers.
5. Fruit - loculicidal capsule.

Synonyms : Tundikeri, Samudranta.

Gana :

Charaka : Brimhaneeya.
Sushruta : Vatasamshamana.

Properties : Rasa - Katu, Kashaya (Root bark), Madhura (Seed); Guna - Laghu, Tikshna (Root bark), Snigdha (Seed); Virya - Atushna (Fruit), Sheeta (R.N.) and Vipaka - Katu (Root bark), Madhura (Seed).

Pharmacological Actions : Vatahara, Mutrala (Leaf), Vrishya (Seed), Sthanyada, Raktavardhaka.

Indications : Mutrakricchra, Karnapeeda, Karnanada, Karnapuya, Kastartava, Anartava (Decoction of root bark).

Therapeutic Uses :

1. Karnasrava : The juice of karpasa fruit is poured into the ears after mixing with sarjarasa twak powder. The juice of tender fruit mixed with honey also arrests karnasrava. (S.S.)
2. Pradara: The root powder is pounded with tandulodhaka and administered internally. (Vrinda)
3. Kapala kushta : The external application of the oil processed with root, bark, leaf and flowers of karpasa relieves kaphaja kushta. (Vaidya Manorama)

Parts Used : Root, Bark, Flower, Seed.

Preparations & Dosage : Decoction 50-100 ml., Seed powder 3-6 gm.

Specific Formulation : Karpasastyadi taila.

कार्पासको लघुः कोष्णो मधुरो वातनाशनः ।
तत्पलाशं समीरघ्नं रक्तकृन्मूत्रवर्धनम् ॥
तत्कर्णपिडकानादपूयस्रावविनाशनम् ।
तद्बीजं स्तन्यदं वृष्यं स्निग्धं कफकरं गुरु ॥ भा०प्र०

38
MUCAKUNDA

Pterospermum diversifolium/P. acerifolium

Family : Sterculiaceae

Chief Characters :

1. Tree.
2. Simple leaf.
3. White coloured flowers, cymose inflorescence.
4. Fruit - capsule.

Synonyms : Kshatravriksha, Chitraka, Prativishnuka.

Properties : Rasa - Kashaya, Katu, Tikta; Guna - Laghu, Ruksha; Virya - Ushna and Vipaka - Katu.

Pharmacological Actions : Pittahara (B.P.), Vishahara, Kaphahara, (R.N.), Tridoshahara (N.R.).

Indications : Sirashoola, Raktavikara, Raktapitta, Raktarshas, Kushta, Vrana, Pama, Shopha.

Therapeutic Uses :

The juice of muchakunda on nasya relieves sirashoola. (C.D.)

Flower of muchakunda relieves headache immediately. (V.M., S.S.)

Parts Used : Flower.

Preparations & Dosage : Powder 3-6 gm.

Specific Formulation : Himanshu taila.

मुचकुन्दः क्षत्रवृक्षश्चित्रकः प्रतिविष्णुकः ।
मुचकुन्दः शिरःपीडापित्तास्रविषनाशनः ॥ भा०प्र०

39
PIŚĀCA KĀRPĀSA

Abroma augusta Family : Sterculiaceae

Chief Characters :

1. It is a perennial plant.
2. Simple leaves, alternate phyllotaxy.
3. Reddish violet coloured flowers, cymose inflorescence.
4. Fruit - capsule.

Synonyms : Peevari, Yoshini.

Properties : Rasa - Katu, Tikta; Guna - Laghu, Ruksha; Virya - Ushna and Vipaka - Katu.

Pharmacological Actions : Kaphavatashamaka, Artavajanana, Rajadoshahara.

Indications : Rajorodha, Kashtartava, Yonivayapat.

Therapeutic Uses :

Juice of the root bark along with black pepper is useful in dysmenorrhoea when given in the dosage of ½ gm.

Parts Used : Root.

Preparations & Dosage : Powder 1-3 gm.; Juice 5-10 ml.

पीवरी योषिणी सा स्याद् योनिव्यापद्विनाशिनी ।
रजोदोषप्रशमनी.................................।। आ०वि०

40
ĀVARTANĪ

Helicteres isora Linn. Family : Sterculiaceae

Chief Characters :

1. Perennial herb grows upto 3 m. height.
2. Oval shaped leaves, alternate phyllotaxy.
3. Red coloured flowers, cyamose inflorescence.
4. Fruit - five fruits occur from each flower and appear as a single fruit.

Synonyms : Avartaphala.

Properties : Rasa - Kashaya; Guna - Laghu, Ruksha; Virya - Sheeta and Vipaka - Katu.

Pharmacological Actions : Kaphapittahara, Grahi

Indications : Udara, Shoola, Krimi, Atisara, Raktapitta.

Therapeutic Uses :

1. Atisara and Pravahika : The fruit powder (3 gm.) relives atisara, pravahika and udara shoola. (N.A.)
2. Madhumeha : The decoction of root bark controls madhumeha. (N.A.)

Parts Used : Root, Bark, Fruit.

Preparations & Dosage : Decoction 50-100 ml.; Fruit powder 3-6 gm.

आवर्तनी लघुः शीता कषाया त्वतिसारनुत् ।
बलासपित्तशूलास्रकृमिरोगविनाशिनी ॥ द्र०गु०वि०

41
PARŪṢAKA

Grewia asiatica Linn. Family : Tiliaceae

Chief Characters :

1. Tree.
2. Simple leaf, alterante phyllotaxy.
3. Yellowish flowers arranged in panicle inflorescence.
4. Fruit - drupe.

Synonyms : Parusha, Alpasthi, Parapara.

Gana :

Charaka : Virechanopaga, Jwarahara, Sramahara.
Sushruta : Parushakadi.

Properties : Rasa - Madhura; Guna - Laghu, Snigdha; Virya - Sheeta and Vipaka - Madhura.

Pharmacological Actions : Pittavatahara, Hridya, Pittakara (Amaphala), Brimhana, Tarpana, Shukrala, Balya, Vishtambhi.

Indications : Daha, Jwara, Kshaya, Krishata, Gulma, Raktapitta.

Therapeutic Uses :

1. Shukradosha : In puyaprakhya shukra, ghrita cooked with parushaka and vata should be given. (S.S.)
2. Rohini : Gargle with decoction of draksha and parushaka is useful. (B.P.)
3. Madatyaya : In alcoholism casued by pitta, intake of saturating soups and drinks prepared from juices of draksha, amalaka, kharjura and parushaka is advised.

Parts Used : Fruit, Leaf.

परूषकं कषायाम्लमामं पित्तकरं लघु ॥
तत्पक्वं मधुरं पाके शीतं विष्टम्भि बृंहणम् ।
हृद्यन्तु पित्तदाहास्रज्वरक्षयसमीरहृत् ॥ भा०प्र०

42
GĀṄGERUKĪ

Grewia populifolia Family : Tiliaceae.

Chief Characters :

1. Shrub growing upto 3 m height.
2. Simple leaf, alterante phyllotaxy, leaf ellipitical with 3-4 veins.
3. Yellow coloured flowers appearing in panicles.
4. Fruit - drupe, orange colour.

Properties : Rasa - Kashaya, Madhura; Guna - Laghu, Ruksha; Virya - Sheeta and Vipaka - Katu.

Pharmacological Actions : kaphavatahara, Stambhana.

Indications : Raktapitta, Pravahika, Sadyovrana.

Therapeutic Uses :

The wound caused by sharp instruments like sword etc. should be filled immediately with the juice of gangeruki root. It relieves pain and promotes healing. (S.S.)

Parts Used : Root, Bark.

Preparations & Dosage : Juice 10-20 ml.; Decoction 50-100 ml.

खड्गारिच्छिन्नगात्रस्य तत्कालं पूरितो व्रण: ।
गाङ्गेरुकीमूलरसैर्जायते गतवेदन: ॥ शा०स०

43
GUḌAŚARKARĀ

Grewia hirsuta Family : Tiliaceae

Chief Characters :

1. Shrub growing upto 3 m. height.
2. Simple leaf, round in shape with serrated margins.
3. Elongated bracts, yellow coloured flowers, 2-4 in number.
4. Fruit - berry, consisting of four seeds.

Properties : Rasa - Madhura, Kashaya; Guna - Guru, Snigdha, Picchila; Virya - Sheeta and Vipaka - Madhura.

Pharmacological Actions : Vatapitta shamaka, Rasayana.

Indications : Raktapitta, Kasa, Shwasa, Kshaya, Mutrakricchra, Shoola.

Parts Used : Root.

Preparations & Dosage : Decoction 50-100 ml.; Powder 3-6 gm.

विदारीत्रिपलाटभीरुशृङ्गाटीगुडशर्करा: ।
काश्मरीफलयष्ट्याह्वपरुषकहिमानि च ।। सु०उ०
गुडशर्करा गाङ्गेटीफलम् । डल्हण

44
DHANWANA

Grewia tiliaefolia Vahl. Family : Tiliaceae

Chief Characters :

1. The tree grows upto the height of 10 mts.
2. Simple leaves with serrated margins.
3. Yellowish flowers arranged in panicle inflorescence.
4. Fruit - drupe.

Synonyms : Dhanwanga, Dhanva vriksha, Gotra vriksha, Suteja.

Gana : Charaka : Amla skandha.

Properties : Rasa - Kashaya, Madhura; Guna - Laghu, Picchila; Virya - Sheeta and Vipaka - Katu.

Pharmacological Actions : Kaphapitta shamaka (CS.), Kaphavatahara (SS.), Vranaropana, Balya, Brimhana.

Indications : Atisara, Pravahika, Raktapitta, Vrana, Kasa, Raktatisara.

Therapeutic Uses :

1. Prameha : Decoction of patha, vidanga, arjuna and dhanvana mixed with honey is prescribed in prameha caused by kapha. (C.S.)
2. Raktasrava : In case of excessive haemorrhage powder of the barks of sala, arimeda, meshasringa, dhava and dhanvana should be applied and the bleeding area is firmly bandaged.

Parts Used : Bark.

Preparations & Dosage : Decoction 50-100 ml.

धन्वङ्गस्तु धनुर्वृक्षो गोत्रवृक्षः सुतेजनः ।
धन्वङ्गः कफपित्तास्रकासहृत्तुवरो लघुः ॥
बृंहणो बलकृद्रूक्षः सान्धिकृद् व्रणरोपणः ॥ भा०प्र०

45

ATASĪ

Linum usitatissimum Linn. Family : Linaceae

Chief Characters :

1. Big shrub grows upto 50 cm. height.
2. Simple leaves, alternate phyllotaxy.
3. Blue coloured flowers.
4. Fruit - septicidal capsule.

Synonyms : Neela pushpi, Uma, Kshuma, Masruna.

Properties : Rasa - Madhura, Tikta; Guna - Guru, Snigdha; Virya - Ushna and Vipaka - Katu.

Pharmacological Actions : Vatahara, Kaphapittakara, Balya, Grahi, Achakshushya, Shukrahara.

Indications : Vrana, Shotha, Vatarakta, Prameha, Vataroga, Kushta, Arshas, Atisara, Grahini, Vranashopha, Hridroga.

Therapeutic Uses :

1. Vrana : The external application of seeds pounded in sour curd hastens suppuration of wounds. (C.S.) The external application of seed oil relieves pain due to wounds. (C.S.)
2. Vatarakta : The seeds pounded in milk relieves pain in vatarakta on external application. (S.S.)
3. Prameha : The oils of kusumbha, sarshapa and atasi are useful in prameha. (S.S.)

Parts Used : Seed, Flower, Oil.

Preparations & Dosage : Powder 3-6 gm.; Oil 5-10 ml.

Specific Formulations : Atasyadilepa.

अतसी मधुरा तिक्ता स्निग्धा पाके कटुर्गुरुः ।
उष्णा दृक्शुक्रवातघ्नी कफपित्तप्रकोपिणी ॥
तैल—
अतसीतैलमाग्नेयं स्निग्धोष्णं कफपित्तकृत् ।
कटुपाकमचक्षुष्यं बल्यं वातहरं गुरु ॥
मलकृद्रसतः स्वादु ग्राहि त्वग्दोषहृद् घनम् ।
बस्तौ पाने तथाभ्यङ्गे नस्ये कर्णस्य पूरणे ॥
अनुपानविधौ चापि प्रयोज्यं वातशान्तये ॥ भा०प्र०

46

CAÑCU

Corchorus fascicularis Family : Tiliaceae

Chief Characters :

1. Annual herb.
2. Simple leaves.
3. Yellow coloured flower.
4. Fruit - capsule.

Synonyms : Chincha, Deerghapatra, Satiktaka.

Properties : Rasa - Madhura, Tikta; Guna - Picchila; Virya - Sheeta and Vipaka - Madhura.

Pharmacological Actions : Tridoshahara, Balya, Medhya, Ruchya.

Indications : Aruchi, Anaha, Shosha, Apasmara, Daha, Mutrakricchra.

Therapeutic Uses :

Sinus : Application of the paste of chanchu fruits is an excellent remedy for sinus (Nadivrana). (A.H.)

Parts Used : Whole plant.

Preparations & Dosage : Decoction 30-50 ml.

चञ्चुः शीता सरा रुच्या स्वाद्वी दोषत्रयापहा ।
धातुपुष्टिकरी बल्या मेध्या पिच्छिलका स्मृता ॥ भा०प्र०

47
KARMARAṄGA

Averrhoa carambola Linn. Family : Oxalidaceae

Chief Characters :

1. Small tree.
2. Paripinnate compound leaf, alternate phyllotaxy.
3. White or violet coloured flowers.
4. Panicle inflorescence.
5. Fruit - berry.

Synonyms : Brihadamla, Rujakara, Sirala, Dharaphala, Peetaphala.

Properties : Rasa - Madhura, Amla; Guna - Laghu; Virya - Ushna and Vipaka - Madhura.

Pharmacological Actions : Kaphavatahara, Grahi, Balya.

Indications : Jwara, Atisara, Raktapitta, Raktarshas.

Therapeutic Uses :

1. Jwara : Its decoction is useful in jwara.
2. Scurvy : Sharbat made from its fruits alleviates scurvy.

Parts Used : Fruit.

Preparations & Dosage : Sharbat (Panaka) 10-20 ml.

कर्मरङ्गं शिरालं च बृहदम्लं रुजाकरम् ।
कर्मरङ्गं हिमं ग्राहि स्वाद्वम्लं कफवातहृत् ॥ भा०प्र०

48
BĪJAPŪRA

Citrus medica Linn. Family : Rutaceae

Chief Characters :

1. Tree.
2. Compound leaf, alternate phyllotaxy.
3. White coloured flowers.
4. Fruit - berry.

Synonyms : Matulunga, Ruchaka, Phalapuraka.

Properties : Rasa - Madhura, Amla; Guna - Laghu, Snigdha; Virya - Ushna and Vipaka - Amla.

Pharmacological Actions : Vatakaphahara, Hridya, Deepana, Grahi.

Indications : Chardi, Raktapitta, Trishna, Shwasa, Kasa, Aruchi, Hikka, Ajirna, Shoola.

Therapeutic Uses :

1. Vomiting : Matulunga rasa with laja, pippali, madhu, sharkara is useful in chardi. (V.S.)
2. Internal haemorrhage : The paste of root and flowers of matulunga should be taken with rice water. (S.S.)
3. Pain in cardiac region : Powdered hingu mixed with one of the salts should be given with juice of matulunga. (C.S.)
   • Matulunga juice mixed with rock salt should be taken. This is the best remedy for cardiac pain. (K.S.)

Parts Used : Fruit.

Preparations & Dosage : Fruit juice 10-20 ml.

Specific Formulations : Matulunga rasayana, Matulungadi yoga, Beejapuradya ghrita.

बीजपूरो मातुलुङ्गो रुचकः फलपूरकः ।
बीजपूरफलं स्वादु रसेऽम्लं दीपनं लघु ॥
रक्तपित्तहरं कण्ठजिह्वाहृदयशोधनम् ।
श्वासकासारुचिहरं हृद्यं तृष्णाहरं स्मृतम् ॥ भा०प्र०

49

SUDDĀVA

Ruta graveolens Linn. Family : Rutaceae

Chief Characters :

1. Fragrant shrub.
2. Compound leaves, alterante phyllotaxy.
3. Light yellow flowers, corymb inflorescence.
4. Fruit - capsule.

Properties : Rasa - Tikta; Guna - Laghu, Ruksha, Tikshna; Virya - Ushna and Vipaka - Katu.

Pharmacological Actions : Kaphavatahara, Deepana.

Indications : Agnimandhya, Shoola, Krimi, Rajorodha, Kashtartava.

Therapeutic Uses :

The leaf juice is internally administered to relive colic.

Parts Used : Whole plant.

Preparations & Dosage : Juice 5-10 ml.; Powder 1-3 gm.

सन्तापं कटूषं परं तिक्तयुक्तं तथैवोग्रगन्धि प्रभूताग्निकारि।
सदाक्षेपशूलक्रिमिघ्नं प्रयुक्तं रजःस्रावकं गर्भपातापकारि ॥ द्र०गु०वि०

50
HARAMALA

Peganum harmala Linn. Family : Rutaceae

Chief Characters :

1. Perennial herb.
2. Simple leaf, alternate phyllotaxy.
3. White coloured flower.
4. Fruit - capsule.

Properties : Rasa - Katu, Tikta; Guna - Laghu, Ruksha; Virya - Ushna and Vipaka - Katu.

Pharmacological Actions : Kaphavatahara, Vrishya, Stanyajanana, Madakari.

Indications : Kushta, Krimi, Vatavyadhi, Shoola.

Therapeutic Uses :

1. Root powder along with sarshapa taila on external application destroys krimi.
2. Leaf decoction relieves amavata.

Parts Used : Seed.

Preparations & Dosage : Powder 1-3 gm.

मतं रूक्षं तिक्तं पचति कटु वीर्योष्णमिति च,
समीरं श्लेष्माणं शमयति तथा पित्तबहुलम् ।
परं वृष्यं स्तन्यं गमयति तथा गर्भशयनम्,
ज्वरं जन्तून् कुष्ठं हरति बहुशूलं हरमलम् ॥ द्र०गु०वि०

51
AMLAVETASA

Garcinia pedunculata Family : Guttiferae

Chief Characters :

1. A tree growing upto 60 ft. in height, stem hallow.
2. Leaf with long petiole.
3. Flower doecious.
4. Fruit - fleshy with 5-10 kidney shaped seeds.

Synonyms : Shatavedhi, Shasranut, Chukra.

Gana :

Charaka : Hridya, Deepaniya, Shwasahara.

Properties : Rasa - Amla; Guna - Laghu, Ruksha; Virya - Ushna and Vipaka - Amla.

Pharmacological Actions : Kaphavatahara, Pittala, Deepana, Bhedana.

Indications : Hridroga, Shoola, Gulma, Pleeha, Udavarta, Hikka, Anaha, Shwasa, Kasa, Chardi.

Therapeutic Uses :

1. Pleeha : The intake of amlavetasa mixed with pippali, maricha, saindhava lavana and sigrupatra kwatha relieves pleehodara. (G.N.)
2. Jalodara : The phalaniryasa should be administered with ghrita. (G.N.)
3. Ashmari : The phalaniryasa administered internally with dadhimantha.
4. Arshas : Vardhamana rasayana prayoga of amlavesta sara relieves arshas and gulma.

Parts Used : Fruit.

Preparations & Dosage : Juice 5-20 ml.

Specific Formulations : Bhaskara lavana.

अम्लवेतसो भेदनीयदीपनीयानुलोमिकवातश्लेष्महराणाम् । च०सू०

52

ARALU

Ailanthus excelsa Roxb. Family : Simaroubaceae

Chief Characters :

1. Tree grows upto 20 m.
2. Paripinnate compound leaf.
3. Light green coloured small flowers.
4. Panicle inflorescence.
5. Fruit - samara.

Synonyms : Katwanga, Putivriksha, Deerghavrinta.

Properties : Rasa - Tikta, Kashaya; Guna - Ruksha; Virya - Sheeta and Vipaka - Katu.

Pharmacological Actions : Kaphahara, Grahi, Deepana.

Indications : Krimi, Kushta, Atisara.

Therapeutic Uses :

1. Atisara : The intake of bark juice with honey relieves atisara. (N.R.)
2. Karna shoola : Luke warm juice of the bark applied locally (as ear drops) in karna shoola (ear ache). (Vagbhata)

Parts Used : Bark.

Preparations & Dosage : Powder 1-3 gm.; Juice 10-20 ml.

Specific Formulations : Araluputapaka.

कट्वङ्गं सांग्राहिकपाचनीयदीपनीयानाम् । च०सू०

53
IṄGUDĪ

Balanites aegyptiaca Linn. Family : Balanitaceae

Chief Characters :

1. Tree grows upto 6 m. height, covered with thorns.
2. Bifoliate compound leaf.
3. White colored small flowers, cyamose inflorescence.
4. Fruit - drupe.

Synonyms : Angara vriksha, Tiktaka, Tapasadruma.

Guna :

Sushrata : Sleshmasamshamana, Arkadi.

Properties : Rasa - Tikta, Katu; Guna - Laghu, Snigdha; Virya - Ushna and Vipaka - Katu.

Pharmacological Actions : Kaphavatashamaka, Rasayana.

Indications : Kushta, Krimi, Visha, Shwitra, Shoola, Bhutagraha, Vataroga, Vrana.

Therapeutic Uses :

1. Freckles : (a) The fruit kernel pounded with cold water and used as paste on face for 21 days makes it free from freckles. (G.N.)
   (b) The fruit pulp is pounded with water and made into a paste. It is applied on face as cosmetic. (V.J.)
2. Chronic ulcer : Oil of ingudi is used in chronic and infected ulcer. (S.S.)
3. Rat poisoning : One should take paste of sirisha and ingudi fruit pulp mixed with honey. (S.S.)

Parts Used : Bark, Fruit, Seed, Seed oil, Leaves.

Preparations & Dosage : Decoction 50-100 ml.; Fruit pulp 3-6 gm.; Seed powder 3-6 gm.; Seed oil 5-10 drops.

कृमिघ्नमिङ्गुदीतैलमीषतिक्तं तथा लघु ।
कुष्ठामयकृमिहरं दृष्टीशुक्रबलापहम् ॥ सु०सु०

54
BOLA

Commiphora myrrha Family : Burseraceae

Chief Characters :

1. Tree growing upto 3 m. height.
2. On incision gum exudes from the trunk. This resinous material is known as bola.

Synonyms : Gandharasa, Pinda, Prana, Goparasa.

Properties : Rasa - Tikta, Katu, Kashaya; Guna - Laghu, Ruksha; Virya - Ushna and Vipaka - Katu.

Pharmacological Actions : Kaphapittahara.

Indications : Pradara, Vatarakta, Parshwashoola, Vataroga.

Therapeutic Uses :

1. Its paste is useful as an ointment in sandhivata, vatarakta and grudhrasi.
2. Dental disorders and stomatitis : It is useful for gargling.

Parts Used : Gum.

Preparations & Dosage : Powder ½-1 gm.

बोलं तु कटुतिक्तोष्णं कषायं रक्तदोषनुत् ।
कफपित्तामयान् हन्ति प्रदरारिरुजापहम् ॥ रा०नि०

55
ŚALLAKĪ

Boswellia serrata Family : Burseraceae

Chief Characters :

1. A big tree.
2. Imparipinnate compound leaf, alternate phyllotaxy.
3. Small white coloured flowers in panicles.
4. Fruit - drupe.

Synonyms : Gajabhakshya, Susrava, Suvaha, Surabhi, Rasa, Maherushna, Kunduruki, Vallaki, Bahusrava.

Guna :

Charaka : Pureeshavirajaneeya.
Sushrata : Nyagrodhadi.

Properties : Rasa - Kashaya, Tikta, Madhura; Guna - Laghu, Ruksha; Virya - Sheeta and Vipaka - Katu.

Pharmacological Actions : Pittasleshmahara, Grahi.

Indications : Atisara, Raktapitta, Vrana, Arshas, Kushta.

Therapeutic Uses :

1. The bark powder taken with madhu and ghrita relieves shwasa. (C. Ch. 21)
2. Shallaki swarasa taken with sharkara and madhu relieve atisara (S.U. 40)
3. Powder of sallaki fruit should be applied to wound and then bandaged. (S.S.)

Parts Used : Bark, Gum.

Preparations & Dosage : Bark decoction 50-100 ml.; Gum 1-3 gm.

Niryasa of shallaki is known as kunduru.

शल्लकी तिक्तमधुरा कषाया ग्राहिणी परा ।
कुष्ठास्रकफवातार्शोव्रणदोषार्त्तिनाशिनी ॥ भा०प्र०

56

KUṄDURU (ŚALLAKĪ)

Boswellia serrata Roxb. Family : Burseraceae

Synonyms : Mukunda, Kunda, Sugandha, Susrava, Gajabhakshya.

Pharmacological Actions : Kaphapittahara, Grahi, Twachya.

Indications : Kushta, Jwara, Mukharoga, Raktapitta, Vrana, Amavata, Atisara.

कुन्दुरुः कटुकस्तिक्तो वातश्लेष्मामयापहः ।
पाने लेपे च शिशिरः प्रदरामयशान्तिकृत् ॥ ध०नि०

57
MĀṀSAROHIṆĪ

Soymida febrifuga Family : Meliaceae

Chief Characters :

1. Tree.
2. Paripinnate compound leaf, opposite phyllotaxy.
3. Green coloured flowers, panicle inflorescence.
4. Fruit - capsule.

Synonyms : Vasa, Atiruha, Vritta, Charmakasa, Tikata, Vikasa, Praharavalli, Viravati.

Properties : Rasa - Kashaya, Katu; Guna - Laghu, Ruksha; Virya - Sheeta and Vipaka - Katu.

Pharmacological Actions : Tridoshahara, Vrishya, Sara.

Indications : Vishama jwara, Atisara, Raktapitta.

Therapeutic Uses :

1. Wounds : Its decoction is useful for cleaning the wounds.
2. Dental disorders : Its decoction is useful for gargling.
3. Malaria : Syrup made from its bark should be given in the dosage of 25 ml. three times a day.
4. Muscular dystrophy : The intake of bark powder (3 gm.) thrice daily controls the disease condition.

Parts Used : Bark.

Preparations & Dosage : Powder 3-6 gm.; Decoction 25-50 ml.

स्यान्मांसरोहिणी वृष्या सरा दोषत्रयापहा ।
रसे पाके तु कटुका तुवरा शीतला च सा ॥ भा० प्र०

58
BADARA

Ziziphus mauritiana Lamk. Family : Rhamnaceae

Chief Characters :

1. Tree grows upto 10 m. height, covered with thorns.
2. Round or oval shaped simple leaf, alternate phyllotaxy.
3. Light yellow coloured flowers arranged in fascicles.
4. Fruit - drupe.

Synonyms : Badari, Ajapriya.

Properties : Rasa - Madhura, Amla; Guna - Guru, Snigdha; Virya - Sheeta and Vipaka - Madhura.

Pharmacological Actions : Vatapittahara, Hridya.

Indications : Jwara, Atisara, Hikka, Pradara, Udarda, Sthoulya.

Therapeutic Uses :

1. Obesity : Liquid gruel mixed with sour gruel and paste of badari leaves alleviates obesity. (C.D.)
2. Daha (Burning sensation) : Paste of the badari seeds should be taken along with water. (V.S.)
3. Pradara : Intake of badara powder with jaggery checks pradara. (V.M.)
4. Raktatisara : Paste of badari root mixed with that of tila and added with honey and milk checks diarrhoea with blood. (S.G.)

Parts Used : Leaf, Fruit, Root, Bark.

Preparations & Dosage : Powder 3-5 gm.; Paste 5-10 gm.

बदरं मधुरं स्निग्धं भेदनं वातपित्तजित् ।
तच्छुष्कं कफवातघ्नं पित्ते न च विरुध्यते ॥ चरक०

59
UNNĀVA

Zizyphus sativa Gaertn. Family : Rhamnaceae

Chief Characters :

1. Tree grows upto 10 m. height consists of small thorns.
2. Simple leaf, alternate phyllotaxy.
3. Light green coloured small flowers.
4. Panicle inflorescence.
5. Fruit - red or black coloured fleshy fruit with single seed.

Synonyms : Rajabadara, Souveera.

Properties : Rasa - Madhura (Pakvaphala); Guna - Guru, Snigdha; Virya - Sheeta and Vipaka - Madhura.

Pharmacological Actions : Vatapittashamaka, Bhedana, Brimhana, Shukrala.

Indications : Daha, Kshaya, Trishna, Jwara, Raktapitta.

Therapeutic Uses :

1. Wound healing : Its root decoction is useful for cleaning the wounds.
2. Daha : Juice made from its leaves should be used as anointment to alleviate daha.
3. Swarabheda : Leaf paste fried with ghrita should be given along with rock salt.

Parts Used : Bark, Leaf, Fruit.

Preparations & Dosage : Decoction 50-100 ml.; Powder 1-3 gm.

सौवीरं बदरं शीतं भेदनं गुरु शुक्रलम् ।
बृहणं पित्तदाहास्रक्षयतृष्णानिवारणम् ॥
सौवीरं लघु सम्पक्वं मधुरं कोलमुच्यते ।
कोलन्द बदरं ग्राहि रुच्यमुष्णोच्च वातहृत् ॥ (भा०प्र०)

60
DRĀKṢĀ

Vitis vinifere Linn. Family : Vitaceae

Chief Characters :

1. It is a creeper, grows upto 15 cms.
2. Simple leaf, alternate phyllotaxy.
3. Green coloured small flowers, cymose inflorescence.
4. Fruit - berry.

Synonyms : Swaduphala, Madhurasa, Mridvika, Harahera, Gostani.

Guna :

Charaka : Kanthya, Snehopaga, Virechanopaga, Kasahara, Jwarahara, Shramahara.
Sushruta : Kakolyadi, Parushakadi.

Properties : Rasa - Madhura; Guna - Guru, Snigdha, Mridu; Virya - Sheeta and Vipaka - Madhura.

Pharmacological Actions : Kaphakara, Pittahara, Chakshushya, Brimhana, Swarya, Mutrala, Vrishya, Virechanopaga.

Indications : Jwara, Trishna, Shwasa, Vatarakta, Kamala, Mutrakricchra, Daha, Shosha, Madatyaya, Raktapitta, Rajayakshma.

Therapeutic Uses :

1. The juice of fruit with honey relieves garbhashoola. (V.M.)
2. The fruit paste taken with water relieves mutrakricchra. (A.H. Ch. 11)

Parts Used : Fruit.

Specific Formulations : Draksharishta, Drakshyadi kwatha, Drakshyadi leha, Drakshadi ghrita, Drakshyadi rasayana.

तृष्णादाहज्वरश्वासरक्तपित्तक्षतक्षयान् ।
वातपित्तमुदावर्तस्वरभेदं मदात्ययम् ॥
तिक्तास्यतामास्यशोषं कासं चाशु व्यपोहति ।
मृद्वीका बृंहणी वृष्या मधुरा स्निग्धशीतला ॥ च०सू०

61
ASTHISAṀHĀRAKA

Cissus quadrangularis Linn. Family : Vitaceae

Chief Characters :

1. Perennial herb (climber) grows upto 10 m. height.
2. Simple leaf, alternate phyllotaxy.
3. Violet coloured flowers.
4. Cymose inflorescence.
5. Pea sized red coloured fruit.

Synonyms : Granthimana, Vajrangi, Vajravalli, Asthishrinkhala.

Properties : Rasa - Madhura; Guna - Laghu, Ruksha; Virya - Ushna and Vipaka - Madhura.

Pharmacological Actions : Vatakaphahara, Sara, Pittala, Vrishya, Balya, Pachana.

Indications : Asthibhagna, Krimi, Arshas, Netraroga, Kushta.

Therapeutic Uses :

1. Kanda bhagna : It acts as best vatahara when used in ghrita form with blackgram. This preparation is very useful in fractures. (B.P.)
2. Urusthambha : It is made in the form of puri or pakodi (fried in oil mixed with wheat flour) and administered in urustambha.

Parts Used : Stem.

Preparations & Dosage : Juice 10-20 ml.

Specific Formulations : Asthisamhara taila.

वज्रवल्ली सरा रूक्षा कृमिदुर्नामनाशिनी ।
दीपन्युष्णा विपाकेऽम्ला स्वाद्वी वृष्या बलप्रदा ॥
अस्थिसंघातजननी वातश्लेष्महरा लघुः ॥ कै०नि०

62
ARIṢṬAKA

Sapindus trifoliatus Linn. Family : Sapindaceae

Chief Characters :

1. Tree grows upto 20 m. height.
2. Compound leaf, alternate phyllotaxy.
3. White coloured hairy flowers.
4. Panicle inflorescence.
5. Fruit - fleshy fruit.

Synonyms : Mangalya, Krishnavarna, Arthashadhana, Raktabeeja, Peetaphena, Phenola, Garbhapatana, Reetakaranja, Shitaphene.

Properties : Rasa - Tikta, Katu; Guna - Laghu, Teekshna; Virya - Ushna and Vipaka - Katu.

Pharmacological Actions : Tridoshaghna, Garbhapatana, Grahajit, Vishahara, Lekhana, Vamaka.

Indications : Kushta, Kandu, Visarpa, Visha, Visphota, Ardhavabhedaka (Nasya karma).

Therapeutic Uses :

1. Daha : The foam of the soapnut fruit on external application relieves daha (Sodhala).
2. Ardhavabhedhaka : Nasal inhalation of the foam (4-5 drops in each nostril) relieves ardhavabhedhaka. (N.A.)

Parts Used : Fruit.

Preparations & Dosage : Powder 3-6 gm.

Specific Formulations : Vatari guggulu.

Vatariguggulu (reetaguggulu) is reported to be effective in worts (charmakeela).

अरिष्टः कटुकः पाके तीक्ष्णोष्णो लेखनोऽगुरुः ।
दोषत्रयहरो गर्भपातनो ग्रहशान्तिकृत् ॥
तज्जलं वामकं पानान्नस्याच्छीर्षरुजापहम् ।
अर्धशीर्षव्यथां हन्ति वमनाद्विषनाशनः ॥ नि॰स॰

63
KOŚĀMRA

Schleichera trijuga Willd. Family : Sapindaceae

Chief Characters :

1. Big tree.
2. Paripinnate compound leaf, alternate phyllotaxy.
3. Light yellow coloured flowers, panicle inflorescence.
4. Dry indehiscent fruit.

Synonyms : Kshudramra, Ghanaskanda, Krimivriksha, Sukoshaka.

Properties : Rasa - Amla; Guna - Guru (Fresh fruit), Laghu (dry fruit); Virya - Ushna and Vipaka - Katu.

Pharmacological Actions : Kaphavatahara, Pittala, Grahi (fruit), Deepana, Ruchya.

Indications : Kushta, Shotha, Raktapitta, Vrana, Krimi, Atisara.

Therapeutic Uses :

1. Palita : The seed oil is applied to the hair. (N. A.)
2. Pama : The bark powder mixed with oil is externally applied to relieve katishoola. (N.A.)

Parts Used : Bark, Seed, Oil.

Preparations & Dosage : Decoction 50-100 ml.; Powder 1-3 gm.; Seed oil 5-10 gm.

कोशाम्र: कुष्ठशोथास्रपित्तव्रणकफापहः ।।
तत्फलं ग्राहि वातघ्नमम्लोष्णं गुरु पित्तलम् ।
पक्वं तु दीपनं रुच्यं लघूष्णं कफवातनुत् ।। भा०प्र०

64
ĀMRA

Mangifera indica Linn. Family : Anacardiaceae

Chief Characters :

1. Tree grows upto 20 m. height.
2. Simple leaf, alternate phyllotaxy.
3. Yellow coloured small flowers.
4. Panicle inflorescence.
5. Fruit - drupe.

Synonyms : Chuta, Rasala, Sahakara, Atisourabha, Kamanga, Pikavallbha, Madhuduta, Makanda.

Guna :

Charaka : Mutrasangrahaniya, Purishasangrahaniya, Chardinigrahana, Hridya, Kashayaskandha, Amlaskandha.
Sushruta : Nyagrodadhi.

Properties : Rasa - Madhura (Pakwa phala), Kashaya, Amla (Ama phala); Guna - Laghu, Ruksha; Virya - Sheeta and Vipaka - Katu.

Pharmacological Actions : Kaphapittahara, (pushpa), Vatahara (Pakwaphala), Hridya, Grahi, Mutra sangrahaniya, Purisha sangrahaniya, Deepana, Shukrala, Varnya, Vrishya.

Indications : Atisara, Chardi, Prameha, Hridroga, Raktapradara, Hridayadaha (Beeja).

Therapeutic Uses :

1. Chardi : Sheetakashaya of jambu and amra leaves taken with honey relieves vomiting. (C.S.)
2. Pleehodara : Fruit juice mixed with honey relieves pleehodara. (V.M.)
3. Darunaka : The external application of seeds of mango and fruits of haritaki are pounded with milk relieves daruna. (S.G.)

Parts Used : Bark, Leaf, Flower, Fruit, Seed.

Preparations & Dosage : Decoction 50-100 ml.; Powder 1-3 gm.; Seed oil 5-10 gm.

आम्रपुष्पमतीसारकफपित्तप्रमेहनुत् ।
असृग्दरहरं शीतं रुचिकृद् ग्राहि वातलम् ॥
आम्रं बालं कषायाम्लं रुच्यं मारुतपित्तकृत् ।
तरुणं तु तदत्यम्लं रूक्षं दोषत्रयास्रकृत् ॥
पक्वं तु मधुरं वृष्यं स्निग्धं बलसुखप्रदम् ।
गुरु वातहरं हृद्यं वर्ण्यं शीतमपित्तलम् ॥
कषायानुरसं वह्निश्लेष्मशुक्रविवर्धनम् ॥
मन्दानलत्वं विषमज्वरं च रक्तामयं बद्धगुदोदरं च ।
आम्रातियोगो नयनामयं च करोति तस्मादति तानि नाद्यात् ॥
शुण्ठ्यम्भसोऽनुपानं स्यादाम्राणामतिभक्षणे ।
जीरकं वा प्रयोक्तव्यं सह सौवर्चलेन च ॥
आम्रबीजं कषायं स्याच्छर्दतीसारनाशनम् ।
ईषदम्लं च मधुरं तथा हृदयदाहनुत् ।
आम्रस्य पल्लवो रुच्यः कफपित्तविनाशनः ॥ भा०प्र०

65

TINTIḌĪKA

Rhus parviflora Roxb. Family : Anacardiaceae

Chief Characters :

1. It is a shrub.
2. Leaves compound, alternate phyllotaxy.
3. Panicle inflorescence with green coloured flowers.
4. Fruit - drupe.

Synonyms : Tintidi

Properties : Rasa - Amla; Guna - Laghu, Ruksha; Virya - Ushna and Vipaka - Amla.

Pharmacological Actions : Vatashamaka, Kaphapitta vardhaka, Deepana, Grahi.

Indications : Agnimandhya, Atisara, Grahani, Pravahika, Hridroga, Vataroga.

Therapeutic Uses :

1. Dental disorders : Its hot infusion is useful for gargling.
2. Conjunctivitis : It is used as eye drops.
3. Oedema : Its paste is useful for external application.

Parts Used : Fruit.

Preparations & Dosage : Powder 3-6 gm.

वातापहं तिन्तिडीकमामं पित्तबलासकृत् ।
ग्राह्युष्णं दीपनं रुच्यं सपक्वं कफवातनुत् ॥ सु०सू०

66
PRIYĀLA

Buchanania latifolia Roxb. Family : Anacardiaceae

Chief Characters :

1. It is a tree grows upto 15 m. height.
2. Simple leaf, alternate phyllotaxy.
3. Greenish flowers arranged in panicle inflorescence.
4. Fruit - drupe.

Synonyms : Kharaskanda, Dhanushpata, Bahuvalkala, Rajadana, Tapaseshta, Sannakadru, Chara, Dhanusphata.

Guna :

Sushruta : Nyagrodhadi.

Properties : Rasa - Madhura; Guna - Guru, Snigdha, Sara; Virya - Sheeta and Vipaka - Madhura.

Pharmacological Actions : Pittakaphahara (B.P.), Vrishya (phalamajja), Hridya, Vishtambhi, Pittavatahara (B.P.), Phalamajja.

Indications : Daha, Jwara, Trishna, Udarda, Siroshoola, Vatavyadhi.

Therapeutic Uses :

1. Bark powder taken with honey and milk relieves raktatisara.
2. Milk boiled with priyala and madhuka, checks haemorrhage. (B.P.)

Parts Used : Fruit, Seed pulp, Bark.

Preparations & Dosage : Bark decoction 50-100 ml.; Seed pulp 10-20 gm.

वातपित्तहरं वृष्यं प्रियालं गुरु शीतलम् ।
प्रियालमज्जा मधुरो वृष्य: पित्तानिलापहः ॥ सु०सू०

67
AṄKOṬA

Alangium salvifolium Linn. F. Family : Alangiaceae

Chief Characters :

1. Small tree grows upto 6-7 m. height.
2. Simple leaf, alternate phyllotaxy.
3. White coloured flowers.
4. Fruit - berry.

Synonyms : Ankola, Nikochaka, Rechi, Tamraphala, Deerghakeelka, Peetasara, Gandhapushpa.

Guna :

Charaka : Shothahara.

Sushruta : Brihat panchamoola.

Properties : Rasa - Katu, Kashaya, Tikta; Guna - Tikshna, Guru, Snigdha, Sara; Virya - Ushna and Vipaka - Katu.

Pharmacological Actions : Kaphavatahara, Vishahara, Rechaka, Balya, Brimhana.

Indications : Mushika-Luta-Alarka-Matysa visha, Visarpa, Krimi, Shoola, Shopha, Kamala, Atisara, Garadosha.

Therapeutic Uses :

1. Atisara : The intake of root powder with rice water in the dose of 5 gm. relieves atisara and grahani. (C.D.)
2. Kamala : Inhalation of root paste processed with rice water relieves kamala. (G.N.)
3. Visha : The internal as well as external application of the root paste processed in goat's urine relieves the poisonous effects of rat bite. (A.H.)

Parts Used : Root, Leaf, Oil.

Preparations & Dosage : Powder 1-2 gm., For emesis 3-6 gm.

Specific Formulation : Ankolyadi kwatha.

अङ्कोटो दीर्घकील: स्यादङ्कोलश्च निकोचक: ।
अङ्कोटक: कटुस्तीक्ष्ण: स्निग्धोष्णस्तुवरो लघु: ।।
रेचन: कृमिशूलामशोफग्रहविषापहा ।
विसर्पकफपित्तास्रमूषिकाहिविषापहा ।।
तत्फलं शीतलं स्वादु श्लेष्मघ्नं बृंहणं गुरु ।
बल्यं विरेचनं वातपित्तदाहक्षयास्रजित् ।। भा०प्र०

68
RUMĪMASTAGĪ

Pistacia lentiscus Linn. Family : Anacardiaceae

Chief Characters :

1. Tree grows upto 3 mts.
2. Gum like substance arises from stem and branches and is known as rumimastagi.
3. Flowers in lateral panicle inflorescence.
4. Fruit - 4-5 mm., black, round.

Synonyms : Ruma

Properties : Rasa - Kashaya, Madhura; Guna - Laghu, Ruksha; Virya - Ushna and Vipaka - Madhura.

Pharmacological Actions : Vatapittahara, Deepana, Grahi, Vrishya, Mutrala.

Indications : Agnimandya, Grahani, Chaladanta, Mutrakricchra.

Therapeutic Uses :

1. Oedema : Its paste is applied externally.
2. Parshwa shoola : Its paste should be applied externally to alleviate pain.

Parts Used : Gum.

Preparations & Dosage : Powder 1-3 gm.

रूमजो मस्तकीगुन्द्रो दशनस्थिरताकरः । सि०भे०म०

69
GUÑJĀ

Abrus precatorius Family : Fabaceae

Chief Characters :

1. Perennial creeper, grows upto 10 mts.
2. Compound leaf. Leaflets - 20-40 in number.
3. Light rose coloured flowers, racemose inflorescence.
4. Fruit - 2 cm.; Seeds - round, red coloured with black spot.

Synonyms : Raktika, Kakananti, Kakapeelu, Kakadani, Kakachirelu, Uchchta, Krishnala (Shweta gunja).

Properties : Rasa - Tikta, Kashaya; Guna - Laghu, Ruksha; Virya - Ushna and Vipaka - Katu.

Pharmacological Actions : Kaphapittahara, Vrishya, Balya, Keshya.

Indications : Kushta, Krimi, Kandu, Shoola, Indragupta, Netra roga, Mukhapaka (Leaf).

Therapeutic Uses :

1. Root grounded with ajamutra and applied as anjana relieves andhatwa or timira. (G.N.)
2. Oil processed with gunja seeds along with bhringaraja juice destroys itching, dandruff and other diseases of scalp. (V.M.)

Parts Used : Seed, Root, Leaf.

Preparations & Dosage : Seed powder 60-180 mg.; Root/Leaf powder 1-3 gm.

Specific Formulation : Gunjabhadra rasa.

गुञ्जाद्वयं तु केश्यं स्याद् वातपित्तज्वरापहम् ।
मुखशोषभ्रमश्वासतृष्णामदविनाशनम् ॥
नेत्रामयहरं वृष्यं बल्यं कण्डूव्रणापहम् ।
कृमीन्द्रलुप्तकुष्ठानि रक्तवद् धवलापि च ॥ भा०प्र०

70
AGASTYA

Sesbania grandiflora Linn. Family : Fabaceae

Chief Characters :

1. Big tree grows upto 10 m. height.
2. Compound leaves, alternate phyllotaxy.
3. Red & white coloured flowers.
4. Panicle inflorescence.
4. Fruit - follicle.

Synonyms : Vangasena, Munidruma, Muniputri, Agastya.

Properties : Rasa - Tikta; Guna - Laghu, Ruksha; Virya - Sheeta and Vipaka - Katu.

Pharmacological Actions : Pittakaphahara, Vatakara, Vishahara.

Indications : Apasmara, Vatarakta, Chaturthika jwara, Shoola, Naktandhya, Kshayaja kasa, Pandu, Gulma, Peenasa, Krimi, Pratishyaya.

Therapeutic Uses :

1. Naktandhya : The intake of leaf fried in ghee cures naktandhya. (A.H.)
2. Chaturthika Jwara : The inhalation with the juice of agastya leaf relieves chaturthika jwara. (Vrinda)
3. Shoola : The intake of decoction of leaf or juice of leaf mixed with hingu and lavana relieves shoola. (V.M.)

Parts Used : Leaf, Flowers.

Preparations & Dosage : Juice 10-20 ml.; Decoction 50-200 ml.

अगस्त्य: पित्तकफजिच्चातुर्थिकहरो हिम: ।
रूक्षो वातकरस्तिक्त: प्रतिश्यायनिवारण: ।।
तत्पुष्पं पीनसंश्लेष्मपित्तनक्तान्ध्यनाशनम् । भा०प्र०

71
JAYANTĪ

Sesbania aegyptiaca Family : Fabaceae

Chief Characters :

1. Perennial herb.
2. Paripinnate compound leaf.
3. Consists of yellow, orange, red, violet coloured flowers.
4. Fruit - legume.

Synonyms : Balamota, Jaya, Sukshma moola, Aparajita.

Properties : Rasa - Katu, Tikta; Guna - Laghu, Ruksha; Virya - Ushna and Vipaka - Katu.

Pharmacological Actions : Kaphapittahara, Vishahara.

Indications : Mutrakricchra, Kushta, Krimi, Atisara, Madhumeha, Pleehodara.

Therapeutic Uses :

Shweta jayanti root grounded in water is used in shwitra kushta. (B.R.)

Parts Used : Root, Seed, Bark, Flower.

Preparations & Dosage : Powder 2-6 gm.; Juice 10-20 ml.; Decoction 50-100 ml.

Specific Formulations : Jaya vati.

श्वेतजयन्तीमूलं पीतं पिष्टञ्च पयसैव ।
श्वित्रं निहन्ति नियतं रविवारे वैद्यनाथाज्ञा ॥ भै०र०

72
NĪLĪ

Indigofera tinctoria Linn. Family : Fabaceae

Chief Characters :

1. It is a perennial plant.
2. Paripinnate compound leaf, alternate phyllotaxy.
3. Red coloured flowers, racemose inflorescence.
4. Fruit - legume.

Synonyms : Neelini, Tuttha, Grameena, Kala, Dola, Neelika, Tuni, Ranjani, Sriphali, Madhuparnika, Kleetaka, Kalakeshi, Neelapushpa.

Properties : Rasa - Tikta; Guna - Laghu, Ruksha; Virya - Ushna and Vipaka - Katu.

Pharmacological Actions : Kaphavatahara, Keshya, Rechana, Vishahara.

Indications : Moha, Bhrama, Udara, Pleeha, Vatarakta, Amavata, Udavarta, Mada.

Therapeutic Uses :

1. Root grinded with goat's milk relieves mutrakricchra (V.M.)
2. Seeds taken with honey relieve symptoms of poisoning. (S.S.)
3. Neelini root taken with cow's milk alleviates Wasting. (G.N.)

Parts Used : Whole plant.

Preparations & Dosage : Decoction 50-100 ml.

Specific Formulations : Neelinyadi ghrita, Neelikadi taila.

नीली तु नीलिनी तूली काला दोला च नीलिका ।
रञ्जनी श्रीफली तुत्था ग्रामीणा मधुपर्णिका ॥
क्लीतिका कालकेशी च नीलपुष्पा च सा स्मृता ।
नीलिनी रेचनी तिक्ता केश्या मोहभ्रमापहा ॥
उष्णा हन्त्युदरप्लीहवातरक्तकफानिलान् ।
आमवातमुदावर्त्तं मदं च विषमुद्धतम् ॥ भा०प्र०

73
AŚMANTAKA

Ficus rumphii Blume. Family : Moraceae

Chief Characters :

1. Big tree.
2. Oval shaped leaves with a long petiole.
3. Hypanthodium inflorescence.
4. Fruit - achene.

Synonyms : Peelupatra, Amlapatrika, Slakshnatwak, Yamalappatraka, Induka, Pashanantaka.

Properties : Rasa - Kashaya; Guna - Laghu, Ruksha; Virya - Sheeta and Vipaka - Katu.

Pharmacological Actions : Pittakaphahara, Grahi, Vamaka (Latex), Lekhana, Mutrasangrahaniya.

Indications : Prameha, Krimi, Medoroga, Chardi, Daha, Trishna, Vishama jwara.

Therapeutic Uses :

1. Prameha : The intake of fruits relieves prameha. (S.S.)
2. Arshas : The sitz bath with the decoction of leaves relieves pain due to arshas.

Parts Used : Bark, Latex, Fruit.

Preparations & Dosage : Decoction 50-100 ml.; Latex 10-20 drops.

अश्मन्तकः कषायस्तु हिमः पित्तकफापहः ।
कषायः शीतसंग्राही कफपित्तास्रदोषनुत् ॥ ध०नि०

74
GORAKṢA

Dalbergia lanceolaria Family : Fabaceae

Chief Characters :

1. Tree.
2. Paripinnate compound leaf.
3. White, blue and rose coloured flowers, panicle inflorescence.
4. Fruit - long, brown colour.

Properties : Rasa - Katu, Kashaya, Tikta; Guna - Laghu; Virya - Ushna and Vipaka - Katu.

Pharmacological Actions : Kaphavata shamaka, Vedana shamaka, Deepana, Pachana, Vedana sthapana.

Indications : Shotha, Amavata, Agnimandhya, Dourbalya.

Therapeutic Uses :

Amavata : The oil prepared from its seeds is useful in amavata and sandhivata.

Parts Used : Whole plant, Seed oil.

Preparations & Dosage : Decoction 50-100 ml.

शिरीषपत्रो गोरक्षः कषायकटुतिक्तकः ।
लघुरुष्णः कटुः पाके कफवातविनाशनः ॥
वेदनास्थापनः शोथहरस्त्वामविपाचनः ।
आमवातेऽग्निमान्द्ये च सदौर्बल्ये प्रशस्यते ॥ द्र०गु०वि०

75
MUDGAPARṆĪ

Phaseolus trilobus Family : Fabaceae

Chief Characters :

1. Annual herb.
2. Paripinnate compound leaf.
3. Yellow coloured flowers, racemose inflorescence.
4. Fruit - legume.

Synonyms : Kakaparni, Suryaparni, Alpika, Saha, Kakamudga, Kshudrasaha.

Gana :

Charaka : Shukrajanana, Jeevaneeya.

Sushruta : Vidarigandhadi, Kakolyadi, Laghu panchamooladi.

Properties : Rasa - Tikta, Madhura; Guna - Laghu, Ruksha; Virya - Sheeta and Vipaka - Madhura.

Pharmacological Actions : Tridoshahara, Shukrala, Chakshushya, Grahi.

Indications : Grahani, Atisara, Arshas.

Therapeutic Uses :

1. Mudgaparni, mashaparni, nirgundi churna with honey is used in rat poisoning. (S.K. 6)
2. Intravaginal application of pichu soaked in oil processed with mudgaparni relieves pradara.

Parts Used : Root, Whole plant.

Preparations & Dosage : Decoction 50-100 ml.

मुद्गपर्णी हिमा रूक्षा तिक्ता स्वाद्वी च शुक्रला ।
चक्षुष्या क्षयशोथघ्नी ग्रहणीज्वरदाहनुत् ।।
दोषत्रयहरी लघ्वी ग्रहण्यर्शोतिसारहृत् ।। भा०प्र०

76
MĀṢAPARṆĪ

Teramnus labialis Family : Fabaceae

Chief Characters :

1. Climber.
2. Paripinnate compound leaf.
3. Red coloured flowers, racemose inflorescence.
4. Fruit - legume.

Synonyms : Kamboji, Hayapuchchika, Pandulomashaparni, Krishnavrinta, Mahasaha.

Guna :

Charaka : Shukrajanana, Jeevaniya.
Sushruta : Vidarigandhadi, Kakolyadi, Laghu panchamula.

Properties : Rasa - Tikta, Madhura; Guna - Ruksha; Virya - Sheeta and Vipaka - Madhura.

Pharmacological Actions : Vatapittahara, Grahi, Shukrala, Jeevaniya, Balya.

Indications : Shotha, Jwara, Raktapitta, Daha, Grahani.

Therapeutic Uses :

Cough : Ghee processed with the paste of sharkara, jivaka, mudgaparni, masaparni and durlabha alleviates cough casued by pitta. (A.H.)

Parts Used : Whole plant, Root.

Preparations & Dosage : Decoction 50-100 ml.; Powder 3-6 gm.

माषपर्णी हिमा तिक्ता स्निग्धा शुक्रबलासकृत् ।
मधुरा ग्राहिणी शोथवातपित्तज्वरास्रजित् ॥ भा०प्र०

77
BĪJAKA

Pterocarpus marsupium Family : Fabaceae

Chief Characters :

1. Tree.
2. Paripinnate compound leaf, alternate phyllotaxy.
3. Yellow coloured flowers, panicle inflorescence.
4. Fruit - legume.

Synonyms : Peetasara, Peetasalaka, Bandukapushpa, Priyaka, Sarvaka, Asana, Peetasala.

Properties : Rasa - Kashaya, Tikta; Guna - Laghu, Ruksha; Virya - Sheeta and Vipaka - Katu.

Pharmacological Actions : Kaphapittahara, Twachya, Keshya, Rasayana.

Indications : Kushta, Visarpa, Shwitra, Prameha, Krimi, Raktapitta, Vrana.

Therapeutic Uses :

1. Kushta : Khadira and bijaka are the drugs of choice for kushta. (S.S.)
2. Obesity : Sesamum oil in the morning or decoction of the heart-wood of asana should be taken mixed with honey. (V.D.)
3. Filaria : Intake of paste of heartwood of khadira, asana and sala with cow's urine mixed with honey alleviates filariasis. (G.N.)

Parts Used : Gum, Heart-wood.

Preparations & Dosage : Decoction 50-100 ml.; Powder 3-6 gm; Gum 1-3 gm.

बीजकः कुष्ठवीसर्पश्वित्रमेहव्रणक्रिमीन् ।
हन्ति श्लेष्मास्रपित्तं च त्वच्यः केश्यो रसायनः ।। भा०प्र०

78
ŚIṀŚAPĀ

Dalbergia sissoo Family : Fabaceae

Chief Characters :

1. Tree.
2. Paripinnate compound leaf.
3. Yellow coloured pedicillate flowers, panicle inflorescence.
4. Fruit - legume.

Synonyms : Krishnasara, Vrittapatra, Bhasmagarbha.

Guna :

Charaka : Kashayaskandha.
Sushruta : Salasaradi, Mushkakadi.

Properties : Rasa - Kashaya, Katu, Tikta; Guna - Laghu, Ruksha; Virya - Ushna and Vipaka - Katu.

Pharmacological Actions : Kaphavatahara, Garbhapataka.

Indications : Shotha, Kushta, Krimi, Vastiroga, Dushtavrana, Shwitra.

Therapeutic Uses :

1. The rasakriya of shimshupa relieves gridhrasi. (V.S.)
2. Ksheerapaka of shimshup and asana relieves all types of jwara. (S.U.)
3. Decoction of shimshupa is the specific remedy for vasameha. (S.S.)

Parts Used : Bark, Heartwood, Root, Leaf.

Preparations & Dosage : Decoction 50-100 ml.; Powder 3-6 gm.

शिंशपा कटुका तिक्ता कषाया शोथहारिणी ।
उष्णवीर्या हरेन्मेदःकुष्ठश्वित्रवमिक्रिमीन् ॥
बस्तिरुग्व्रणदाहास्रबलासान् गर्भपातिनी ॥ भा०प्र०

79
PĀRIBHADRA

Erythrina indica Lamk. Family : Fabaceae

Chief Characters :

1. Tree grows to a height of 10 m. and its shoot is spiny.
2. Trifoliate leaves.
3. Red coloured flowers, racemose inflorescence.
4. Fruit - dry follicle.

Synonyms : Nimbataru, Mandara, Parijataka, Kantakipalasha, Raktapushpa.

Properties : Rasa - Katu, Tikta; Guna - Laghu; Virya - Ushna and Vipaka - Katu.

Pharmacological Actions : Vatasleshmahara, Pittahara (Leaf), Deepana.

Indications : Shotha, Krimi, Medoroga, Karnavyadhi, Agnimandya.

Therapeutic Uses :

1. Fresh juice taken with honey is used in krimi. (S.U.)
2. The leaves & amlaki decoction is used in amlapitta. (H.S.)
3. Juice of paribhadra root should be used for avabahuka. (G.N.)

Parts Used : Leaf, Bark.

Preparations & Dosage : Bark decoction 50-100 ml; Leaf juice 5-10 ml.

Specific Formulations : Paribhadravaleha.

पारिभद्रोऽनिलश्लेष्मशोफमेदः कृमिप्रणुत् ।
तत्पत्रं पित्तरोगघ्नं कर्णव्याधिविनाशनम् ॥ भा०प्र०

80
VĪRATARU

Dichrostachys cinerea Family : Mimosaceae

Chief Characters :

1. Perennial shrub.
2. Bipinnate compound leaves.
3. Red, yellow, white coloured flowers, spike inflorescence.
4. Fruit - legume.

Synonyms : Vellantara.

Properties : Rasa - Tikta, Katu; Guna - Laghu; Virya - Ushna and Vipaka - Tikta (B.P.), Katu.

Pharmacological Actions : Kaphavatahara, Grahi.

Indications : Ashmari, Sharkara, Mutrakricchra, Mutraghata, Mut-radosha, Vatajapeeda, Trishna, Yoniroga.

Therapeutic Uses :

1. Calculus : Veeratarvadi group of drugs alleviates disorders of vata, calculus, gravels, dysuria, retention of urine. (S.S.)
2. Eye diseases : In anyatovata, ghee processed with meshasringi or veerataru along with milk should be used. (S.S.)

Parts Used : Root.

Preparations & Dosage : Decoction 50-100 ml.

Specific Formulation : Viratarvadi kwatha.

Note : Bhavamishra mentions virataru's vipaka as tikta.

बेल्लन्तरो जगति वीरतरुः प्रसिद्धः,
बेल्लन्तरो रसे पाके तिक्तस्तृष्णाकफापहः ।
मूत्राघाताश्मजिद् ग्राही योनिमूत्रानिलार्त्तिजित् ॥ भा०प्र०

81
AMLIKĀ

Tamarindus indica Family : Caesalpinaceae

Chief Characters :

1. Tree grows upto 20 m.
2. Paripinnate compound leaf, opposite phyllotaxy.
3. Yellow coloured flowers with red stripes.
4. Racemose inflorescence.
5. Fruit - legume.

Synonyms : Chukrika, Amli, Chukra, Dantasata, Chinchika, Chincha, Tintidi, Tintidika.

Properties : Rasa - Amla, Madhura; Guna - Guru, Ruksha; Virya - Ushna and Vipaka - Amla.

Pharmacological Actions : Vatahara, Deepana, Sara, Pittakaphahara, Kaphavatahara (Pakwa).

Indications : Gulma, Shoola, Agnimandya, Shotha, Kamala, Vatavyadi.

Therapeutic Uses :

1. Pratishyaya : The intake of gruel prepared with the fruits relieves pratishyaya. (C.D.)
2. Dadru : The external application of leafy juice relieves itching in dadrukushta. (V.M.)
3. Asthibhaghna : The fomentation of the gingely oil mixed with the fruit pulp of amlika relieves the pain of the fractured area. (B.P.)

Parts Used : Leaf, Flower, Seed, Bark, Kshara, Fruit.

Preparations & Dosage : Powder 1-3 gm.; Alkali 1-2 gm.; Decoction 50-200 ml.

Specific Formulations : Shankha vati, Chinchyadi lehya.

अम्लिकाऽम्ला गुरुर्वातहरी पित्तकफास्रकृत् ।
पक्वा तु दीपनी रूक्षा सरोष्णा कफवातनुत् ॥ भा०प्र०

82
ŚAMĪ

Prosopis cineraria Family : Mimosaceae

Chief Characters :

1. Tree.
2. Bipinnate compound leaves.
3. Yellow coloured small flowers, spikes inflorescence.
5. Fruit - legume.

Synonyms : Keshahantri, Tunga, Shivaphala, Lakshmi, Mangalya, Sameera.

Properties : Rasa - Tikta, Katu, Kashaya; Guna - Guru, Ruksha; Virya - Sheeta and Vipaka - Katu.

Pharmacological Actions : Kaphahara, Rechana, Keshaghna.

Indications : Kasa, Bhrama, Shwasa, Kushta, Arshas, Krimi.

Therapeutic Uses :

1. As depilatory agent : Ash of kadali and shyonaka, orpiment salt and seeds of shami—all are pounded together with cold water and applied as paste which acts as a good depilatory agent. (S.S.)
2. Piles : Haemorrhoids should be fumigated with arka root and shami leaves.

Parts Used : Bark, Fruit.

Preparations & Dosage : Decoction 50-100 ml.; Fruit powder 3-6 gm.

शमी तिक्ता कटु: शीता कषाया रोचनी लघु: ।
कफकासभ्रमश्वासकुष्ठार्श:क्रिमिजित् स्मृता ॥ भा०प्र०

83
PATRĀṄGA

Caesalpinia sappan Linn. Family : Caesalpinaceae

Chief Characters :

1. It is a spiny plant.
2. Paripinnate compound leaves.
3. Reddish flowers arranged in panicle inflorescence.
4. Fruit - legume.

Synonyms : Patanga, Raktasara, Suranga, Ranjana, Pattura, Patt-aranjaka, Kuchandana.

Properties : Rasa - Madhura, Kashaya, Tikta; Guna - Ruksha; Virya - Sheeta and Vipaka - Katu.

Pharmacological Actions : Kaphapittahara, Vranaropana.

Indications : Jwara, Daha, Trishna, Chardi, Raktapitta, Vrana, Vyanga.

Therapeutic Uses :

1. Rohini : Patranga mixed with sugar and honey should be applied locally in paittika type of rohini. (S.S.)
2. Skin disorders : Anointing its paste in skin disorders and wounds alleviates the condition.
3. Haemorrhage : Its powder when used as dusting powder acts as haemostatic.

Parts Used : Heartwood.

Preparations & Dosage : Decoction 50-100 ml.

Specific Formulation : Patrangasava.

पतङ्गं मधुरं शीतं पित्तश्लेष्मव्रणास्रनुत् ।
हरिचन्दनवद् वेद्यं विशेषाद् दाहनाशनम् ।। भा०प्र०

84
CAKRAMARDA

Cassia tora Family : Caesalpinaceae

Chief Characters :

1. Annual herb.
2. Paripinnate compound leaf, alternate phyllotaxy.
3. Yellow coloured flowers.
4. Fruit - legume.

Synonyms : Prapunnata, Dadrughna, Meshalochana, Edagaja, Punnata, Chakri.

Properties : Rasa - Katu, Madhura; Guna - Laghu, Ruksha; Virya - Sheeta, Ushna (Phala) and Vipaka - Katu.

Pharmacological Actions : Pittavatahara (B.P.), Hridya, Medhohara, Kaphavatahara (D.N.).

Indications : Dadrukushta, Kandu, Krimi, Kasa, Shwasa, Gulma.

Therapeutic Uses :

1. Dadrukushta : Seeds of edagaja and mulaka applied externally in dadrukushta.
2. Sidhma kushta : External application of cakramarda, sarjarasa etc. mixed with sour gruel is a remedy for sidhma kushta. (C.S.)

Parts Used : Root, Leaf.

Preparations & Dosage : Seed powder 1-3 gm.; Leaf juice 5-10 ml.

Specific Formulations : Dadrughni vati.

हन्त्युष्णं तत्फलं कुष्ठकण्डूदद्रुविषानिलान् ।
गुल्मकासकृमिश्वासनाशनं कटुकं स्मृतम् ॥ भा०प्र०

85
KĀSAMARDA

Cassia occidentalis Linn. Family : Caesalpinaceae

Chief Characters :

1. Herb grows upto 2 m. height.
2. Paripinnate compound leaf, alternate phyllotaxy.
3. Yellow coloured flowers, corymb inflorescence.
4. Fruit - ash coloured legume.

Synonyms : Kasari, Karkasa, Arimarda.

Gana :

Sushruta : Surasadigana.

Properties : Rasa - Tikta, Madhura, Katu; Guna - Laghu, Ruksha; Virya - Ushna and Vipaka - Katu.

Pharmacological Actions : Kaphapittahara, Anulomana, Deepana, Pachana, Vrishya.

Indications : Prameha, Kushta, Krimi, Jwara, Hikka, Kasa, Shwasa, Sidhma, Shlipada, Vicharchika.

Therapeutic Uses :

1. Hikka & Shwasa : The gruel prepared with leaves relieves hiccough and breathlessness. (C.S.)
2. Dadru-Kitibha : The root pounded with souveera is externally applied. (C.D.)
3. Vataja sleepada : The root powder should be internally administered with milk. (Vangasena)

Parts Used : Leaf, Seed, Bark, Leaf.

Preparations & Dosage : Decoction 40-80 ml.; Seed powder 3-6 gm.; Leaf juice 10-20 ml.

कासमर्दः सुतिक्तः स्यान्मधुरः कफवातजित् ।
विशेषतः पित्तहरः पाचनः कण्ठशोधनः ।। ध०नि०

86
METHIKĀ

Trigonella foenumgraecum Family : Fabaceae

Chief Characters :

1. Annual herb.
2. Trifoliate compound leaf.
3. Yellow coloured flowers, racemose inflorescence.
4. Fruit - legume.

Synonyms : Peetabheeja, Methi, Methini, Deepani, Bahupatrika, Bahubeeja, Jyoti, Gandhaphala, Vallari, Chandrika, Mantha, Mishrapushpa, Kairavi, Bahuparni.

Properties : Rasa - Katu; Guna - Laghu, Snigdha; Virya - Ushna and Vipaka - Katu.

Pharmacological Actions : Vatakaphahara, Deepana, Raktapittaprakopaka.

Indications : Jwara, Aruchi, Shoola.

Therapeutic Uses :

1. Pravahika : Methika soaked in curd relieves pravahika.
2. Diabetes : In recent researches methika is found to process hypoglycaemic action. Methika powder (25 gm/ day) controls diabetes mellitus.

Parts Used : Seed, Whole plant.

Preparations & Dosage : Seed powder 1-3 gm.

मेथिका वातशमनी श्लेष्मघ्नी ज्वरनाशिनी ।
ततः स्वल्पगुणा वन्या वाजीनां सा तु पूजिता ॥ भा०प्र०

87
RAKTACANDANA

Pterocarpus santalinus Family : Fabaceae

Chief Characters :

1. Tree.
2. Paripinnate compound leaf.
3. Yellow coloured flowers, panicle inflorescence.
4. Fruit - leegume.

Synonyms : Raktanga, Kshudrachandana, Tilaparna, Raktasara, Pravalaphala.

Properties : Rasa - Tikta, Madhura; Guna - Guru, Ruksha; Virya - Sheeta and Vipaka - Katu.

Pharmacological Actions : Pittahara, Chakshushya, Vrishya.

Indications : Chardi, Trishna, Raktapitta, Jwara, Vrana, Visha, Kasa, Bhrama, Daha.

Therapeutic Uses :

1. Hiccough : Raktacandana pounded with breast milk, warm ghee, powdered rocksalt with water checks hiccough by taking as snuff. (S.S.)
2. Freckles : Raktacandana, manjistha, kushta, lodhra, priyangu, buds of vata and masura—as an external application destroy freckles etc. and promote lustre of face. (A.H.)
3. Defects of vision : Raktacandana pounded with water, ghee, honey and oil each for a week and applied as collyrium alleviates defects of vision. (B.S.)

Parts Used : Heartwood.

Preparations & Dosage : Powder 3-6 gm.

रक्तं शीतं गुरु स्वादु च्छर्दितृष्णास्रपित्तहृत् ।
तिक्तं नेत्रहितं वृष्यं ज्वरव्रणविषापहम् ॥ भा०प्र०

88
VIDĀRĪ

Pueraria tuberosa DC. Family : Fabaceae

Chief Characters :

1. Perennial climber.
2. Paripinnate compound leaf, oval leaflets lower surface covered with white hairs.
3. Blue coloured flowers, racemose inflorescence.
4. Fruit - legume.

Synonyms : Ikshugandha, Swadukanda.

Properties : Rasa - Madhura; Guna - Guru, Snigdha; Virya - Sheeta and Vipaka - Madhura.

Pharmacological Actions : Vatapittashamaka, Balya, Brimhaniya, Shukrala, Stanyajanana, Mutrala, Varnya.

Indications : Vishmajwara, Daha, Shukrameha, Kshaya, Mutrakricchra.

Therapeutic Uses :

1. As aphrodisiac : Intake of the powder of vidari impregnated with its own juice and mixed with ghee and honey acts as aphrodisiac. (S.S. Ci.)
2. Colic : Juice of vidari mixed with juice of trayamana, draksa and sugar removes pittaja shoola immediately. (V.M.)
3. Dysuria : Ghee and milk cooked with vidari is useful in discolouration of urine and dysuria. (C.S. Ci.)

Parts Used : Tuber.

Preparations & Dosage : Powder 3-6 gm.

Specific Formulations : Shatavaryadi churna, Vidari churna.

विदारी मधुरा स्निग्धा बृंहणी स्तन्यशुक्रदा ।
शीता स्वर्या मूत्रला च जीवनी बलवर्णदा ॥
गुरुः पित्तास्रपवनदाहान् हन्ति रसायनम् ॥ भा०प्र०

89
CAKṢUṢYA

Cassia absus Family : Caesalpinaceae

Chief Characters :

1. Annual herb.
2. Paripinnate compound leaf, alternate phyllotaxy.
3. Reddish yellow coloured flowers, racemose inflorescence.
4. Fruit - legume.

Synonyms : Prapaundarika, Paudarya, Kuluthika, Kulali.

Properties : Rasa - Madhura, Tikta, Kashaya; Guna - Laghu, Ruksha; Virya - Sheeta and Vipaka - Katu, Madhura.

Pharmacological Actions : Pittakaphahara, Varnya, Chakshushya, Shukrala.

Indications : Arshas, Vibandha, Shoola, Kandu, Vispota, Visha.

Therapeutic Uses :

Cakshushya seeds are put in a cloth-pouch and steamed in cow dung juice. Then they are dehusked and powdered. This powder used as collyrium in night alleviates inflammation of eyes. (A.H.)

Parts Used : Seed.

Preparations & Dosage : Powder 1-3 gm.

चक्षुष्या दृक्प्रसादा च सैव प्रोक्ता कुलत्थिका ।
कुलाली लोचनहिता कुम्भकारी मलापहा ॥
हिमा प्रोक्ता कषाया च विषं स्थावरजङ्गमम् ।
छिनत्ति योजिता सम्यक् नेत्रस्रावाननेकशः ॥
सा च विस्फोटकण्ड्वर्तिव्रणदोषनिबर्हणी ॥ ध०नि०

90
KULATTHA

Dolichos biflorus Linn. Family : Fabaceae

Chief Characters :

1. Annual herb, grows upto 1 m. height.
2. Trifoliate compound leaf.
3. Light yellow coloured flowers.
4. Fruit - legume.

Synonyms : Kuluthika, Tamrabeeja.

Gana :

Charaka : Swedopaga.

Properties : Rasa - Tikta, Kashaya; Guna - Laghu, Ruksha; Virya - Ushna and Vipaka - Katu.

Pharmacological Actions : Kaphavatahara, Vidahi, Medhohara, Sweda sangrahika, Shukrahara.

Indications : Ashmari, Shwasa, Kasa, Hikka, Krimi, Jwara, Peenasa, Medoroga.

Therapeutic Uses :

1. Sikatameha : Kulatha kashaya is useful in ashmari, sharkara and shukrashmari. (Vagbhata)
2. Sitapitta : Kulatha should be given as food supplement. (C.D.)
3. Amavata : The gruel prepared with kulatha is administered. (Vangasena)
4. Annadrava shoola : The flower of kulatha mixed with curd relieves pain. (Vangasena)
5. Atisweda : Severe sweating in fever can be stopped with the intake of powder. (C.D.)

Parts Used : Seed.

Preparation & Dosage : Powder 3-6 gm.; Decoction 50-100 ml.

Specific Formulations : Dhanwantari taila.

कुलत्थः कटुकः पाके कषायः पित्तरक्तकृत् ।
लघुर्विदाही वीर्योष्णः श्वासकासकफानिलान् ॥
हन्ति हिक्काऽश्मरीशुक्रदाहानाहान् सपीनसान् ।
स्वेदसंग्राहको मेदोज्वरक्रिमिहरः सरः ॥ भा०प्र०

91
TINIŚA

Ougeinia dalbergioides Benth. Family : Fabaceae

Chief Characters :

1. Tree grows upto the height of 13 m.
2. Leaves are trifoliate with serrated margins.
3. Consists of white or rose coloured flowers.
4. Fruit - legume.

Synonyms : Syandana, Rathadru, Vanjula, Nemi.

Properties : Rasa - Kashaya; Guna - Laghu, Ruksha; Virya - Sheeta and Vipaka - Katu.

Pharmacological Actions : Sleshma-pittaghna, Medohara.

Indications : Kushta, Prameha, Shwitra, Daha, Vrana, Pandu, Krimi.

Therapeutic Uses :

1. Raktatisara : The bark of tinisha and shallaki grinded with milk and taken with honey relieve raktatisara. (S.U.)
2. Kushta : Decoction of tinisha is one of the eight remedies for kushta and used as bath and internal medication. (C.S.)
3. Rasayana : Decoction of tinisha should be taken according to the method as prescribed in case of nagabala for rasayana action. (C.S.)

Parts Used : Bark, Heartwood.

Preparations & Dosage : Decoction 50-100 ml.

तिनिशः श्लेष्मपित्तास्रमेदःकुष्ठप्रमेहजित् ।
तुवरः श्वित्रदाहघ्नो व्रणपाण्डुक्रिमिप्रणुत् ॥ भा०प्र०

92
IRIMEDA

Acacia farnesiana Willd. Family : Mimosaceae

Chief Characters :

1. Tree, grows upto 7-8 m. height covered with small thorns.
2. Paripinnate compound leaf, alternate phyllotaxy.
3. Yellow coloured small flowers. Head inflorescence.
4. Fruit - legume.

Synonyms : Vitkhadira, Arimedaka, Kalaskanda.

Properties : Rasa - Tikta, Kashaya; Guna - Laghu, Ruksha; Virya - Ushna and Vipaka - Katu.

Pharmacological Actions : Kaphavata shamaka, Pachana.

Indications : Mukhadantaroga, Kandu, Krimi, Kushta, Vrana, Visha, Kasa, Prameha, Shotha.

Therapeutic Uses :

1. Disease of mouth : Vagbhata has prescribed the uses of the rasakriya (semisolid extract) of arimeda like that of daruharidra, patola, nimba, madhuyashti, vasa, jati, khadira and triphala. (A.H.)
2. Excessive haemorrhage : The powder of the bark of sala, sarja, arjuna, arimeda, mesashringa, dhava and dhanvana should be applied on the part to arrest bleeding. (S.S.)

Parts Used : Bark.

Preparations & Dosage : Powder 1-3 gm.; Decoction 50-100 ml.

Specific Formulations : Irimedadi taila.

इरिमेदः कषायोष्णो मुखदन्तगदास्त्रजित् ।
हन्ति कण्डूविषश्लेष्मकृमिकुष्ठविषव्रणान् ॥ भा०प्र०

93

MĀRKAṆḌIKĀ

Cassia angustifolia Family : Caesalpinaceae

Chief Characters :

1. Perennial herb.
2. Paripinnate compound leaf.
3. Alternate phyllotaxy.
4. Yellow coloured flowers, corymb inflorescence.
5. Fruit - legume.

Synonyms : Markandi, Mridurechani, Bhumivalli, Sonamukhi.

Properties : Rasa - Kashaya, Tikta; Guna - Ruksha; Virya - Ushna and Vipaka - Katu.

Pharmacological Actions : Vatakaphahara, Rechaka, Vamaka.

Indications : Kushta, Kasa, Gulma, Udara, Krimi.

Therapeutic Uses :

Regular use of markandika alleviates kushta. It also relieves constipation.

Parts Used : Leaf, Fruit.

Preparations & Dosage : Leaf powder 3-6 gm.

मार्कण्डीका भूमिवल्ली मार्कण्डी मृदुरेचनी ॥
मार्कण्डिका कुष्ठहरी ऊर्ध्वाध:कायशोधिनी ।
विषदुर्गन्धकासघ्नी गुल्मोदरविनाशिनी ॥ भा०प्र०

94
ĀVARTAKĪ

Cassia auriculata Linn. Family : Caesalpinaceae

Chief Characters :

1. Perennial herb grows upto ½ m. height.
2. Compound leaf, alternate phyllotaxy.
3. Yellow coloured flowers.
4. Corymb inflorescence.
5. Fruit - legume.

Synonyms : Charmaranga, Pitakalika, Akulya, Talapota.

Properties : Rasa - Kashaya, Tikta; Guna - Laghu, Ruksha; Virya - Sheeta and Vipaka - Katu.

Pharmacological Actions : Kaphapittashamaka, Stambhana, Chakshushya.

Indications : Atisara, Raktapitta, Krimi, Kushta, Prameha, Madhumeha (seed).

Therapeutic Uses :

1. Visuchi & Atisara : The juice of root mixed with salt checks cholera and diarrhoea. (Vanaspati Shastra)
2. Bahumutra : The decoction of flowers checks bahumutra.
3. Madhumeha : The intake of seed powder controls madhu-meha. (Kapotabhatta)

Parts Used : Flower, Seed, Bark.

Preparations & Dosage : Bark decoction 50-100 ml.; Seed powder 3-6 gm.

Specific Formulations : Akulyadi putapaka (Basavarajeeyam).

आवर्त्तकी कषायातिस्तम्भनी तिक्तशीतला ।
रक्तपित्तातिसारघ्नी कृमिकुष्ठविनाशिनी ॥
नेत्ररोगे प्रमेहे च तत्पुष्पं तु प्रयुज्यते ॥ द्र०गु०वि०

95
BABBŪLA

Acacia arabica Family : Mimosaceae

Chief Characters :

1. Thorny small tree.
2. Bipinnate compound leaf, alternate phyllotaxy.
3. Yellow coloured flowers, corymb inflorescence.
4. Fruit - legume.

Synonyms : Kimkirata, Kinkirata, Sapeetaka, Abhasatpadamodini, Yugmakanta.

Properties : Rasa - Kashaya; Guna - Guru, Ruksha; Virya - Sheeta and Vipaka - Katu.

Pharmacological Actions : Kaphahara, Pittavatahara (Gum), Grahi, Lekhana (Phala).

Indications : Atisara, Kushta, Krimi, Visha, Pravahika, Raktapitta, Asthibhagna, Prameha, Pradara.

Therapeutic Uses :

1. Diarrhoea : Paste of tender leaves of babbula checks diarrhoea. (C.D.)
2. Guinea worm : Paste of babbula seeds applied locally. (B.P.)
3. Colic : Powder of babbula fruit is slightly heated with in an earthen saucer and then taken with boiled water. It relieves pain in the abdomen. (S.B.)

Parts Used : Fruit, Bark, Gum.

Preparations & Dosage : Bark decoction 50-100 ml.; Fruit powder 3-6 gm.; Gum 3-6 gm.

Specific Formulations : Babbularishta, Lavangadi vati, Abhaguggulu.

बब्बूलस्य तु निर्यासो ग्राही पित्तानिलापहः ।
रक्तातिसारपित्तास्रमेहप्रदरनाशनः ॥
भग्नसन्धानकः शीतः शोणितस्रुतिवारणः ॥ आ०वि०

96
LAJJĀLU

Mimosa pudica Family : Mimosaceae

Chief Characters :

1. Perennial herb.
2. Biparipinnate compound leaf.
3. Light pink coloured flowers, racemose inflorescence.
5. Fruit - legume.

Synonyms : Namaskari, Samanga, Shamipatra, Jalakarika, Raktapadi, Khadiraka.

Properties : Rasa - Tikta, Kashaya; Guna - Laghu, Ruksha; Virya - Sheeta and Vipaka - Katu.

Pharmacological Actions : Kaphapittahara, Sandhaneeya, Pureesha sangrahaneeya.

Indications : Raktapitta, Atisara, Yoniroga, Shwasa, Kushta, Shotha, Vrana.

Therapeutic Uses :

1. Scrotal enlargement : Paste of lajjalu root and vulter's excreta applied externally alleviate enlargement of scrotum and disorders of female genital tract. (B.S.)
2. Snake poison : Intake of lajjalu root counteracts snake poison. (R.M.)
3. Accidental wound : Oil processed with fresh lajjalu root is applied hot on the wound which helps to heals up fastly. (R.M.)

Parts Used : Whole plant, Root.

Preparations & Dosage : Juice 10-20 ml.

लज्जालु: शीतला तिक्ता कषाया कफपित्तजित् ।
रक्तपित्तमतिसारं योनिरोगान् विनाशयेत् ॥ भाव०प्र०

97
TARUṆĪ

Rosa indica Family : Rosaceae

Chief Characters :

1. Thorny shrub.
2. Alternate phyllotaxy.
3. Rosed coloured flowers.
4. Fruit - achene.

Synonyms : Shatapatri, Charukeshara, Laksha, Karnika, Mahakumari, Gandhaddya, Atimanjula.

Properties : Rasa - Katu, Tikta, Kashaya; Guna - Laghu; Virya - Sheeta and Vipaka - Madhura.

Pharmacological Actions : Tridoshahara, Hridya, Grahi, Shukrala, Pachana, Varnya.

Indications : Vibandha, Hridroga, Raktapitta, Daha.

Therapeutic Uses :

1. Wounds : The powder is useful for dusting the wounds. Its paste can be used as anointment in pitta predominant wounds.
2. Perspiration : Its paste when applied externally helps in removing the foul smell from the body.

Parts Used : Flower.

Preparations & Dosage : Powder 3-6 gm.; Gulkanda 10-20 gm.; Ark 20-40 ml.

Specific Formulations : Gulkanda, Ark gulab.

शतपत्री तरुण्युक्ता कर्णिका चारुकेशरा ।
महाकुमारी गन्धाढ्या लाक्षा पुष्पातिमञ्जुला ॥
शतपत्री हिमा हृद्या सारिणी शुक्रला लघु ।
वातपित्तास्रजिद् वर्ण्या कषाया स्वादुतिक्तका ॥ द्र०गु०वि०

98
VĀTĀDA

Prunus amygdalus Family : Rosaceae

Chief Characters :

1. Small tree.
2. Simple leaves, alternate phyllotaxy.
3. Pink coloued flowers, racemose inflorescence.
4. Fruit - drupe.

Synonyms : Vatavairi, Netropamaphala.

Properties : Rasa - Madhrua; Guna - Guru, Snigdha; Virya - Ushna and Vipaka - Madhura.

Pharmacological Actions : Pittavatahara, Vrishya.

Contraindication : Raktapitta (B.P.)

Indications : Vataroga, Prameha, Katishoola, Shwetapradara.

Terminalia catappa (Combretaceae) is known as country almond and being used as a substitute for vatada.

वाताद उष्ण: सुस्निग्धो वातघ्न: शुक्रकृद् गुरु: ।
वातादमज्जा मधुरो वृष्य: पित्तानिलापह: ।।
स्निग्धोष्ण: कफकृन्नेष्टो रक्तपित्तविकारिणाम् ।। भा०प्र०

99
PADMAKA

Prunus puddum Roxb. ex Wall. Family : Rosaceae

Chief Characters :

1. It is a big tree.
2. Simple leaves with alternate phyllotaxy.
3. Rod coloured flowers, umbel inflorescence.
4. Fruit - drupe.

Synonyms : Padmagandhi.

Gana :

Charaka : Varnya, Purishasangrahaneeya, Mutravirajaneeya.

Sushruta : Kakolyadi, Sarivadi, Priyangwadi, Guduchyadi, Ambastadi.

Properties : Rasa - Kashaya, Tikta, Madhura; Guna - Laghu, Ruksha; Virya - Sheeta and Vipaka - Katu.

Pharmacological Actions : Kaphapittahara, Ruchya, Vatala, Garbhasthapana, Vrishya, Varnya.

Indications : Visarpa, Daha, Vishphota, Kushta, Chardi, vrana, Trishna.

Therapeutic Uses :

1. The powder taken with ghee relieves hikka and shwasa. (A.H.Ch.)
2. Its paste can be used as anointment. It relieves kushta, kandu, visarpa and daha.

Parts Used : Bark, Seed pulp.

Preparations & Dosage : Powder 1-3 gm.

पद्मकं तुवरं तिक्तं शीतलं वातहृल्लघु ।
विसर्पदाहविस्फोटकुष्ठश्लेष्मास्रपित्तनुत् ॥
गर्भसंस्थापनं वृष्यं वमिव्रणतृषाप्रणुत् ॥ भा०प्र०

100
PĀṢĀṆABHEDA

Bergenia lingulata Family : Saxifragaceae

Chief Characters :

1. It is a perennial plant.
2. Radical leaves.
3. Red coloured flowers, corymb inflorescence.
4. Fruit - berry.

Synonyms :Ashmaghna.

Gana :

Charaka : Mutravirechaneeya.
Sushruta : Viratarvadi.

Properties : Rasa - Kashaya, Tikta; Guna - Laghu, Snigdha; Virya - Sheeta and Vipaka - Katu.

Pharmacological Actions : Tridoshahara, Vastishodhana, Mutravirechaneeya, Hridya.

Indications : Ashmari, Mutrakricchra, Shoola, Pleeharoga, Yoniroga, Vrana, Hridruja.

Therapeutic Uses :

Calculus, retention of urine and dysuria : One should take nala, pashanabheda, darbha, ikshu and seeds of trapusa and ervaru boiled in milk and added with ghee. (S.S.)

Parts Used : Root.

Preparations & Dosage : Powder 3-6 gm.; Decoction 50-100 ml.

Specific Formulations : Pashanabhedadya ghrita.

अश्मभेदो हिमस्तिक्तः कषायो बस्तिशोधनः ।
भेदनो हन्ति दोषार्शोगुल्मकृच्छ्राश्महृद्रुजः ॥
योनिरोगान् प्रमेहाँश्च प्लीहशूलव्रणानि च ॥ भा०प्र०

101

PARṆABĪJA

Bryophyllum calycinum Salsib. (or) ***Kalanchoe pinnata*** Pers. Family : Crassulaceae

Chief Characters :

1. It is a perennial plant.
2. Reddish flowers arranged in panicle inflorescence.
3. Simple leaves, alternate phyllotaxy.
4. Fruit - follicle.

Properties : Rasa - Kashaya, Amla; Guna - Laghu, Ruksha; Virya - Sheeta and Vipaka - Madhura.

Pharmacological Actions : Vatapittahara, Vrana shodhana, Raktastambhana.

Indications : Raktapravahika, Raktarshas, Raktapradara, Vrana.

Therapeutic Uses :

1. External application of juice heals vrana.
2. External application stops the bleeding.

Parts Used : Leaf.

Preparations & Dosage : Juice 10-20 ml.

पर्णबीजं कषायाम्लं मधुरं शीतमेव च ।
वातपित्तहरं रक्तस्तम्भनं व्रणरोपणम् ॥ द्र०गु०वि०

102
SILHAKA

Altingia excelsa Family : Hamamelidaceae

Chief Characters :

1. Tree.
2. Simple leaves, alternate phyllotaxy.
3. Head inflorescence.
4. Consists of yellow coloured flowers.
5. Fruit - capsule.

Synonyms : Turushka, Kapitaila.

Gana :

Sushruta : Eladi.

Properties : Rasa - Katu, Madhura, Tikta; Guna - Laghu, Snigdha; Virya - Ushna and Vipaka - Katu.

Pharmacological Actions : Kaphavata shamaka, Kanthya, Vrishya.

Indications : Kushta, Ashmari, Mutraghata, Shwasa, Jwara.

Therapeutic Uses :

1. Vata vyadhi : The oil is useful for massaging the affected part. The oil is also useful in skin diseases.
2. Accidental wounds : The paste on external use acts as wound healer.

Parts Used : Gum.

Preparations & Dosage : Powder ½-1 gm.

Specific Formulations : Panchaguna taila.

सिल्हकस्तु तुरुष्कः स्याद्यतो यवनदेशजः ।
कपितैलं स चाख्यातं तथा च कपिनामकः ॥
सिल्हकः कटुकः स्वादुः स्निग्धोष्णः शुक्रकान्तिकृत् ।
वृष्यः कण्ठ्यः स्वेदकुष्ठज्वरदाहग्रहापहः ॥ भा०प्र०

103
DHAVA

Anogeissus latifolia Family : Combretaceae

Chief Characters :

1. Tree grows upto the height of 20 m.
2. Simple leaf, alternate phyllotaxy.
3. Green coloured small flowers, racemose infloresence.
4. Fruit - drupe.

Synonyms : Nanditaru, Dhata, Sthira, Goura, Dhurdhara.

Gana :

Sushruta : Mushkakadi.

Properties : Rasa - Madhura, Kashaya; Guna - Laghu, Ruksha; Virya - Sheeta and Vipaka - Katu.

Pharmacological Actions : Kaphapittahara.

Indications : Prameha, Arashas, Pandu, Kushta.

Therapeutic Uses :

1. External application of oleoresin relieves kushta. (C.Ch.)
2. The bark powder relieves visarpa. (C.Ch.)

Parts Used : Bark, Oleoresin (Gum), Heartwood.

Preparations & Dosage : Decoction 50-100 ml.; Oleoresin 1-2 gm.

धवः शीतः प्रमेहार्शःपाण्डुपित्तकफापहः ।
मधुरस्तुवरस्तस्य फलं तु मधुरं मनाक् ॥ भा०प्र०

104
TILAPARṆA

Eucalyptus globulus Labill. Family : Myrtaceae

Chief Characters :

1. It is a tree.
2. White coloured flowers, umbel inflorescence.
3. Simple leaf with alternate phyllotaxy.
4. Fruit - capsule.

Synonyms : Ekalipta, Malayaja, Girija bhandhava, Sarvatobhadra, Haridruma, Haritaparna, Neelaniryasa, Sugandhapatra.

Properties : Rasa - Katu, Kashaya, Tikta; Guna - Laghu, Snigdha; Virya - Ushna and Vipaka - Katu.

Pharmacological Actions : Kaphavatashamaka, Vedana sthapana, Balya, Ruchya.

Indications : Sirahshoola, Agnimandya, Vataroga, Krimi, Kasa, Pratishyaya, Swarabheda, Vishamajwara, Atisara, Pravahika.

Therapeutic Uses :

1. Fever : The hot infusion or powder of the leaves is useful in fever, especially in chronic fever and malaria.
2. Sandhivata : Its oil along with sarshapa taila is useful for massage in sandhivata.
3. Its steam inhalation is useful in chronic respiratory disorders, chronic cough, tuberculosis etc.

Parts Used : Leaf, Gum, Oil.

Preparations & Dosage : Powder 1-2 gm.; Gum 1-2 gm.; Oil 1-3 drops.

तिलपर्णी पूतिगन्धाऽत्युग्रगन्धा च रोमशा ।
तिलपर्णी कटूष्णा स्यात्तीक्ष्णा विस्फोटकारिणी ॥
विदाहिकृमिशूलघ्नी स्वेदला कफवातनुत् ॥ द्र०गु०वि०

105
HIJJALA

Barringtonia acutangula Family : Barringtoniaceae

Chief Characters :

1. Tree.
2. Rose coloured flowers, racemose inflorescence.
3. Simple leaves, alternate phyllotaxy.
4. Fruit - berry.

Synonyms : Ijjala, Nichula, Ambuja.

Properties : Rasa - Katu, Tikta; Guna - Laghu, Ruksha; Virya - Sheeta and Vipaka - Katu.

Pharmacological Actions : Vatahara, Vishahara.

Indications : Kushta, Atisara, Krimi, Udara, Jeernajwara, Vatavyadhi.

Therapeutic Uses :

1. Diarrhoea : Intake of the juice of hijjala leaves mixed with honey alleviates amatisara. (V.M.)
2. Goitre : Nicula, shigru seeds or dashamula—these are applied as warm paste in galganda caused by vata. (S.G.)
3. Eye disease : The fruit of hijjala applied with water as anjana cures netra srava. (V.S.)

Parts Used : Root, Bark, Leaf, Fruit .

Preparations & Dosage : Leaf juice 10-20 ml.; Fruit powder 3-6 gm. for emesis.

फलं समुद्रस्य कटूष्णकारि वातापहं भूतनिरोधकारि ।
त्रिदोषदावानलदोषहारि कफामयभ्रान्तिविरोधकारि ॥ नि०आ०

106
MADAYANTIKĀ

Lawsonia inermis Family : Lythraceae

Chief Characters :

1. Perennial herb.
2. Simple leaves, opposite phyllotaxy.
3. White coloured small flowers, panicle inflorescence.
4. Fruit - capsule.

Synonyms : Mehandi, Heena.

Properties : Rasa - Tikta, Kashaya; Guna - Laghu, Ruksha; Virya - Sheeta and Vipaka - Katu.

Pharmacological Actions : Kaphapittahara.

Indications : Kushta, Kandu, Kamala, Raktatisara, Mutrakricchra, Vrana.

Therapeutic Uses :

1. Prameha : In raktameha, paste of madayanti mixed with honey should be taken with cold water. (A.S.)
2. Consumption : Intake of the juice of leaves of madayanti for a month alleviates consumption. (B.S.)
3. Intrinsic haemorrhage : Decoction of madayanti added with sugar and honey checks intrinsic haemorrhage. (G.N.)

Parts Used : Flower, Seed, Leaf.

Preparations & Dosage : Juice 5-10 ml.; Seed powder 1-3 gm.

मदयन्ती लघू रूक्षा कषाया तिक्तशीतला ।
कफपित्तप्रशमनी कुष्ठघ्नी सा प्रकीर्त्तिता ॥
निहन्ति ज्वरकण्डूतिदाहासृक्पित्तकामला: ।
रक्तातीसारहद्रोगमूत्रकृच्छ्रभ्रमव्रणान् ॥ द्र०गु०वि०

107
SṚṄGĀṬAKA

Trapa bisponosa Family : Trapaceae

Chief Characters :

1. Shrub.
2. Radicle and cauline leaves.
3. White coloured flowers.
4. Fruit - capsule.

Synonyms : Jalaphala, Trikonaphala, Singhada.

Properties : Rasa - Madhura, Kashaya; Guna - Guru; Virya - Sheeta and Vipaka - Madhura.

Pharmacological Actions : Pittahara, Vrishya, Grahi, Shukrala, Kaphavatakara.

Indications : Daha, Raktapitta, Shukra dourbalya, Garbhasrava.

Therapeutic Uses :

1. Habitual abortion : To prevent abortion, the pregnant woman should be given to eat sringataka, lotus seeds and kasheruka. (C.S.)
2. As Galactogogue : Kasheruka, sringataka, lotus stem, vidari tubes etc. should be taken to increase lactation. (S.S.)
3. Intrinsic haemorrhage : One should take powder of sringataka, prached paddy, musta, kharjura and lotus stamens with honey. (C.S)

Parts Used : Seed.

Preparations & Dosage : Powder 5-10 gm.

शृङ्गाटकं जलफलं त्रिकोणफलमित्यपि ।
शृङ्गाटकं हिमं स्वादु गुरु वृष्यं कषायकम् ॥
ग्राहि शुक्रानिलश्लेष्मप्रदं दाहास्रपित्तनुत् ॥ भा०प्र०

108
SAPTACAKRĀ

Salacia roxburghii Family : Hippocrataceae

Chief Characters :

1. Perennial climber.
2. Simple leaves, opposite phyllotaxy.
3. Consists of yellow coloured flowers.
4. Fruit - berry.

Synonyms : Swarnamoola.

Properties : Rasa - Kashaya, Tikta; Guna - Laghu, Ruksha, Tikshna; Virya - Ushna and Vipaka - Katu.

Pharmacological Actions : Kapahpittashamaka.

Indications : Madhumeha, Yakritroga, Kashtartava, Rajorodha.

Parts Used : Root.

Preparations & Dosage : Decoction 50-100 ml.

सप्तचक्रा लघू रूक्षा तीक्ष्णा तिक्तकषायका ।
वीर्योष्णा मधुमेहघ्नी यकृद्रोगहरा परम् ।
रजोरोधं रजःकृच्छ्रं कफं पित्तं च नाशयेत् ॥ द्र०गु०वि०

109
ERAṆḌAKARKAṬĪ

Carica papaya Linn. Family : Caricaceae

Chief Characters :

1. Tree grows upto 6 m. height.
2. Big leaves with long petiole.
3. Light yellow coloured male & female flowers occur on different plants.
4. Fruit - round or oval shaped.

Synonyms : Madhukarkati, Erandachirbhati, Nalaparni.

Properties : Rasa - Katu, Tikta; Guna - Laghu, Ruksha; Virya - Ushna and Vipaka - Katu.

Pharmacological Actions : Kaphavatashamaka, Pachana, Hridya, Grahi.

Indications : Agnimandya, Shoola, Arshas, Shotha, (Leaf) Mutra-kricchra, Krimi, Hridroga, Jwara.

Therapeutic Uses :

1. Mutrakricchra : Its leaf infusion is useful.
2. Hepatospleenomegaly : The milk extracted from unripen fruit should be taken regularly.
3. Vatavyadhi : Its seed and milk should be given internally.
4. Skin disorders : Its milk should be used as anointment in pama, kushta, dadru and other skin diseases.

Parts Used : Fruit, Latex, Seed, Leaf.

Preparations & Dosage : Decoction 40-50 ml.; Latex 3-6 gm.; Seed powder ½-1 gm.

एरण्डकर्कटी लघ्वी तीक्ष्णा कट्वी सतिक्तका ।
वीर्योष्णा पाचनी हृद्या ग्राहिणी कफवातनुत् ॥
एरण्डकर्कटीक्षीरं पाचनं परमं स्मृतम् ।
फलं सतिक्तमधुरं पक्वं तु मधुरं लघु ॥ द्र०गु०वि०

110
TRAPUṢA

Cucumis sativus Linn. Family : Cucurbitaceae

Chief Characters :

1. It is an annual creeper.
2. Monocieous plant.
3. Consists of yellow coloured flowers.
4. Fruit - pepo.

Synonyms : Kantakiphala, Sudhavasa, Susheetala.

Properties : Rasa - Madhura; Guna - Laghu, Ruksha; Virya - Sheeta, Ushna (Ripe fruit) and Vipaka - Madhura.

Pharmacological Actions : Pittahara, Kaphavatahara, (Ripe fruit), Mutrala (Seed).

Indications : Raktapitta, Trishna, Mutrakricchra, Shotha.

Therapeutic Uses :

1. Powder with grape juice relieves caliculus. (C.S.)
2. Retention of urine : Seeds of trapusa 10 gm. mixed with sour gruel and salt should be taken. It relieves severe retention of urine. (K.K.)
3. Intrinsic haemorrage : Paste of trapusa root mixed with honey should be taken with rice water. (S.S.)

Parts Used : Seed, Fruit, Root.

Preparations & Dosage : Juice 25-50 ml.; Seed powder 3-6 gm.

स्वादु पित्तापहं शीतं रक्तपित्तहरं परम् ।
तद्बीजं मूत्रलं शीतं रूक्षं पित्तास्रकृच्छ्रजित् ॥ भा०प्र०

111
KAṬUTUMBĪ
(IKṢVĀKU)

Lagenaria leucantha Duch. Family : Cucurbitaceae

Chief Characters :

1. Annual climber grows upto 10 m.
2. Heart shaped simple leaf, alternate phyllotaxy.
3. White coloured large flowers.
4. Fruit - round or oval shaped with many seeds.

Synonyms : Ikshwaku, Mahaphala, Tumbi, Tiktalabu, Pindaphala.

Properties : Rasa - Tikta; Guna - Laghu, Ruksha; Virya - Sheeta and Vipaka - Katu.

Pharmacological Actions : Kaphapittahara, Hridya, Vamaka.

Indications : Jwara, Kasa, Krimi, Shoola, Kushta, Sotha, Shwasa, Dushtavrana.

Therapeutic Uses :

1. Ashmari : The seed powder mixed with honey and sheep's milk administered for 7 days dissolves ashmari. (Vagbhat)
2. Pradara : The fruit powder mixed with honey and sugar relieves pradara. (B.P.)
3. Padasuptata : The fruit pulp applied externally for 3 days relieves padasuptata. (Shodhala)

Parts Used : Fruit, Root, Leaf.

Preparations & Dosage : Juice 10-20 ml.

कटुतुम्बी हिमाऽहृद्या पित्तकासविषापहा ।
तिक्ता कटुर्विपाके च वातपित्तज्वरान्तकृत् ।। भा०प्र०

112
KOŚĀTAKĪ

Luffa acutangula Linn. Family : Cucurbitaceae

Chief Characters :

1. Annual climber grows upto 6 m. height.
2. Simple leaf, alternate phyllotaxy.
3. Yellow coloured male and female flowers.
4. Fruit - pepo.

Synonyms : Mridangaphala, Jalini, Kritavedhana, Rajimatphala.

Properties : Rasa - Tikta; Guna - Laghu, Ruksha, Tikshna; Virya - Ushna and Vipaka - Katu.

Pharmacological Actions : Kaphavatahara, Deepana, Vamaka.

Indications : Krimi, Kushta, Pandu, Shotha, Prameha, Gulma, Pleehodara, Garavisha.

Therapeutic Uses :

1. Mushika visha : The internal administration of koshataki panchanga kashaya relieves mushika visha. (G.N.)
2. Kushta : Koshataki beeja taila is used for abhyanga. (C.S.)

   The intake of cold infusion of the fruit at dose of one tola every day relieves any type of kushta. (Sodhala)
3. Yoniromasatana : The hairs on the yoni should be plucked and seed oil is applied which acts as permanent hair remover. (Rajamartanda)

Parts Used : Fruit, Leaf, Root.

Preparations & Dosage : Juice 5-10 ml.; Powder 3-6 gm.

कृतवेधन... तैलानि तीक्ष्णानि लघून्युष्णवीर्याणि कटूनि कटुविपाकानि सराण्यनिलकफकृमिकुष्ठप्रमेहशिरोरोगापहराणि च । सु०सू०

113
JĪMŪTAKA

Luffa echinata Family : Cucurbitaceae

Chief Characters :

1. Climber.
2. Simple leaf, alternate phyllotaxy.
3. White coloured flowers, racemose inflorescence.
4. Fruit - pepo.

Synonyms : Devadali, Garagari, Devatadaka.

Properties : Rasa - Katu, Tikta; Guna - Laghu, Ruksha; Virya - Ushna and Vipaka - Katu.

Pharmacological Actions : Tridoshahara, Vamaka.

Indications : Jwara, Shwasa, Kasa, Hikka, Shotha, Kamala, Pandu.

Therapeutic Uses :

1. Jaundice : The cold infusion of jimuta used as snuff alleviates jaundice. (R.M., V.J.)
2. Kushta : Devadali fruit is impregnated with snuhi latex seven times and taken in the dose of 125 mg. with milk should be kept on salt free diet. (S.B.)
3. Poison : Devadali fruit should be taken with curd to induce vomiting. This is an excellent remedy for all types of poisons rat bite.

Parts Used : Fruit.

Preparations & Dosage : Powder 1-3 gm.

देवदाली तु तिक्तोष्णा कटु: पाण्डुकफापहा ।
दुर्नामश्वासकासघ्नी कामलाशोथनाशिनी ।। रा०नि०

114
DHĀMĀRGAVA

Luffa aegyptiaca Mill ex Hook f. Family : Cucurbitaceae

[Syn : Luffa cylindrica]

Chief Characters :

1. Annual creeper.
2. Simple leaf, alternate phyllotaxy.
3. Yellow coloured flowers.
4. Fruit - Pepo.

Synonyms : Mahakoshataki, Mahajalini, Mahaphala, Hastighosha, Ghoshaka.

Properties : Rasa - Tikta; Guna - Snigdha, Laghu, Ruksha, Tikshna; Virya - Ushna and Vipaka - Katu.

Pharmacological Actions : Kaphapittashodhaka, Vamaka, Vishahara, Vatahara.

Indications : Raktapitta, Gulma, Udara, Kasa.

Parts Used : Fruit, Leaf.

Preparations & Dosage : Juice 10-20 ml.

गरे गुल्मोदरे कासे वाते श्लेष्माशयस्थिते ।
कफे च कण्ठवक्त्रस्थे कफसञ्चयजेषु च ।
रोगेष्वेषु प्रयोज्यं स्यात् स्थिराश्च गुरवश्च ये ॥ च०क०

115
BIMBĪ

Coccinia grandis Linn. Family : Cucurbitaceae

Chief Characters :

1. It is a creeper.
2. Simple leaf, alternate phyllotaxy.
3. White coloured flowers.
4. Fruit - berry.

Synonyms : Raktaphala, Tundi, Tundikeri, Bimbika, Peduparni.

Gana :

Sushruta :Varunadi.

Properties : Rasa - Madhura (B.P.), Tikta, Katu (R.N.); Guna - Laghu, Ruksha, Tikshna, Guru (B.P.); Virya - Ushna/Sheeta (B.P.) and Vipaka - Katu.

Pharmacological Actions : Pittavatahara, Stambhana, Lekhana, Ruchya, Vamaka, Vibandhakaraka.

Indications : Shotha, Kamala, Pandu, Raktapitta, Madhumeha, Kasa, Shwasa, Jwara.

Therapeutic Uses :

1. Madhumeha : Root, leaves are useful in madhumeha.
2. Lockjaw : Ripe fruit of bimbi along with jaggery should be put in mouth and the jaw should be set in position followed by oleation and fomentation. (B.S.)
3. Worms : Intake of bimbighrita destroys worms located in gastrointestinal tract. (G.N.)

Parts Used : Leaf, Root.

Preparations & Dosage : Juice 10-20 ml.

तुण्डिका कफपित्तासृक्शोथपाण्डुज्वरापहा ।
श्वासकासापहं स्तन्यं फलं वातकफापहम् ॥
तिक्तं प्रसूनं पित्तघ्नं तत्परं कामलापहम् ॥ कै०नि०

116
KĀRAVELLAKA

Momordica charantia Linn. Family : Cucurbitaceae

Chief Characters :

1. Annual creeper grows upto 5 m. height.
2. Simple leaf, alternate phyllotaxy.
3. Yellow coloured male & female flowers.
4. Fruit - berry.

Synonyms : Katilla, Karavelli, Sushavi.

Properties : Rasa - Katu, Tikta; Guna - Laghu, Ruksha; Virya - Sheeta and Vipaka - Katu.

Pharmacological Actions : Kaphapittahara, Bhedana, Deepana.

Indications : Jwara, Pandu, Krimi, Prameha, Madhumeha.

Therapeutic Uses :

1. Vatarakta : The decoction mixed with oil is internally administered. (S.S.)
2. Yoninirgamana : The pounded root is applied intravaginally. (Rajamartanda)
3. Jwara : The intake of fruit is useful in febrile condition. (C.D.)
4. Masurika : The leafy juice mixed with haridra churna is taken internally. (C.D.)
5. Vishuchi : The juice of leaf mixed with oil relieves vishuchika. (B.P.)

Parts Used : Pericarp, Whole plant.

Preparations & Dosage : Juice 10-20 ml.

कारवेल्लं सकटुकं कटुपाकमवातलम् ।
दीपनं भेदनं तिक्तमवृष्यमहिमं लघु ॥
हन्त्यरोचकपित्तास्रकफपाण्डुव्रणक्रिमीन् ।
श्वासकासप्रमेहाश्मकोठकुष्ठज्वरानपि ॥ कै०नि०

117
GARJARA

Daucus carota Family : Umbelliferae (Apiaceae)

Chief Characters :

1. Annual plant.
2. Paripinnate compound leaf, alternate phyllotaxy.
3. White flowers, umbel inflorescence.
4. Fruit - cremocarp.

Synonyms : Grinjanaka, Naranga varnaka, Gajara.

Properties : Rasa - Madhura, Tikta; Guna - Laghu, Tikshna; Virya - Ushna and Vipaka - Madhura.

Pharmacological Actions : Kaphavatahara, Deepana, Grahi, Garbhapataka (Seed).

Indications : Raktapitta, Arsas, Grahani, Atisara, Shotha.

Therapeutic Uses :

1. Asthma : It should be pounded with water and should be given as nasya. (C.S.)
2. Piles : The curry cooked with garjara, dadima and curd and fried in ghee and oil should be taken. It is very useful in piles. (C.S.)
3. Diarrhoea : Yusha prepared from garjara is useful. (C.S.)

Parts Used : Root, Seed.

Preparations & Dosage : Powder 1-3 gm.

गृञ्जनं गाजरं प्रोक्तं तथा नारङ्गवर्णकम् ।
गाजरं मधुरं तीक्ष्णं तिक्तोष्णं दीपनं लघु ।
संग्राहि रक्तपित्तार्शोग्रहणीकफवातजित् ॥ भा०प्र०

118
CORAKA

Angelica glauca Family : Umbelliferae

Chief Characters :

1. Shrub.
2. Paripinnate compound leaf, alternate phyllotaxy.
3. Light voilet coloured flowers, umbel inflorescence.
4. Fruit - cremocarp.

Synonyms : Kshemaka, Taskara.

Gana :

Charaka : Sanjnasthapana.
Sushruta : Eladi.

Properties : Rasa - Katu, Tikta; Guna - Laghu, Tikshna; Virya - Ushna and Vipaka - Katu.

Pharmacological Actions : Kaphavatahara, Sanjnasthapana, Hri-dya.

Indications : Kushta, Kandu, Vrana, Krimi, Vatahara.

Therapeutic Uses :

1. Insanity : Ghee cooked with brahmi, hingu and coraka is useful. (C.S.)
2. Epilepsy : Ghee cooked with vacha, aragvadha, kaitarya, brahmi, hingu, coraka and jatamamsi is useful in epilepsy caused by vata and kapha. (C.S.)
3. Headache : Aguru, eraka, padmaka and coraka all together are powdered and mixed with ghee. This balm applied to the forehead relieves headache. (C.S.)

Parts Used : Root.

Preparations & Dosage : Powder 1-3 gm.

Specific Formulations : Mahapaisachika ghrita, Rasnadi churna.

चोरको मधुरस्तिक्तः कटुः पाके कटुर्लघुः ।
तीक्ष्णो हृद्योऽहिमो हन्ति कुष्ठकण्डूकफानिलान् ॥
रक्षोऽश्रीस्वेदमेदोऽस्रज्वरगन्धविषव्रणान् । भा०प्र०

119
NĀḌĪHIṄGU

Gardenia gummifera Linn. Family : Rubiaceae

Chief Characters :

1. It is a tree and grows upto 6 m. height.
2. Simple leaves, opposite phyllotaxy.
3. White coloured flowers.
4. Fruit - oval in shape with persistent calyx.

Synonyms : Dikamali.

Properties : Rasa - Katu, Tikta; Guna - Laghu, Ruksha; Virya - Ushna and Vipaka - Katu (B.P.), Ushna (R.N.).

Pharmacological Actions : Kaphavatahara, Deepana, Pachana, Vishtambhahara, Vibandhahara.

Indications : Anaha, Gulma, Shwasa, Kasa, Krimi, Dantashoola, Vibandha, Vishamajwara.

Therapeutic Uses :

Wounds : The external application on the wound with its paste alleviates pain. It is also useful in toothache.

Parts Used : Gum.

Preparations & Dosage : Powder ¼-½ gm.

नाडीहिङ्गुकटूष्णं च कफवातार्त्तिशान्तिकृत् ।
विष्ठाविबन्धदोषघ्नमानाहामयहारि च ॥ रा०नि०

120
KADAMBA

Anthocephalus indicusa Family : Rubiaceae

Chief Characters :

1. Big deciduous tree.
2. Simple leaf, opposite phyllotaxy.
3. Orange coloured small flowers.
4. Head inflorescence.
5. Fruit - berry.

Synonyms : Neepa, Halipriya, Vrittapushpa.

Gana :

Caraka : Vedanasthapana, Shukrashodhana, Vamanopaga, Kasayaskandha.
Sushruta : Nyagrodhadi, Rodhradi.

Properties : Rasa - Tikta, Kashaya; Guna - Guru, Ruksha; Virya - Sheeta and Vipaka - Katu.

Pharmacological Actions : Tridoshahara, Vedana sthapana, Vama-nopaga, Kashaya skandha, Shukra sodhana.

Indications : Shopha, Vrana, Daha, Kasa, Visha.

Therapeutic Uses :

1. Raktatisara : The bark and shunthi are made into decoction and administered for 3 days. (V.M.)
2. Mutrakricchra : The milk or ghee processed with decoction of root bark in mutrakricchra or mutra vaivarnya. (C.S.)

Parts Used : Bark Fruit.

Preparations & Dosage : Powder 3-6 gm.; Juice 10-20 ml.

Specific Formulations : Kalyana lavana.

कदम्बस्तिक्तकटुक: कषायो वातनाशन: ।
शीतल: कफपित्तार्तिनाशन: शुक्रवर्धन: ।।
त्रिकदम्बा: कटुवर्ण्या विषशोफहरा हिमा: ।
कषायास्तिक्तपित्तघ्ना वीर्यवृद्धिकरा: परा: ।। रा०नि०

121
HARIDRĀ

Adina cordifolia Family : Rubiaceae

Chief Characters :

1. Tree.
2. Simple leaf, alternate phyllotaxy.
3. Yellow coloured flowers, panicle inflorescence.
4. Fruit - capsule.

Synonyms : Peetadaru, Kadambaka, Vrittadala, Haridraka.

Properties : Rasa - Tikta; Guna - Laghu, Ruksha; Virya - Sheeta and Vipaka - Katu.

Pharmacological Actions : Kaphapittahara, Balya, Varnya.

Indications : Kushta, Krimi, Vrana.

Therapeutic Uses :

Kushta : The paste is useful for external application.

Parts Used : Bark.

Preparations & Dosage : Decoction 50-100 ml.

हरिद्रा तु रसे तिक्ता रूक्षोष्णा विषकुष्ठनुत् ।
मेहकण्डूव्रणान् हन्ति देहवर्णविधायिनी ॥
विशोधनी कृमिहरा पीनसारुचिनाशिनी ॥ ध०नि०

122
TAGARA

Valeriana wallichii Family : Valerianaceae

Chief Characters :

1. Perennial shrub.
2. Radicle leaves.
3. White coloured flowers, corymb inflorescence.
4. Fruit - achene.

Synonyms : Kalanusarya, Kutila, Nata, Nahusha.

Properties : Rasa - Titka, Katu, Kashaya; Guna - Snigdha, Laghu; Virya - Ushna and Vipaka - Katu.

Pharmacological Actions : Tridoshahara, Vishahara.

Indications : Apasmara, Shoola, Netraroga.

Therapeutic Uses :

1. The root grounded in takra relieves sandhivata.
2. Its cold infusion alleviates pain and helps in wound healing fastly.

Parts Used : Root.

Preparations & Dosage : Powder 1-3 gm.

तगरं कटुकं तिक्तं कटुपाकरसं लघु ।
स्निग्धोष्णं तुवरं भूतमदापस्मारनाशनम् ॥
विषचक्षुःशिरोरोगरक्तदोषामयापहम् । कै०नि०

123
DAMANAKA

Artemisia vulgaris Linn. Family : Asteraceae

Chief Characters :

1. Perennial herb.
2. Paripinnate compound leaves, alternate phyllotaxy.
3. Yellow coloured small flowers, corymb inflorescence.
4. Fruit - achene.

Synonyms : Danta, Muniputra, Tapodhana, Gandhotkata, Bhramajata, Vinita, Kalapatraka.

Properties : Rasa - Tikta, Kashaya; Guna - Laghu, Ruksha, Tikshna; Virya - Ushna and Vipaka - Katu.

Pharmacological Actions : Tridoshahara, Hridya, Vrishya, Vishahara.

Indications : Kushta, Raktavikara, Kandu, Grahani.

Therapeutic Uses :

1. Dysuira : Its alkali alleviates the condition.
2. Wound : Anointing the wound with its paste alleviates the condition.

Parts Used : Whole plant.

Preparations & Dosage : Juice 5-10 ml.; Powder ½-1 gm.

दमनस्तुवरस्तिक्तो हृद्यो वृष्य: सुगन्धिक: ।
ग्रहणीविषकुष्ठास्रक्लेदकण्डुत्रिदोषजित् ॥ भा०प्र०

124
CAUHĀRA

Artemisia maritima Family : Asteraceae

Chief Characters :

1. Annual herb.
2. Paripinnate compound leaf, alternate phyllotaxy.
3. Red coloured flowers, homogamous head.
4. Fruit - achene.

Synonyms : Kitamani yavani, Jantunashana.

Properties : Rasa - Katu, Tikta; Guna - Laghu, Ruksha; Virya - Ushna and Vipaka - Katu.

Pharmacological Actions : Kaphavatahara, Deepana, Krimighna.

Indications : Krimi, Agnimandhya, Adhmana.

Therapeutic Uses :

1. Wounds : Its oil is useful for external application.
2. Inflammatory conditions : Its paste is used for external application.
3. Alopecia : Its ash mixed with oil should be applied.
4. Worms : One should take one pill made of it on empty stomach. It acts as antihelminthic. In chronic condition, the same dosage should be repeated after one week.

Parts Used : Whole plant.

Preparations & Dosage : Powder 3-6 gm.

यवानिका यवानी स्याच्चौहारो जन्तुनाशनः ।
चौहारस्तद्गुणः प्रोक्तो विशेषात् कृमिनाशनः ॥ रा०नि०

125
SAHADEVĪ

Vernonia cinerea Family : Asteraceae

Chief Characters :

1. Annual plant.
2. Simple leaves, alternate phyllotaxy.
3. Rose or violet coloured flowers, homogamous head.
4. Fruit - cypsela.

Properties : Rasa - Tikta; Guna - Laghu, Ruksha; Virya - Ushna and Vipaka - Katu.

Pharmacological Actions : Kaphavatashamaka.

Indications : Jwara, Sidhma, Vispota, Anidra.

Therapeutic Uses :

1. Eruptive boils : Paste of sahadevi destroys all types of eruptive boils. (G.N.)
2. Accidental wounds : The wound should be filled up with the juice of sahadevi and bandage be applied for quicker healing. (G.N.)
3. Filariasis : By application of paste of the root of sahadevi and tala, filariasis gets alleviated. (B.S.)

Parts Used : Root.

Preparations & Dosage : Juice 10-20 ml.; Decoction 50-100 ml.

दण्डोत्पला सहदेवी विषमज्वरनाशिनी ।
सहदेवी द्विधा प्रोक्ता श्वेता नीला च पुष्पतः ॥
द्रयं चैकान्तरं हन्ति भक्षणात् धारणादपि ।
निद्राकरा धृता शीर्षे नीला सिध्मविनाशिनी ॥
सहदेवीकृता पिण्डी सर्वविस्फोटनाशिनी ॥ शोढल०

126
MUṆḌĪ

Spheranthus indicus Family : Asteraceae

Chief Characters :

1. Annual shrub.
2. Simple leaf, alternate phyllotaxy.
3. Violet coloured flowers, homogeneous head.
4. Fruit - achene.

Synonyms : Bikshu, Sravani, Tapodhana, Mundatika, Sravanashirshaka.

Properties : Rasa - Madhura (B.P.); Katu, Tikta (D.N.); Kashaya (R.N.); Guna - Laghu, Ruksha (M.N.); Virya - Ushna and Vipaka - Katu.

Pharmacological Actions : Tridoshahara, Medhya.

Indications : Galaganda, Apachi, Mutrakricchra, Krimi, Yonishula, Pandu, Shleepada, Aruchi, Apasmara, Pleeha, Medoroga, Gudashula, Suryavarta, Ardhavabhedhaka.

Therapeutic Uses :

1. Scrofula, cervical adenitis and jaundice : By taking the juice of mundi leaves 50 ml. scrofula, cervical adenitis and jaundice are relieved. (S.G., V.M., B.S.)
2. Suryavarta : Juice and pepper taken with the first bolus of food relieve suryavarta and ardhavabhedaka. (Shodhala)

Parts Used : Whole plant.

Preparations & Dosage : Juice 10-20 ml.; Decoction 50-100 ml.

Specific Formulations : Mundi ark.

मुण्डी तिक्ता कटु: पाके वीर्योष्णा मधुरा लघु: ।
मेध्या गण्डापचीकुष्ठकृमियोन्यर्त्तिपाण्डुनुत् ॥
श्लीपदारुच्यपस्मारप्लीहमेदोगुदार्त्तिहृत् ।
महामुण्डी च तत्तुल्या गुणैरुक्ता महर्षिभि: ॥ भा०प्र०

127
ĀKĀRAKARABHA

Anacyclus pyrethrum DC. Family : Asteraceae

Chief Characters :

1. Hairy shrub consisting of small glands on the stem.
2. White or yellow coloured flowers.

Synonyms : Akallaka, Kallaka.

Properties : Rasa - Katu; Guna - Ruksha, Tikshna; Virya - Ushna and Vipaka - Katu.

Pharmacological Actions : Kaphavata shamaka, Balya.

Indications : Pratishyaya, Shotha, Vataroga, Phirangiroga, Dwajabhanga.

Therapeutic Uses :

Phirangi roga : Parada (½ tola), khadirasara (½ tola), akarakarabha (1 tola) and honey (1½ tola) are to be mixed and made into seven pills. These pills are to be administered in the dose of one pill a day with water to relieve phirangiroga. The individual should avoid foods consisting of salt and sour tastes.

Parts Used : Root.

Preparations & Dosage : Powder ½-1 gm.

Specific Formulations : Akarakarabhadi churna, Akarakarabhadi vati.

आकारकरभश्चैव कल्लकोऽथ ह्यकल्लकः ।
अकल्लकोष्णो वीर्येण बलकृत् कटुको मतः ॥
प्रतिश्यायं च शोथं च वातं चैव विनाशयेत् ॥ शा०नि०

128
ARAṆYAJĪRAKA

Centratherum anthelminticum Willd. Family : Asteraceae

Chief Characters :

1. Annual herb grows upto 2 m.
2. Simple leaf, alternate phyllotaxy.
3. Light voilet coloured flowers.
4. Homogamous head inflorescence.
4. Fruit - achene.

Synonyms : Vanajeeraka, Somaraji.

Properties : Rasa - Katu, Tikta; Guna - Laghu, Tikshna; Virya - Ushna, Sheeta (R.N.) and Vipaka - Katu.

Pharmacological Actions : Kaphavatahara, Krimighna.

Indications : Krimi, Vrana, Kandu, Jwara, Visha, Kushta, Adhmana.

Therapeutic Uses :

1. Kushta : The regular intake of somaraji for a period of one year relieves kushta. (B.R.)
2. Galactogogue : The drug is prescribed for chronic fevers and supposed to be the medicine administered to women after delivery for increasing lactation. (Watt)

Parts Used : Seed.

Preparations & Dosage : Powder 1-3 gm.

सोमराजी कटुस्तिक्ता कृमिकुष्ठकफापहा ।
तीक्ष्णोष्णा विषकण्डूतिज्वरप्रशमनी च सा ॥ द्र०गु०वि०

129
KUKUNDARA

Blumea lacera DC. Family : Asteraceae

Chief Characters :

1. Annual herb.
2. Oval shaped simple leaf, alternate phyllotaxy.
3. Yellow coloured flowers, head inflorescence.
4. Fruit - achene.

Synonyms : Tamrachuda, Sukshmapatra, Mruduchchda.

Properties : Rasa - Tikta, Kashaya; Guna - Laghu, Ruksha; Virya - Ushna and Vipaka - Katu.

Pharmacological Actions : Kaphapittashamaka, Raktahara.

Indications : Jwara, Trishna, Daha, Mukhashosha, Raktaja vikaras.

Therapeutic Uses :

1. Coryza & headache : Its leaf juice or powder when used as nasya alleviates the condition.
2. Inflammation : The hot leaves should be tied over the inflammatory area.
3. Wounds : Leaf juice or paste can be used as anointment.
4. Conjunctivitis : Its leaf juice should be used as eye-drops.

Parts Used : Root, Leaf.

Preparations & Dosage : Juice 10 ml.; Paste 3-6 gm.

कुकुन्दरस्ताम्रचूडः सूक्ष्मपत्रा मृदुच्छदः ।
कुकुन्दरः कटुस्तिक्तो ज्वररक्तकफावहः ॥
तन्मूलमार्द्रं निक्षिप्तं वदने मुखशोषहृत् ॥ भा०प्र०

130
JHAṆḌU

Tagetus erecta Family : Asteraceae

Chief Characters :

1. Annual herb.
2. Alternate phyllotaxy.
3. Yellow coloured flowers, head inflorescence.
4. Fruit - achene.

Synonyms : Sthulapushpa, Jhanduka.

Properties : Rasa - Katu, Kashaya; Guna - Laghu, Ruksha; Virya - Sheeta and Vipaka - Katu.

Pharmacological Actions : Kaphapittashamaka, Grahi.

Indications : Jwara, Raktapitta, Raktatisara, Raktapradara, Shotha, Vrana.

Therapeutic Uses :

1. Bleeding piles : One should take the paste of the leaves of nimba, mahanimba and sahasrasuma in quantity of 40 gm. It alleviates bleeding piles. (S.B.)
2. Gonorrhoea : Tender leaves of jhandu plant pounded with some grains of marica should be taken with water in gonorrhoea and bleeding piles. (S.B.)

Parts Used : Flower, Leaf.

Preparations & Dosage : Juice 5-10 ml.

झण्डुः कटुकषाया स्यात्तिक्ता शीता च वीर्यतः ।
कफपित्तप्रशमनं रक्तसांग्राहिकं परम् ॥ द्र०गु०वि०

131
ĀYĀPĀNA

Eupatorium triplinerve Vahl. Family : Asteraceae

Chief Characters :

1. Perennial shrub grows upto 1 m height.
2. Simple leaf, opposite phyllotaxy.
3. Blue colored flowers.
4. Head inflorescence.
5. Fruit - achene.

Synonyms : Ajaparna.

Properties : Rasa - Tikta, Kashaya; Guna - Laghu, Ruksha; Virya - Ushna and Vipaka - Katu.

Pharmacological Actions : Kaphapittashamaka, Hridya, Vranashodhana, Vranaropana.

Indications : Vishamajwara, Raktapitta, Prameha, Vrana, Raktapradara.

Therapeutic Uses :

1. Vrana : A poultice prepared with leaves is externally applied on wounds for preventing bleeding. (Dravyaguna Vijnana)
2. Rakta pradara : The decoction of the whole plant is adminstered internally in the treatment of raktapradara. (Dravyaguna Vijnana)

Parts Used : Whole plant

Preparations & Dosage : Juice 5-20 ml.

अजापर्णं तु तुवरं तिक्तं वीर्योष्णमेव च ।
कफपित्तहरं हृद्यं ज्वरघ्नं रक्तरोधकम् ॥ द्र०गु०वि०

132
DUGDHAPHENĪ

Taraxacum officinale Weber Family : Asteraceae

Chief Characters :

1. It is a latex yeilding plant.
2. Radicle leaves.
3. Yellow coloured small flowers, homogamous head.
4. Fruit - achene with pappus.

Synonyms : Lutari, Payaswini

Properties : Rasa - Tikta, Katu; Guna - Laghu, Ruksha; Virya - Ushna and Vipaka - Katu.

Pharmacological Actions : Kaphapittahara, Vishahara, Vranaropana, Rasayana.

Indications : Agnimandhya, Yakritroga, Kamala, Kushta, Jeernajwara.

Therapeutic Uses :

Chronic ulcer : Its juice is useful in chronic ulcers.

Parts Used : Root, Rhizome.

Preparations & Dosage : Powder ½-1 gm.; Decoction 50-100 ml.

दुग्धफेनी कटुस्तिक्ताऽशिशिरा विषनाशिनी ।
व्रणापसारिणी रुच्या युक्त्या चैव रसायनी ॥ रा०नि०

133
CHIKKIKĀ

Centipeda minima Family : Asteraceae

Chief Characters :

1. Annual shrub.
2. Simple leaf, alternate phyllotaxy.
3. Yellow coloured flowers, heterogamous head.
4. Fruit - achene.

Synonyms : Kshawaka, Chikkani, Tikshna, Ghranadukhada.

Properties : Rasa - Katu; Guna - Tikshna; Virya - Ushna and Vipaka - Katu.

Pharmacological Actions : Vatakaphahara, Deepana.

Indications : Kushta, Krimi, Vatarakta.

Parts Used : Seed.

Preparations & Dosage : Powder 1-3 gm.

छिक्कनी क्षवकृत्तीक्ष्णा छिक्किका घ्राणदु:खदा ।
छिक्कनी कटुका रुच्या तीक्ष्णोष्णा वह्निपित्तकृत् ॥
वातरक्तहरी कुष्ठक्रिमिवातकफापहा । भा०प्र०

134
KĀSANĪ

Cichorium intybus Linn. Family : Cichoriaceae.

Chief Characters :

1. Annual shrub grows upto 1 m height.
2. Rectangular shaped leaves.
3. Blue coloured flowers, head inflorescence.
4. Fruit - achene.

Properties : Rasa - Tikta; Guna - Laghu, Ruksha; Virya - Ushna and Vipaka - Katu.

Pharmacological Actions : Kaphapittahara, Deepana.

Indications : Yakritroga, Mutrakricchra, Hridroga.

Therapeutic Uses :

Insomnia : Sharbat made from its seeds should be given.

Parts Used : Leaf, Root, Seed.

Preparations & Dosage : Juice 10-20 ml.; Powder 3-6 gm.

Specific Formulations : Arka kasan.

कासनी लघुतिक्तोष्णा कफपित्तहरी कटुः ।
यकृद्विकारे हृद्रोगे मूत्रकृच्छ्रे च शस्यते ॥ द्र०गु०वि०

135

RĀSNĀ

Pluchea lanceolate Family : Asteraceae

Chief Characters :

1. Perennial herb.
2. Simple leaves, alternate phyllotaxy.
3. White coloured flowers, compound leaves.
4. Fruit - achene.

Synonyms : Yuktarasa, Rasya, Suvaha, Rasana, Rasa, Elaparni, Surasa, Sugandha, Sreyasi, Yukta.

Properties : Rasa - Tikta; Guna - Guru; Virya - Ushna and Vipaka - Katu.

Pharmacological Actions : Kaphavatahara, Amapachana, Vishahara, Vayahsthapana.

Indications : Shotha, Vatarakta, Shwasa, Shoola, Kasa, Jwara, Sidhma, Asitivatavyadhi.

Therapeutic Uses :

1. Vatarakta : Decoction of rasna, guduci and aragvadha mixed with castor oil should be taken. (V.M.)
2. Psoriasis : In psoriasis caused by vata paste of rasna, sugandha (gandhanakuli) and nakuli should be applied. (K.S.)
3. Piles : Haemorrhoides should be fomented with warm lump of rasna. (C.S.)

Parts Used : Leaf.

Preparations & Dosage : Decoction 50-100 ml.

Specific Formulations : Rasnadi kwatha, Rasnadi taila, Rasnadi ghrita, Rasna saptaka kwatha.

रास्नाऽऽमपाचनी तिक्ता गुरूष्णा कफवातजित् ।
शोथश्वाससमीरामवातशूलोदरापहा ॥
कासज्वरविषाशीतिवातिकामयसिध्महृत् ॥ भा०प्र०

136
MADHŪKA

Madhuca longifolia Family : Sapotaceae

Chief Characters :

1. Tree.
2. Simple leaves.
3. Yellow coloured flowers.
4. Fruit - berry.

Synonyms : Gudapushpa, Madhupushpi, Madhusrava, Vanaprastha, Madhustheela.

Properties : Rasa - Madhura, Kashaya; Guna - Guru, Snigdha; Virya - Sheeta and Vipaka - Madhura.

Pharmacological Actions : Vatapittahara, Brimhana, Balya, Shukrala.

Indications : Trishna, Daha, Shwasa, Kshaya, Raktapitta, Grahani.

Therapeutic Uses :

1. The gum along with honey used as anjana is used in shukravaivarnya of netra. (S.U.)
2. The kshara of madhuka and bijaka cures raktapitta. (C.S.)
3. Scrofula : Seeds of shigru or apamarga or madhuka sara are useful as nasal inhalation. (S.S.)
4. Poisoning : Snuff of the paste of madhuka sara impregnated with cow's urine should be used as snuff and paste. (G.N.)

Parts Used : Flower, Seed, Oil.

Preparations & Dosage : Flower juice 10-20 ml.; Bark decoction 50-200 ml., Powder 1-3 gm.

Specific Formulations : Madhukasava.

मधूकपुष्पं मधुरं शीतलं गुरु बृंहणम् ।
बलशुक्रकरं प्रोक्तं वातपित्तविनाशनम् ॥
फलं शीतं गुरु स्वादु शुक्रलं वातपित्तनुत् ।
अहृद्यं हन्ति तृष्णास्रदाहश्वासक्षतक्षयान् ॥ भा०प्र०

137
BAKULA

Mimusops elengi Linn. Family : Sapotaceae

Chief Characters :

1. Tree.
2. Simple leaf, alternate phyllotaxy.
3. White coloured flowers.
4. Fleshy fruit.

Synonyms : Madhugandha, Simhakesara, Chirapushpa, Brihat vakula, Shivamalli, Pashupata, Ekashtila, Vaka, Vasu.

Properties : Rasa - Kashaya, Katu; Guna - Guru, Snigdha; Virya - Sheeta, Anushna and Vipaka - Katu.

Pharmacological Actions : Kaphapittahara, Vishahara, Dantya, Grahi, Hridya.

Indications : Shwitra, Krimidanta, Atisara, Chaladanta.

Therapeutic Uses :

1. Seed powder is used as tooth powder. (Sodhala)
2. Bark on chewing chaladanta (loose teeth) become strong and stable. (V.M.)

Parts Used : Bark, Flower, Fruit.

Preparations & Dosage : Bark decoction 50-100 ml.; Flower powder 1-2 gm.

Specific Formulations : Bakuladya taila.

बकुलस्तुवरोऽनुष्णं कटुपाकरसो गुरुः ।
कफपित्तविषश्वित्रकृमिदन्तगदापहः ॥ भा०प्र०

138
PĀRIJĀTA

Nyctanthes arbortristis Linn. Family : Nyctanthaceae

Chief Characters :

1. It is a tree grows upto 10 m.
2. Simple leaf, opposite phyllotaxy.
3. White coloured flowers, cymose inflorescence.
4. Fruit - capsule.

Synonyms : Shephalika, Ragapushpi, Kharapatraka.

Properties : Rasa - Tikta; Guna - Laghu, Ruksha; Virya - Ushna and Vipaka - Katu.

Pharmacological Actions : Kaphavatahara, Anulomana.

Indications : Gridhrasi, Sandhivata, Kasa, Jwara, Shotha.

Therapeutic Uses :

1. Decoction of parijata leaf relieves gridhrasi.
2. Patraswarasa is useful in krimi & jwara.
3. Udakameha : Decoction of parijata is the specific remedy. (S.S, V.M.)
4. Ringworms :Ringworms emerged due to indigestion is alleviated immediately by rubbing with leaves of shephali and applying the juice of the same. (G.N.)

Parts Used : Leaf, Bark.

Preparations & Dosage : Juice 10-20 ml.; Powder 1-3 gm.

शेफालिः कटुतिक्तोष्णा रूक्षा वातक्षयापहा ।
स्यादङ्गसन्धिवातघ्नो गुदवातादिदोषनुत् ॥ रा०नि०

139
JĀTĪ

Jasminum grandiflorum Family : Oleaceae

Chief Characters :

1. Perennial shrub.
2. Paripinnate compound leaves, opposite phyllotaxy.
3. White flowers, cymose inflorescence.
4. Fruit - berry.

Synonyms : Sumana, Chetika, Hridyagandha, Malati.

Properties : Rasa - Tikta, Kashaya; Guna - Laghu; Virya - Ushna and Vipaka - Katu.

Pharmacological Actions : Tridoshahara, Vranashodhana, Ropana, Vishahara.

Indications : Siroroga, Netraroga, Mukharoga, Kushta, Vrana.

Therapeutic Uses :

1. The leaf of jatipatra relieves mukharoga. (B.P.)
2. The juice of patra proocessed in the oil is used in putikarna (CSOM). (B.P.)

Parts Used : Leaf, Root, Flower.

Preparations & Dosage : Decoction 50-100 ml.; Powder 1-3 gm.

Specific Formulations : Jatyadi taila, Jatyadi ghrita, Jatyadi vati.

मालती तु वरा तिक्ता कटूष्णा दोषनाशिनी ।
शिरोऽक्षिमुखदन्तार्त्तिविषकुष्ठव्रणास्रजित् ॥ कै०नि०

140
YŪTHIKĀ

Jasminum auriculatum Family : Oleaceae

Chief Characters :

1. It is a perennial climbing shrub.
2. Both simple and compound leaves present; simple—oval shaped and compound—trifoliate.
3. White coloured flowers, panicle inflorescence.
4. Fruit - berry.

Synonyms : Ganika, Ambashta, Sumana, Jati, Punyagandha.

Properties : Rasa - Madhura, Tikta, Kashaya; Guna - Laghu; Virya - Sheeta and Vipaka - Katu.

Pharmacological Actions : Pittahara, Kaphavatala, Vishahara, Hridya, Mutrala.

Indications : Vrana, Mukharoga, Dantaroga, Siroroga, Akshiroga, Sharkara, Ashmari, Mutraghata, Mutrakricchra.

Therapeutic Uses :

1. Calculus : The root and goat's milk together relieves mutraghata sharkara and ashmari. (G.N.)
2. Diarrhoea : Yuthika cooked with curd should be taken. (S.S.)

Parts Used : Root.

Preparations & Dosage : Decoction 50-100 ml.

यूथिका गणिकाऽम्बष्ठा सा पीता हेमपुष्पिका ।
यूथीयुगं हिमं तिक्तं कटुपाकरसं लघु ॥
मधुरं तुवरं हृद्यं पित्तघ्नं कफवातलम् ।
व्रणास्रमुखदन्ताक्षिशिरोरोगविषापहम् ॥ भा०प्र०

141
TINDUKA

Diospyros tomentosa Roxb. Family : Ebenaceae

Chief Characters :

1. Deciduous tree.
2. Simple leaf, alternate and opposite phyllotaxy.
3. Consists of white coloured flowers.
4. Cymose inflorescence.
5. Fruit - berry.

Synonyms : Sfurjaka, Kalaskandha, Asitakaraka.

Properties : Rasa - Madhura; Guna - Laghu (Amaphala)/Guru (Pakvaphala), Ruksha; Virya - Sheeta and Vipaka - Katu.

Pharmacological Actions : Vatala-grahi (Amaphala), Pitta sleshmahara.

Indications : Udarada, Kushta, Prameha, Atisara, Grahini, Pravahika.

Therapeutic Uses :

1. Diarrhoea : Bark of tinduka is wrapped with kasmari leaves, covered with paste of earth and cooked in mild fire. The juice so extracted is mixed with honey and taken. It controls all types of diarrhoea. (H.S.)
2. Burns : The paste of tinduka bark mixed with ghee should be applied locally. It is an excellent healing remedy for all sorts of burn. (B.P.)

Parts Used : Bark, Fruit, Seed, Seed oil.

Preparations & Dosage : Decoction 50-100 ml.; Seed powder 1-3 gm.; Seed oil 10-20 drops.

तिन्दुक स्फूर्जक: कालस्कन्धश्चासितकारक: ।
स्यादामं तिन्दुकं ग्राहि वातलं शीतलं लघु ॥
पक्वं पित्तप्रमेहास्त्रश्लेष्मघ्नं मधुरं गुरु ॥ भा०प्र०

142
PĪLU

Salvadora persica Linn. Family : Salvadoraceae

Chief Characters :

1. Tree.
2. Simple leaves, opposite phyllotaxy.
3. Greenish flowers arranged in panicle inflorescence.
4. Fruit - drupe.

Synonyms : Gudaphala, Sransi, Sitaphala.

Gana :

Charaka : Virechanopaga, Jwarahara.

Properties : Rasa - Madhura, Tikta; Guna - Laghu, Snigdha; Virya - Ushna and Vipaka - Katu.

Pharmacological Actions : Sleshmavatahara, Pittala, Bhedi.

Indications : Gulma, Arshas, Udara, Raktapitta, Mutrakricchra, So-tha.

Therapeutic Uses :

1. Piles : Fruits of peelu should be taken with buttermilk for a fortnight or a week. (A.S., A.H.)
2. Gulma : Fried peelu fruits mixed with salt should be taken. (S.S.)
3. Udara : Ghrita processed with the paste of peelu breaks hardness of bowels and is efficacious in gulma, poisoning and udara roga. (C.S.)

Parts Used : Fruit, Seed, Leaf, Root bark.

Preparations & Dosage : Seed powder 1-3 gm.; Decoction 50-100 ml.

Specific Formulations : Peelu taila, Peelu asava.

तिक्तं पित्तकरं तेषां सरं कटुविपाकि च ।
तीक्ष्णोष्णं कटुकं पीलु सस्नेहं कफवातजित् ॥ सु०सू०

143
KARAMARDA

Carissa carandas Linn. Family : Apocyanaceae

Chief Characters :

1. Perennial, big thorny shrub.
2. Simple leaf, opposite phyllotaxy.
3. Rose coloured flowers, cyamose inflorescence.
4. Fruit -berry.

Synonyms : Krishnapakaphala, Sushena, Kantaki, Ksheeraphala.

Guna :

Charaka : Hridya, Amlaskandha.
Sushrata : Kantaka panchamoola.

Properties : Rasa - Amla, Madhura (Pakwaphala); Guna - Guru, Laghu (Pakwaphala); Virya - Ushna and Vipaka - Amla.

Pharmacological Actions : Vatahara, Vishahara, Hridya, Pittakaphakara, Tridoshahara (Pakwaphala).

Indications : Trishna, Mutrakricchra, Vishamajwara.

Therapeutic Uses :

1. Its leaf decoction alleviates jwara.
2. It is proved to be useful in scurvy.

Parts Used : Fruit, Leaf, Root.

Preparations & Dosage : Decoction 50-100 ml.; Juice 10-20 ml.

Specific Formulations : Karamarda panaka.

करमर्दद्वयं त्वाममम्लं गुरु तृषाहरम् ।
उष्णं रुचिकरं प्रोक्तं रक्तपित्तकफप्रदम् ।
तत्पक्वं मधुरं रुच्यं लघु पित्तसमीरजित् ॥ भा०प्र०

144
JĪVANTĪ

Leptadenia reticulata Family : Asclepiadaceae

Chief Characters :

1. Perennial climber.
2. Simple leaf, opposite phyllotaxy.
3. Green or yellow coloured flowers.
4. Fruit - follicle.

Synonyms : Jivani, Jiva, Jivaniya, Madhusrava, Shakasreshta, Payasarini.

Gana :

Charaka : Madhuraskandha, Jivaniya, Snehopaga.
Sushruta : Kakolyadi.

Properties : Rasa - Madhura; Guna - Laghu, Snigdha; Virya - Sheeta and Vipaka - Madhura.

Pharmacological Actions : Tridoshahara, Chakshushya, Grahi, Balya, Rasayana.

Indications : Grahani, Atisara, Pandu, Raktapitta.

Therapeutic Uses :

1. Diarrhoea : Putapaka (juice extracted by closed heating) of jivanti, meshasringa and should be administered. (S.S.)
2. Wound : Paste of jivanti should be applied locally for three days. It promotes healing. (V.D.)

Parts Used : Root.

Preparations & Dosage : Powder 3-6 gm.; Decoction 50-100 ml.

Specific Formulations : Jeerakadya ghrita, Jeevaniyadi taila.

जीवन्ती शीतला स्वादुः स्निग्धा दोषत्रयापहा ।
रसायनी बलकरी चक्षुष्या ग्राहिणी लघुः ॥ भा०प्र०

145

MEṢAŚṚṄGĪ

Gymnema sylvestre Family : Asclepiadaceae

Chief Characters :

1. Perennial creeper.
2. Simple leaf, opposite phyllotaxy.
3. Light green coloured small flowers, cymose inflorescence.
4. Fruit - follicle.

Synonyms : Vishani, Meshavalli, Ajasringika.

Guna :

Sushruta : Salasaradi, Varunadi.

Properties : Rasa - Kashaya, Tikta; Guna - Laghu, Ruksha; Virya - Ushna and Vipaka - Katu.

Pharmacological Actions : Pittakaphahara, Vatala, Deepana, Samsrana.

Indications : Shwasa, Kasa, Vrana, Netrashoola, Kushta, Prameha, Krimi (Phala).

Therapeutic Uses :

1. The flowers of meshasringi and neelanjana cure kacha on application as anjana. (S.U.)
2. Oil cooked with bark of mesashringi promotes wound healing. (S.S.)

Parts Used : Leaf, Root.

Preparations & Dosage : Leaf powder 3-6 gm.; Root decoction 50-100 ml.

In recent researches G. sylvestre has shown insulinotrophic action and found to be useful in diabetes.

मेषशृङ्गीदलं तिक्तं कुष्ठमेहकफप्रणुत् ।
दीपनं स्रंसनं कासक्रिमिव्रणविषापहम् ॥ द्र०गु०वि०

146
MŪRVĀ

Marsdenia tenacissima Family : Asclepiadaceae

Chief Characters :

1. Perennial creeper.
2. Simple leaf, opposite phyllotaxy.
3. Pale violet or yellow coloured flowers, cymose inflorescence.
4. Fruit - follicle.

Synonyms : Madhurasa, Devi, Morata, Tejani, Sruva, Madhulika, Madhusreni, Gokarni, Peeluparni.

Gana :

Charaka : Stanyashodhana.
Sushruta : Aragwadhadi, Patoladi.

Properties : Rasa - Kashaya, Tikta (R.N., B.P.), Madhura (D.N., B.P.); Guna - Guru (B.P.), Ruksha; Virya - Ushna and Vipaka - Katu.

Pharmacological Actions : Tridoshahara (B.P.), Sara, Kapha-vatahara (D.N., R.N.)

Indications : Prameha, Trishna, Hridroga, Kandu, Kushta, Jwara, Chardi.

Therapeutic Uses :

1. Bhavana of the powder of murva, haridra and amalaki in gomutra is used in pandu. (S.S.)
2. Murva should be taken with rice water to arrest vomiting.

Parts Used : Root.

Preparations & Dosage : Decoction 50-100 ml.

मूर्वा तिक्ता कषायोष्णा हृद्रोगकफवातहृत् ।
वमिप्रमेहकुष्ठारिर्विषमज्वरहारिणी ॥ रा०नि०

147
KATAKA

Strychnos potatorum Linn. Family : Loganiaceae

Chief Characters :

1. Tree grows upto 15 m. height.
2. Simple leaf, opposite phyllotaxy.
3. Light green coloured flowers, cymose inflorescence.
4. Fruit - berry.

Synonyms : Payaprasadi, Nirmali, Chakshushya.

Gana :

Charaka : Vishaghna.
Sushruta : Parushakadi.

Properties : Rasa - Madhura, Kashaya, Tikta; Guna - Guru (B.P.), Visada, Laghu (K.N.); Virya - Sheeta and Vipaka - Madhura.

Pharmacological Actions : Vatakaphahara, Lekhana, Vamaka, Vishahara, Chakshushya, Jala nirmalikarana.

Indications : Mutrakricchra, Ashmari, Sarkara, Kushta, Kamala, Pandu, Shotha, Pratishyaya, Prameha, Netraroga.

Therapeutic Uses :

1. Kushta : Its root is useful in the management of skin diseases. (Kaiyadeva Nighantu)
2. Prameha : The seeds pounded in buttermilk and mixed with honey should be administered to relieve all pramehas. (Y.R.)
3. Raktabhishyanda : The seed pounded in water and mixed with honey and rocksalt should be applied to the eyes to relieve the inflammation. (S.S.)

Parts Used : Seed.

Preparations & Dosage : Powder 1-3 gm., 6 gm. for emesis.

Specific Formulations : Swarnamuktadi gutika.

पय:प्रसादी कतक: कतकं तत्फलं च तत् ।
कतकस्य फलं नेत्र्यं जलनिर्मलताकरम् ।।
वातश्लेष्महरं शीतं मधुरं तुवरं गुरुम् ।। भा०प्र०

148
TRĀYAMĀṆĀ

Gentiana kurro Royle. Family : Gentianaceae

Chief Characters :

1. It is a perennial plant.
2. Radicle and cauline leaves present, opposite phyllotaxy.
3. Blue coloured flowers, racemose inflorescence.
4. Fruit - rectangular

Synonyms : Trayanthi, Girija, Anuja, Balabhadra, Girirasanuja.

Gana :

Sushruta : Lakshadi.

Properties : Rasa - Tikta, Kashaya; Guna - Laghu, Ruksha; Virya - Ushna and Vipaka - Katu.

Pharmacological Actions : Pittakaphahara, Rechana, Vishahara.

Indications : Jwara, Hridroga, Gulma, Arshas, Bhrama, Shoola.

Therapeutic Uses :

1. The paste of trayamana with milk relieves jwara.
2. Trayamana mixed with profuse quantity of honey and sugar should be used in raktapitta. (C.S.)

Parts Used : Root.

Preparations & Dosage : Powder 1-3 gm.

बलभद्रा त्रायमाणा त्रायन्ती गिरिजाऽनुजा ।
त्रायन्ती तुवरा तिक्ता सरा पित्तकफापहा ॥
ज्वरहृद्रोगगुल्मार्शोभ्रमशूलविषप्रणुत् ॥ भा०प्र०

149
SLEṢMĀTAKA

Cordia dichotoma Family : Boraginaceae

Chief Characters :

1. Tree.
2. Simple leaf, alternate phyllotaxy.
3. Light green whitish flowers, corymb inflorescence.
4. Fruit - berry.

Synonyms : Uddalaka, Selu, Bahuvara, Sheela, Bhuta vrikshaka, Picchila.

Properties : Rasa - Madhura, Tikta, Kashaya; Guna - Guru, Snigdha, Picchila; Virya - Sheeta and Vipaka - Madhura.

Pharmacological Actions : Kaphapittahara, Keshya, Vishaghna.

Indications : Vishpota, Vrana, Visarpa, Kushta.

Therapeutic Uses :

1. The external application of kalka relieves all luthavisha. (S.K.)
2. Nasya karma with oil of shleshmaka prevents greying of hair. (C.D.)

Parts Used : Bark, Fruit.

Preparations & Dosage : Bark decoction 50-100 ml.; Sharbat 10-20 ml.

Specific Formulation : Sleshmataka panaka.

बहुवारो विषस्फोटव्रणवीसर्पकुष्ठनुत् ।
मधुरस्तुवरस्तिक्तः केश्यश्च कफपित्तहृत् ।।
फलमामन्तु विष्टम्भि रूक्षं पित्तकफास्रजित् ।
तत्पक्वं मधुरं स्निग्धं श्लेष्मलं शीतलं गुरु ।। भा०प्र०

150
GOJIHWĀ

Onosma bracteatum Family : Boraginaceae

Chief Characters :

1. Hairy shrub.
2. Radicle and cauline leaves present.
3. Small violet coloured flowers, head inflorescence.
4. Fruit - nutlet.

Synonyms : Gojika, Gobhi, Darvika, Kharaparni.

Properties : Rasa - Madhura, Tikta, Kashaya; Guna - Laghu, Snigdha; Virya - Sheeta and Vipaka - Madhura.

Pharmacological Actions : Kaphapittahara, Vatala, Hridya, Mutrala.

Indications : Prameha, Kasa, Vrana, Jwara, Raktavikara.

Therapeutic Uses :

1. The paste of gojihwa root taken with tandulodaka relieves sheetalatwa (chilly feeling). (R.M.)

Parts Used : Leaf, Flowers.

Preparations & Dosage : Leaf powder 3-6 gm.; Flower powder 3-6 gm.

Specific Formulation : Arka gavajabana, Banfshadi kwatha.

गोजिह्वा गोजिका गोभी दार्विका खरपर्णिनी ।
गोजिह्वा वातला शीता ग्राहिणी कफपित्तनुत् ॥
हृद्या प्रमेहकासास्रव्रणज्वरहरी लघुः ।
कोमला तुवरा तिक्ता स्वादु पाकरसा स्मृता ॥ भा०प्र०

151
ADHAḤPUṢPĪ

Trichodesma indicum R.Br. Family : Boraginaceae

Chief Characters :

1. Annual shrub grows upto 40 m. height.
2. Simple leaf.
3. Light blue coloured flowers.
4. Racemose inflorescence.
5. Fruit - carcerulus consisting of nutlets.

Synonyms : Avakpushpi, Romalu.

Properties : Rasa - Katu, Tikta; Guna - Laghu; Virya - Ushna and Vipaka - Katu.

Pharmacological Actions : Kaphavatashamaka, Deepana, Grahi, Vishaghna, Chakshushya.

Indications : Agnimandya, Grahini, Sarpavisha, Shotha, Mudhagarbha.

Therapeutic Uses :

1. Shotha : The decoction of the root acts as diuretic and relieves oedema.
2. Sarpavisha : The intake of juice of the root acts as an antidote for snake poison. (Anubhuta)

Parts Used : Root, Leaf, Stem, Flower.

Preparations & Dosage : Juice 10-20 ml.; Powder 3-6 gm.

Specific Formulations : Avakpushpighrita (Gada Nigraha).

अध:पुष्पी रसे तिक्ता कट्वी लघ्वी प्रशस्यते ।
वीर्योष्णा कफवातघ्नी व्रणशोथहरा परम् ॥ द्र०गु०वि०

152
VṚDDHADĀRUKA

Argyreia nervosa Family : Convolvulaceae

Chief Characters :

1. Perennial herb, climber.
2. Simple leaf, alternate phyllotaxy.
3. Pink, rose and violet coloured flowers.
4. Fruit - round with 1-4 seeds.

Synonyms : Avegi, Chagantri, Vrishya gandhika.

Properties : Rasa - Tikta, Katu, Kashaya; Guna - Laghu, Snigdha; Virya - Ushna and Vipaka - Madhura.

Pharmacological Actions : Kaphavatahara, Rasayana, Vrishya, Shukrala, Balya, Medhya, Deepana, Swarya, Sara.

Indications : Amavata, Shotha, Arshas, Prameha.

Therapeutic Uses :

1. Klaibya : Aswagandha and vridhadaru powders taken with milk act as vajikara. (S.S.)
2. Filaria : Powder of vriddhadaruka should be taken with sour gruel. (V.M.; B.S.)
3. Urustambha : Powder of vriddhadaruka and shunthi should be taken with hot water. (G.N.)

Parts Used : Root.

Preparations & Dosage : Powder 3-6 gm.

Specific Formulations : Vriddhadarukasama churna.

वृद्धदारु: कषायोष्ण: कटुस्तिक्तो रसायन: ।
वृष्यो वातामवातार्श: शोथमेहकफप्रणुत् ॥
शुक्रायुर्बलमेधाग्निस्वरकान्तिकर: सर: ॥ भा०प्र०

153

KṚṢṆABĪJA

Ipomoea hederaceae Jacq. Family : Convolvulaceae
(I. nil, Convolvulus nil.)

Chief Characters :

1. Climber with a weak stem.
2. Simple leaf.
3. Rose coloured or blue coloured flowers.
4. Fruit - capsule.

Synonyms : Shyamabeeja.

Properties : Rasa - Katu, Madhura; Guna - Laghu, Ruksha, Tikshna; Virya - Ushna and Vipaka - Katu.

Pharmacological Actions : Kaphavatahara, Rechana.

Indications : Udavarta, Malabaddhata, Krimi, Shiroroga, Shotha, Jwara.

Therapeutic Uses :

1. Oligomenorrhoea & dysmenorrhoea : It is useful in inducing menstruation.
2. Lohagandhi nishwasa & dhumagandhi udgara : It should be given in the dosage of ¼ tola along with ¼ tola of mishreya.
3. Uterine involution and lactation : It should be given after delivery to the puerperal woman for proper uterine involution and lactation.

Parts Used : Seed.

Preparations & Dosage : Powder 1-3 gm.

Specific Formulations : Krishnabeejadi churna.

रेचनं श्यामबीजं स्याच्छोथोदरविनाशनम् ।
ज्वरे पुरिषसङ्गे च दारुणे सिरसो गरे ॥
उदावर्त्ते तथानाहे बुधैरेतत् प्रयुज्यते ॥ आ०वि०

154

ĀKHUPARṆĪ

Merremia emarginata Hall. Family : Convolvulaceae

Chief Characters :

1. Procumbent herb grows to 1 m. length.
2. Simple leaf, alternate phyllotaxy.
3. Yellow coloured flowers.
4. Fruit - small capsule.

Synonyms : Akhukarni, Parnika, Bhudaribhava.

Gana :

Charaka : Krimighna.
Sushruta : Surasadi.

Properties : Rasa - Kashaya, Katu, Tikta; Guna - Laghu, Ruksha, Tikshna; Virya - Sheeta and Vipaka - Katu.

Pharmacological Actions : Kaphavatahara, Rechana.

Indications : Krimi, Mutraroga, Kaphajaroga, Kushta, Shoola, Prameha, Vandhyatwa, Apasmara, Jwara.

Therapeutic Uses :

1. Vandhyatwa : The root of akhuparni should be inserted locally into vagina to relieve garbha dosha. (G.N.)
2. Apasmara : The juice of akhuparni, shankapushpi, kushta and vacha should be boiled with ghee and administered internally to treat apasmara and unmada. (Chikitsakalika)

Parts Used : Whole plant.

Preparations & Dosage : Juice 10-20 ml.

Specific Formulations : Akhuparni kwatha, Karpasadi taila.

आखुकर्णी कटुस्तिक्ता लघ्व्युष्णा कफवातहृत् ।
कुष्ठामज्वरशूलार्तिप्रमेहा क्रिमिनुत् सरा ॥ द्र०गु०वि०

155
AMARAVALLĪ

Cuscuta reflexa Roxb. Family : Convolvulaceae

Chief Characters :

1. Leafless parasitic plant, climber.
2. Yellow coloured plant with branches.
3. White or rose coloured flowers arranged in groups.
4. Fruit - dehiscent capsule.

Synonyms : Khavalli, Akashavalli, Vrishyavalli.

Properties : Rasa - Tikta, Kashaya; Guna - Picchila; Virya - Sheeta and Vipaka - Katu.

Pharmacological Actions : Pittakaphahara, Deepana, Grahi, Amahara, Hridya.

Indications : Netraroga, Agnimandya, Grahini, Pravahika, Amlapitta, Krimi, Amavata.

Therapeutic Uses :

1. Sotha : The seed powder is externally applied to relieve colic. (N.A.)
2. Vibandha : The intake of cold infusion of seeds relieves constipation. (Stuwart)

Parts Used : Whole plant.

Preparations & Dosage : Juice 10-20 ml.

Cassytha filifrrmis Linn. is also considered as amaravalli in certain parts of India.

खवल्ली ग्राहिणी तिक्ता पिच्छिलाक्ष्यामयापहा ।
तुवराग्निकरी हृद्या पित्तश्लेष्मामनाशिनी ॥ भा०प्र०

156
KĀKAMĀCĪ

Solanum nigrum Linn. Family : Solanaceae

Chief Characters :

1. Annual shrub grows upto 1½ m. height.
2. Simple leaf, alternate phyllotaxy.
3. White coloured small flowers, umbel inflorescence.
4. Fruit - berry.

Synonyms : Kakahwa, Vayasi, Dwankshamachi.

Properties : Rasa - Tikta; Guna - Laghu, Snigdha; Virya - Ushna and Vipaka - Katu.

Pharmacological Actions : Tridoshahara, Vrishya, Bhedana, Swarya, Rasayana, Sukrada, Netrahita.

Indications : Sotha, Kushta, Arshas, Prameha, Jwara, Hikka, Chardi, Hridroga, Urusthambha, Sosha.

Therapeutic Uses :

1. Kushta : The external application of the juice relieves kushta. (C.S.)
2. Palita : The oil extracted from the seeds of kakamachi and tila is administered through nose cures the grey hair. (Rasaratnakara)
3. Sotha and urusthambha : The leaves cooked in water and processed in oil without adding salt is suggested. (C.S.)

Parts Used : Fruit, Whole plant.

Preparations & Dosage : Juice 10-20 ml.; Fruit powder 1-3 gm.; Arka 20-50 ml.

Specific Formulations : Kakamachi arka, Hridayarnava rasa.

काकमाची त्रिदोषघ्नी स्निग्धोष्णा स्वरशुक्रदा ।
तिक्ता रसायनी शोथकुष्ठार्शोज्वरमेहजित् ।।
कटु नेत्रहिता हिक्काछर्दिहृद्रोगनाशिनी ।। भा०प्र०

157
KAṬUVĪRA

Capsicum annum Linn. Family : Solanaceae

Chief Characters :

1. Perennial shrub grows upto 60 m.
2. Simple leaf, alternate phyllotaxy.
3. White coloured flowers.
4. Fruit - berry.

Synonyms : Lanka, Rakta-maricha, Pittakarni, Kshupaja maricha, Jwalamukhi.

Properties : Rasa - Katu; Guna - Laghu, Ruksha, Tikshna; Virya - Ushna and Vipaka - Katu.

Pharmacological Actions : Kaphavatahara, Pittakara, Deepana, Vidahakara.

Indications : Ajeerna, Visuchi, Moha, Pralapa, Medoroga, Swarbheda, Alarkavisha, Akhuvisha.

Therapeutic Uses :

1. Dog-bite : Its paste can be used as anointment at the region of dog-bite.
2. Aruchi, agnimandya and anaha : Pills made of katuveera along with hingu and camphor should be given.
3. Pralapa : It should be given in the form of pills in the dosage of 20-30 (grains) along with honey.

Contradictions : Arshas, Prameha.

Parts Used : Fruit.

Preparations & Dosage : 30-60 mg.

Specific Formulations : Lankasava, Vishamajwaraghni vati.

कटुवीरोज्ज्वला तीक्ष्णा तीव्रशक्त्यजडे तथा ।
कटुवीराग्निजननी बलासघ्नी च दाहिनी ॥
हन्त्यजीर्णं विसूचीं च व्रणं क्लित्रं सुदारुणम् ।
तन्द्रां मोहं प्रलापं च स्वरभेदमरोचकम् ॥
नरं लुप्तधरं क्षीणं सन्निपातनिपीडितम् ।
नष्टेन्द्रियगणं तीक्ष्णं मृत्योराकृष्य जीवयेत् ॥ आ०वि०

158
TĀMRAPARṆA

Nicotiana tobaccum Family : Solanaceae

Chief Characters :

1. Annual herb.
2. Simple leaf.
3. White coloured flowers, panicle inflorescence.
4. Fruit - capsule.

Synonyms : Kalanja, Gucchaphala, Tamala, Brihatpatra, Bahubeeja, Bahuphala.

Properties : Rasa - Tikta, Katu; Guna - Laghu, Tikshna; Virya - Ushna and Vipaka - Katu.

Pharmacological Actions : Kaphavatashamaka, Pittavardhaka, Rechana, Shukraghna, Ahridya, Anulomana, Vastishodhana.

Indications : Dantashoola, Shwasa, Kasa, Krimidanta, Krimi, Kandu.

Therapeutic Uses :

1. Arthritis & orchitis : Its leaves when tied to the inflammatory region alleviate inflammation and pain.
2. Dental caries : Its powder is useful for cleaning the tooth, it alleviates pain and kills the causative organism.

Parts Used : Leaf.

Preparations & Dosage : Leaf powder 3-6 gm.

Specific Formulations : Shwasagajankusha, Shwashantakavaleha.

तस्य पत्रं तु तीक्ष्णोष्णं कफवातहरं परम् ।
श्वासकासहरं चैव कोष्ठवातहरं तथा ॥
वातानुलोमनकरं बस्तिशोधनमुत्तमम् ।
दन्तरुक्शमनं चैव क्रिमिकण्ड्वादिनाशनम् ॥
मदपित्तभ्रमकरं वमनं रेचनं स्मृतम् ।
दृष्टावन्धकरं चैव तीक्ष्णशुक्रकरं तथा ॥
तस्यैव धूमपानं तु विशेषाद् हृदि शुक्रहृत् ।
देशान्तरप्रभेदेन तीक्ष्णं चार्त्तवपित्तलम् ॥
वमनस्य प्रभावेण वृश्चिकादिविषं हरेत् ।
रेचनत्वाद् हरेद् वातं श्लेष्माणं च नियच्छति ॥ योगरत्नाकर

159
HṚTPATRĪ

Digitalis purpurea Family : Scrophulariaceae

Chief Characters :

1. Annual herb.
2. Simple leaf, alternate phyllotaxy.
3. Big flowers, racemose inflorescence. Flowers are whitish violet, yellowish violet in colour.
4. Fruit - capsule.

Synonyms : Tilapushpi.

Properties : Rasa - Tikta; Guna - Laghu, Ruksha; Virya - Sheeta and Vipaka - Katu.

Pharmacological Actions : Kaphavatahara, Hridya.

Indications : Hridayorbalyajanya shotha, Shwasa, Kasa.

Therapeutic Uses :

1. Hritpatri churna 1 part, mrigasringa bhasma 2 part taken together is used in heart diseases. (S.Y.S.)
2. Odema in cardiac diseases is relieved by taking hritpatri with arogyavardhini rasa. (S.Y.S.)

Parts Used : Leaf.

Preparations & Dosage : Powder 200 mg -1 gm.

Specific Formulations : Hritpatra churna.

160
ROHITAKA

Tecoma undulata Family : Bignoniaceae

Chief Characters :

1. Shrub.
2. Simple leaves, opposite phyllotaxy.
3. Corymb inflorescence.
4. Fruit - loculicidal capsule.
5. Consists of red or orange coloured flowers.

Synonyms : Rohi, Dadimapushpaka, Pleehagati, Dadimacchada, Raktaghna.

Properties : Rasa - Katu, Tikta, Kashaya; Guna - Laghu, Ruksha; Virya - Sheeta and Vipaka - Katu.

Pharmacological Actions : Raktaprasadana, Ruchya, Kapha-pittashamaka.

Indications : Udara, Pleeha, Yakritroga, Gulma.

Therapeutic Uses :

1. Root paste cures leucorrhea. (C.S.)
2. Root & haritaki processed in gomutra cures kamala, pleeharoga. (Y.R.)

Parts Used : Bark.

Preparations & Dosage : Powder 1-3 gm.; Decoction 50-100 ml.

Specific Formulations : Rohitakarishta, Rohitaka ghrita, Rohitakadya churna, Rohitakaleha.

रोहीतकौ कटुस्निग्धौ कषायौ च सुशीतलौ ।
कृमिदोषव्रणप्लीहरक्तनेत्रामयापहौ ॥ रा०नि०

161
TILA

Sesamum indicum Family : Pedaliaceae.

Chief Characters :

1. Annual herb.
2. Consists of flowers of light pink colour with yellow striped.
3. Leaves are simple with alternate phyllotaxy.
4. Fruit - capsule.

Gana :

Charaka : Pureeshaviranjaneeya.

Properties : Rasa - Katu, Tikta, Kashaya, Madhura; Guna - Guru, Snigdha; Virya - Ushna and Vipaka - Madhura (S.S.)/Katu (B.P. & A.H.).

Pharmacological Actions : Kaphapittakara (C.S. & D.N.), Keshya Balya, Twachya, Grahi, Dantya, Vranaropana, Kaphavatahara. (R.N.)

Indications : Vrana, Vataroga, Agnimandya, Grahani.

Therapeutic Uses :

1. Indigestion : Tilaksahara relieves ajirna. (B.P.)
2. Hair fall : Tilapushpa and gokshura, honey and ghee promote hair growth. (B.P.)
3. Fistula-in-ano :Paste of tila mixed with ghee should be applied locally. (S.S.)

Parts Used : Seed, Seed oil.

Preparations & Dosage : Seed powder 3-6 gm., Seed oil 10-20 ml.

Specific Formulations : Tiladi gutika, Tiladi lepa, Tilashtaka.

तिल: कृष्ण: सितो रक्त: स वन्योऽल्पतिल: स्मृत:।
तिलो रसे कटुस्तिक्तो मधुरस्तुवरो गुरु: ॥
विपाके चापि मधुर: स्निग्धोष्ण: कफपित्तकृत् ।
बल्य: केश्यो हिमस्पर्शस्त्वच्य: स्तन्यो व्रणे हित: ॥
दन्त्योऽल्पमूत्रकृद् ग्राही वातघ्नोऽग्निमतिप्रद: ।
कृष्ण: श्रेष्ठतमस्तेषु शुक्रलो मध्यम: सित: ॥
अन्ये हीनतरा: प्रोक्तास्तज्ज्ञै: रक्तादयस्तिला: ॥ भा०प्र०

162
SAIREYAKA

Barleria prionitis Family : Acanthaceae

Chief Characters :

1. It is a perennial plant.
2. Simple leaves, opposite phyllotaxy.
3. Yellow flowers in spike inflorescence.
4. Fruit - capsule.

Synonyms : Sahachara, Saireya, Katasarika (Shweta), Kuranta, Kurabaka (Rakta); Bana-dasi, Artagala (Neela).

Gana :

Sushruta : Varunadi

Properties : Rasa - Tikta, Madhura, Amla; Guna - Laghu; Virya - Ushna and Vipaka - Katu.

Pharmacological Actions : Kaphavatahara, Kesharanjana.

Indications : Kushta, Vataratka, Kandu.

Therapeutic Uses :

1. Root paste of saireyaka taken with madhu and tanduloda-ka relieves rat poisoning. (A.H.)
2. Oil processed with decoction of sahacara, devadaru and sunthi is useful in vatavyadhi. (A.H.)

Parts Used : Whole plant, Leaf.

Preparations & Dosage : Juice 10-20 ml.; Decoction 50-100 ml.

Specific Formulations : Sahacharadi taila.

सैरेयक: श्वेतपुष्प: सैरेय: कटसारिका ।
सहाचर: सहचर: स च भिन्द्यपि कथ्यते ॥
कुरण्टकोऽत्रपीते स्याद्रक्त कुरबक: स्मृत: ।
नीले बाणाद्वयोरुक्तो दासी चार्त्तगलश्च स: ॥
सैरेय: कुष्ठवातास्रकफकण्डूविषापह: ।
तिक्तोष्णो मधुरोऽनम्ल: सुस्निग्ध: केशरञ्जन: ॥ भा०प्र०

163
KOKILĀKṢA

Asteracantha longifolia Nees. Family : Acanthaceae

Chief Characters :

1. Tall thorny plant.
2. Dagger shaped simple leaf.
3. Light blue coloured flowers.
4. Fruit - capsule.

Synonyms : Kakekshu, Ikshura, Kshuraka, Kshura, Bikshu, Kandaekshu, Ikshugandha, Ikshuvalika.

Gana :

Charaka : Sukrasodhana, Stanyajanana, Madhura skandha.

Properties : Rasa - Madhura, Amla, Tikta; Guna - Snigdha, Picchila; Virya - Sheeta and Vipaka - Madhura.

Pharmacological Actions : Vatapittahara, Vrishya, Balya, Shukrashodhana, Amahara.

Indications : Vatarakta, Amavata, Shotha, Trishna, Ashmari, Netraroga.

Therapeutic Uses :

1. Vatarakta : Intake of whole plant decoction and leaves as curry in the diet relieves vatarakta. (A.H.)
2. Vajeekarana : The powdered fruits of kapikacchu and kokilaksha taken with freshly collected milk (dharoshna kshira) acts as a powerful aphrodisiac. (S.S.)
3. Sopha : Its kshara is administered internally along with gomutra or water. (C.D.)

Parts Used : Root, Seed, Whole plant, Alkali.

Preparations & Dosage : Decoction 5-10 ml.; Seed powder 3-6 gm.; Alkali 1-2 gm.

Specific Formulations : Poushtika churna.

क्षुरकः शीतलो वृष्यः मधुरः पिच्छिलो हिमः ।
स्निग्धपित्तामशोथाश्मतृष्णादृष्ट्यनिलास्रजित् ॥ द्र०गु०वि०

164
KĀLAMEGHA

Andrographis paniculata (Burm. f.) Wall. Ex Nees

Family : Acanthaceae

Chief Characters :

1. Annual herb grows upto 1 m. height.
2. Simple leaf, opposite phyllotaxy.
3. White coloured with violet striped flowers.
4. Panicle inflorescence.
5. Fruit - capsule.

Synonyms : Bhunimba.

Properties : Rasa - Tikta; Guna - Laghu, Ruksha; Virya - Ushna and Vipaka - Katu.

Pharmacological Actions : Kaphapittahara, Deepana, Swedala, Pittasaraka.

Indications : Jwara, Krimi, Pandu, Kamala, Shotha, Kushta, Vrana, Yakritroga.

Therapeutic Uses :

Vishamajwara : Its powder should be given along with pepper or its juice should be given along with pepper.

Parts Used : Whole plant.

Preparations & Dosage : Powder 1-3 gm.; Juice 5-10 ml.

Specific Formulations : Kalamegha churna, Kalamegha, navayasa churna.

कालमेघस्तु भूनिम्बो यवाकारफलस्तथा ।
सुतिक्तः लघुरूक्षोष्णः कफपित्तविनाशनः ॥
दीपनस्वेदनो ज्ञेयः कृमिघ्नः पित्तसारकः ।
यकृद्रोगे क्रिमौ कुष्ठे ज्वरे चासौ प्रशस्यते ॥ द्र०गु०वि०

165
UṬAṄGANA

Blepharis edulis Pers. Family : Acanthaceae

Chief Characters :

1. Herb grows upto 50 cm. height.
2. Simple leaf, opposite phyllotaxy.
3. Blue coloured flowers, head inflorescence.
4. Fruit - capsule.

Properties : Rasa - Tikta, Madhura; Guna - Guru, Snigdha, Picchila; Virya - Ushna and Vipaka - Madhura.

Pharmacological Actions : Vatahara, Mutrala, Vrishya.

Indications : Mutrakriccha, Shukrakshaya, Vataroga.

Therapeutic Uses :

Aphrodisiac :It should be taken along with cow's milk.

Parts Used : Seed.

Preparations & Dosage : Powder 3-6 gm.

उटङ्गनस्य बीजं तु गुरुस्निग्धं सुपिच्छिलम् ।
मधुरं तिक्तमुष्णं च वृष्यं मूत्रलमुच्यते ॥ द्र०गु०वि०

166
BHĀṆḌĪRA

Clerodendurm infortunatum Family : Verbenaceae

Chief Characters :

1. Perennial shrub.
2. Simple leaf, alternate phyllotaxy.
3. Pale violet coloured flowers, panicle inflorescence.
4. Fruit - drupe.

Synonyms : Bhandi, Tiktabhantaka, Tiktavara.

Properties : Rasa - Tikta; Guna - Laghu, Ruksha; Virya - Ushna and Vipaka - Katu.

Pharmacological Actions : Kaphavatahara, Sara.

Indications : Madhumeha, Kushta, Krimi, Jwara, Amavata.

Parts Used : Leaf.

Preparations & Dosage : Juice 10-20 ml.; Powder 1-3 gm.

भाण्डीरः तिक्तभण्टाकः भाण्डी तिक्तवरा स्मृता ।
भाण्डीरः लघुतिक्तोष्णः कफवातविनाशकृत् ॥
पित्तरेची कृमिघ्नश्च सरो ज्वरनिषूदनः ।
कुष्ठे ज्वरे त्वामवाते मधुमेहे प्रशस्यते ॥ द्र०गु०वि०

167
PRIYAṄGU

Callicarpa macrophylla vahl. Family : Verbenaceae

Chief Characters :

1. It is a perennial plant.
2. Simple leaves, opposite phyllotaxy.
3. Violet or red coloured flowers, cymose inflorescence.
4. Fruit - berry.

Synonyms : Anganapriya, Gandhaphali, Phalini, Kanta, Lata, Mahilahwaya, Gundra, Shyama, Priya.

Gana :

Charaka : Sandhaniya, Purishasangrahaniya, Mutravirajaneeya, Shonitasthapana.

Sushruta : Eladi, Anjanadi, Priyangwadi.

Properties : Rasa - Kashaya, Tikta, Madhura (Phala); Guna - Guru, Ruksha; Virya - Sheeta and Vipaka - Katu.

Pharmacological Actions : Vatapittahara (B.P.), Vishahara, Grahi, Vibandha, Adhmanakara, Purishsangrahaniya, Mutravirajaneeya.

Indications : Raktatisara, Daha, Jwara, Chardi, Atisara, Mukharoga, Gulma, Trishna.

Therapeutic Uses :

1. The powder of the flowers taken with honey is used in Raktapitta. (C.S.)
2. Paste of priyangu mixed with honey and taken with rice water checks bleeding immediately. Diarrhoea with blood patient should be kept on diet of meat soup of wild animals. (C.S.; A.S.)

Parts Used : Flower, Fruit.

Preparations & Dosage : Powder 3-6 gm.

Specific Formulations : Priyangwadi taila.

प्रियङ्गु शीतला तिक्ता तुवरानिलपित्तहृत् ।
रक्तातीसारदौर्गन्ध्यस्वेददाहज्वरापहा ॥
गुल्मतृड्विषमेहघ्नी तद्वद् गन्धप्रियङ्गुका । भा०प्र०

168
PŪTIHĀ

Mentha piperata Linn. Family : Lamiaceae

Chief Characters :

1. It is a perennial plant.
2. Simple leaf, opposite phyllotaxy.
3. Violet coloured flowers, spike inflorescence.
4. Fruit - nutlet.

Synonyms : Rochani, Podinaka.

Properties : Rasa - Katu; Guna - Laghu, Ruksha, Tikshna; Virya - Ushna and Vipaka - Katu.

Pharmacological Actions : Kaphavatashamaka, Deepana, Balya.

Indications : Arochaka, Chardi, Krimi, Rajorodha.

Therapeutic Uses :

Indigestion : Arka extracted from the juice of pudina, ardraka, nimbuka and kumari added with jiraka and trijata promotes digestion. (S.B.)

Parts Used : Leaf, Oil.

Preparations & Dosage : Juice 5-10 ml.; Oil 1-3 drops; Infusion 20-40 ml.

अरोचवैरस्यकृद्वमिक्रिमिप्रभञ्जनश्लेष्मगदप्रभञ्जनः ।
रूक्षस्तथोष्णः सुरभीरजप्रदः पोदीनकः कल्कविधौ प्रशस्यते ॥ सि०भे०म०

169
JŪPHĀ

Hyssopus officinalis Family : Laminaceae

Chief Characters :

1. Perennial shrub.
2. Simple leaf, opposite phyllotaxy.
3. Blue and light violet coloured flowers, spike inflorescence.
4. Fruit - nutlet.

Properties : Rasa - Katu, Tikta; Guna - Laghu, Ruksha; Virya - Ushna and Vipaka - Katu.

Pharmacological Actions : Kaphavatashamaka, Pittashamaka, Lek-hana.

Indications : Krimi, Udara, Shotha, Kasa, Shwasa.

Therapeutic Uses :

Oedema : Its paste is useful as external application to relieve swelling.

Parts Used : Whole plant.

Preparations & Dosage : Powder 3-6 gm.

Specific Formulations : Sarbhata jupha, Dayakunja.

जूफा तीक्ष्णा कटुस्तिक्ता वीर्योष्णा कफवातनुत् ।
शोथघ्नी लेखनी पित्तसारणी कृमिनाशिनी ।। द्र०गु०वि०

170
PARṆAYAVĀNĪ

Coleus amboinicus Lour. (or) Family : Lamiaceae
Coleus aromaticus Benth.

Chief Characters :

1. It is a perennial plant.
2. Simple leaf, alternate phyllotaxy.
3. Pale violet coloured flowers, racemose inflorescence.
4. Fruit - nutlets.

Synonyms : Gandhaparnika.

Properties : Rasa - Tikta, Katu; Guna - Laghu, Ruksha, Tiksha; Virya - Ushna and Vipaka - Katu.

Pharmacological Actions : Kaphavatahara, Deepana, Pacahana, Grahi.

Indications : Ashmari, Agnimandhya, Mutrakricchra, Grahani, Visuchi, Udara, Yakridroga, Krimi.

Therapeutic Uses :

The fresh juice in the dosage of 1 tola is useful in atisara.

Parts Used : Leaf.

Preparations & Dosage : Juice 5-10 ml.

ख्याता पर्णयवानी तु यवानी गन्धपर्णिका ।
जाता पूर्वीयद्वीपेषु भारते प्रसृता भृशम् ॥
तीक्ष्णा पर्णयवान्युष्णा कटुस्तिक्ता रसे लघुः ।
दीपनी पाचनी रुच्या मलसंग्राहिणी परम् ॥
अग्निमान्द्ये यकृद्रोगे ग्रहण्यामुदरक्रिमौ ।
विषूचिकायामश्मर्यां मूत्रकृच्छ्रे च शस्यते ॥ द्र०गु०वि०

171
AŚVAGOLA

Plantago ovata Forsk. Family : Plantaginaceae

Chief Characters :

1. Scapigerous annual herb.
2. Radical leaves are seen.
3. Spike inflorescence.
4. Green coloured small flowers.
5. Fruit - cymbiform dehiscent.

Synonyms : Sheetabeeja, Ashwakarnabeeja, Eshadgola, Eswarabola.

Properties : Rasa - Madhura, Kashaya; Guna - Snigdha, Pichchila, Guru; Virya - Sheeta and Vipaka - Madhura.

Pharmacological Actions : Kaphapittahara, Vatakara, Grahi, Balya, Mutrajanana.

Indications : Raktatisara, Raktapitta, Jwara, Trishna, Kasa, Pravahika, Atisara, Mutrakriccha.

Therapeutic Uses :

Constipation : Intake of one spoonful of seeds with water at bed time; relieves constipation. This acts as a bulk increasing laxative.

Parts Used : Seed.

Preparations & Dosage : Powder 5-10 gm.

अश्वगोलमश्वकर्णबीजं च स्निग्धजीरकम् ।
अश्वगोलं गुरु स्वादु स्निग्धं शीतं च पिच्छिलम् ॥
स्नेहनं मूत्रजननं श्लेष्मनि:सारणं परम् ।
दाहतृष्णाहरं बल्यं ज्वरघ्नं चाथ शस्यते ॥
प्रवाहिकातिसारामदाहतृष्णाज्वरादिषु ।
वातपित्तामये कासे दौर्बल्ये मूत्रकृच्छ्रजे ॥ द्र०गु०वि०

172
GORAKṢAGUÑJĀ

Aerva lanata Family : Amaranthaceae

Chief Characters :

1. Perennial herb.
2. Simple leaf.
3. Small white flowers, spikes inflorescence.
5. Fruit - utricle.

Properties : Rasa - Tikta, Kashaya; Guna - Laghu, Tikshna; Virya - Ushna and Vipaka - Katu.

Pharmacological Actions : Kaphavatashamaka, Mutrala, Ashmaribhedana, Mutravirechaneeya.

Indications : Ashmari, Mutrakricchra.

Parts Used : Root.

Preparations & Dosage : Decoction 50-100 ml.

गोरक्षगुञ्जा तुवरा सतिक्ता लघ्वी च तीक्ष्णा परमोष्णवीर्या ।
कफार्त्तिहृन् मूत्रविरेचनीया प्रभावतोऽप्यश्मरिनाशिनी स्यात् ॥

द्र०गु०वि०

173
CUKRIKĀ (CUKRA)

Rumex vesicarius Linn. Family : Polygonaceae

Chief Characters :

1. Annual herb.
2. Simple leaf.
3. White coloured small flowers, racemose inflorescence.
4. Fruit - nutlet.

Synonyms : Patramla, Rochani, Jatavedhini.

Properties : Rasa - Amla, Madhura; Guna - Laghu; Virya - Ushna and Vipaka - Amla.

Pharmacological Actions : Vatahara, Kaphapittakara, Ruchya, Deepana.

Indications : Aruchi, Agnimandya, Atisara, Shopha.

Therapeutic Uses :

1. Bleeding piles : Liquid gruel of parched paddy cooked with cukrika, nagakeshara and utpala checks bleeding immedi-ately.
2. Diarrhoea : In case of diarrhoea, quath made of cangeri, cukrika and dugdhika added with fatty layer of curd, ghee and pomegranate seeds should be given. (C.S.)

Parts Used : Leaf, Seed, Whole plant.

Preparations & Dosage : Powder 1-3 gm.; Juice 10-20 ml.

चुक्रमत्यम्लमुष्णञ्च दीपनं पाचनं परम् ।
शूलगुल्मविबन्धामवातश्लेष्महरं सरम् ।
वमितृष्णाऽऽस्यवैरस्यहृत्पीडावह्निमान्द्यहृत् ॥ भा०प्र०

174
PĪTAMULĪ

Rheum emodi Family : Polygonaceae

Chief Characters :

1. Plant grows upto a height of 2 m.
2. Panicle inflorescence.
3. Simple leaves.
4. Flowers are dark violet in colour.
5. Fruit - nut.

Synonyms : Amlaparni, Revatika, Gandhini.

Properties : Rasa - Tikta, Katu; Guna - Laghu, Ruksha; Virya - Ushna and Vipaka - Katu.

Pharmacological Actions : Kaphapittahara, Mridurechana, Vranaropana.

Indications : Atisara, Agnimandhya, Shitapitta, Dushtavrana, Ud-ara, Yaktritroga, Vitsanga.

Parts Used : Rhizome.

Preparations & Dosage : Powder 0.1-2.0 gm.

गन्धिनी पीतमूली च बल्या सा मृदुरेचनी ।
हन्त्यजीर्णमतीसारं वह्निमान्द्यमरोचकम् ॥
विट्सङ्गं शीतपित्तञ्च दुष्टव्रणविरोहिणी ॥ आ०वि०

175
ĪŚWARĪ

Aristolochia indica Linn. Family : Aristolochiaceae

Chief Characters :

1. Perennial herb grows upto 6 m. height.
2. Simple leaf, alternate phyllotaxy.
3. Light green or violet colored followers.
4. Cyamose inflorescence.
5. Fruit - capsule.

Synonyms : Gandhanakuli, Nakuli.

Properties : Rasa - Tikta, Kashaya, Katu; Guna - Laghu, Ruksha; Virya - Ushna and Vipaka - Katu.

Pharmacological Actions : Kaphavatahara, Vishaghna.

Indications : Sarpavisha, Vrisuchika visha, Akhu visha, Jwara, Krimi, Vrana.

Therapeutic Uses :

1. Vishamajwara : The intake of root powder relieves vishama jwara and sutika jwara. (N.A.)
2. Amavata : The root powder relieves jeerna amavata.
3. Kashta prasava : The internal administration of ishwari and pippali roots facilitates delivery in delayed labour. (N.A.)

Parts Used : Root, Leaf.

Preparations & Dosage : Root powder 1-3 gm.; Leaf juice 5-10 ml.

नाकुली तुवरा तिक्ता कटुकोष्णा नियच्छति ।
भोगिलूतावृश्चिकाखुविषज्वरकृमिव्रणान् ॥ भा०प्र०

176

KĪṬAMĀRĪ

Aristolochia bracteolata Lamk. Family : Aristolochiaceae

Chief Characters :

1. Procumbent perennial plant grows upto a length of 1m.
2. Heart shaped simple leaf, alternate phyllotaxy.
3. Dark violet coloured flowers.
4. Fruit - inverted umbrella shaped.

Synonyms : Dhumapatra, Kitari.

Properties : Rasa - Tikta; Guna - Laghu, Ruksha, Tikshna; Virya - Ushna and Vipaka - Katu.

Pharmacological Actions : Kaphavatashamaka, Rechana.

Indications : Krimi, Shotha, Vishamajwara, Kashtartava.

Therapeutic Uses :

1. Urticaria : The powder or juice of leaves is useful in urticaria.
2. Krimi : Decoction of root should be given.
3. Vishamajwara : It should be given along with black pepper.
4. Chronic ulcers & vicharchika : Its leaf juice should be used as anointment.

Parts Used : Leaf, Root.

Preparations & Dosage : Powder 1-3 gm.; Juice 5-10 ml.; Decoction 50-100 ml.

वातश्लेष्मज्वरहरा संध्यस्थीनि प्राशारिणी । शोढल
तिक्ताकृकृमिघ्नीशोफघ्नी हि उष्णा रुच्या य दीपनी कासघ्नी । रा०नि०

177
SUGANDHAVĀSTUKA

Chenopodium ambrosiodes Family : Chenopodiaceae

Chief Characters :

1. Fragrant annual plant.
2. Simple leaves, alternate phyllotaxy.
3. Green coloured flowers, spike inflorescence.
4. Fruit - utricle.
5. Consists of green coloured flowers.

Properties : Rasa - Madhura; Guna - Laghu; Virya - Ushna and Vipaka - Katu.

Pharmacological Actions : Tridoshahara, Deepana, Pachana.

Indications : Krimi, Arsas, Raktapitta, Pleehodara.

Parts Used : Seed, Oil.

Preparations & Dosage : Seed powder ½ - 2 gm.; Oil 5-20 drops.

वास्तूकद्वितीयं स्वादु क्षारपाके कटूदितम् ।
दीपनं पाचनं रुच्यं लघु शुक्रबलप्रदम् ।
सरं प्लीहास्रपित्तार्शः कृमिदोषत्रयापहम् ॥ भा०प्र०

178
KAṄKOLA

Piper cubeba Linn. Family : Piperaceae

Chief Characters :

1. Twinner grows upto 10-12 cm.
2. Leaf resembles leaf of piper betel.
3. Unisexual flowers.
4. Fruit - resembles black pepper with a tail.

Synonyms : Kolaka, Koshaphala, Gondhamaricha, Kankolaka.

Properties : Rasa - Tikta; Guna - Laghu; Virya - Sheeta (B.P.), Ushna (R.N.) and Vipaka - Katu.

Pharmacological Actions : Kaphavatashamaka, Deepana, Pachana, Hridya, Ruchya, Vrishya.

Indications : Trishna, Aruchi, Kasa, Shwasa, Hridroga, Andhatwa, Asyadaurgandhya.

Therapeutic Uses :

1. Shopha : It can be used as anointment in places where inflammation and pain are present.
2. Sirahshoola and shirogata sleshma : It is used in nasya karma.

Parts Used : Fruit.

Preparations & Dosage : Powder 1-3 gm.; Oil 1-3 drops.

Specific Formulations : Khadiradi vati.

कङ्कोलकं लवङ्गञ्च तिक्तं कटु कफापहम् ।
लघु तृष्णापहं वक्त्रक्लेददौर्गन्ध्यनाशनम् ॥ सु०सू०

179
PATRAKA
(TEJAPATRA)

Cinnamomum tamala Ness. Family : Lauraceae

Chief Characters :

1. Tree with simple leaves and alternate phyllotaxy.
2. Panicle inflorescence.
3. Flowers - pale yellowish in colour.
4. Fruit - Small, oval or elliptical in shape.

Synonyms : Tamalapatra, Patranamaka.

Properties : Rasa - Madhura, Katu; Guna - Picchila, Laghu, Tikshna; Virya - Ushna and Vipaka - Katu.

Pharmacological Actions : Kaphavatahara, Ruchya.

Indications : Arsas, Aruchi, Hrillasa, Pinasa.

Therapeutic Uses :

Obesity : Anointment of patra, balaka, aguru, usheera and candana removes foul smell of the body. (V.M.)

Parts Used : Leaf.

Preparations & Dosage : Powder 1-4 gm.

Specific Formulations : Trijatakadi vati.

पत्रं तमालपत्रञ्च तथा स्यात्पत्रनामकम् ।
पत्रकं मधुरं किञ्चित्तीक्ष्णोष्णं पिच्छिलं लघु ॥
निहन्ति कफवाताशोंर्हृल्लासारुचिपीनसान् ॥ भा०प्र०

180
MEDĀSAKA

Litsea chinensis Family : Lauraceae.

Chief Characters :

1. Deciduous tree.
2. Simple leaf, alternate phyllotaxy.
3. Consists of yellow coloured flowers.
4. Fruit - drupe.

Properties : Rasa - Katu, Tikta, Kashaya; Guna - Laghu, Snigdha; Virya - Ushna and Vipaka - Katu.

Pharmacological Actions : Kaphavatahara, Deepana, Stambhana, Vedanasthapana.

Indications : Agnimandhya, Atisara, Shotha, Shoola, Vatavyadhi.

Therapeutic Uses :

Its paste is useful as external application in fractures, accidental wounds, arthritis and joint stiffness.

Parts Used : Bark.

Preparations & Dosage : Powder 1-3 gm.

मेदासकः सदापर्णः गन्धपर्णश्च स स्मृतः ।
मध्यमाकृतिवृक्षश्च वन्यदेशोद्भवोऽपि च ॥
मेदासको लघुः स्निग्धः कटुस्तिक्तः कषायकः ।
उष्णौ वातकफौ हन्ति शोथशूलविनाशनः ॥
दीपनः स्तम्भनश्चैव सर्ववातविकारनुत् ।
अग्निमान्द्येऽतिसारे च रक्तस्रावे च युज्यते ॥ द्र०गु०वि०

181
BANDĀKA

Dendrophthoe falcata Linn. Family : Loranthaceae

Chief Characters :

1. It is a perennial plant, parasite.
2. Simple leaf, opposite phyllotaxy.
3. Red coloured flowers.
4. Fruit - berry.

Synonyms : Vrikshadani, Vriksharuha, Bandaka.

Properties : Rasa - Kashaya, Tikta, Madhura; Guna - Laghu, Ruksha; Virya - Sheeta and Vipaka - Katu.

Pharmacological Actions : Kaphapittahara, Vishahara.

Indications : Ashmari, Raktapittahara, Vrana, Vandhyatwa.

Therapeutic Uses :

The bark powder of badanika and udumbara churna taken with goat's milk cures vandhyatwa. (V.M.)

Parts Used : Whole plant.

Preparations & Dosage : Juice 10-20 ml.

बन्दाकः स्याद्धिमः तिक्तः कषायो मधुरो रसे ।
माङ्गल्यः कफपित्तास्ररक्षोव्रणविषापहः ॥ भा०प्र०

182
SNUHĪ

Euphorbia neriifolia Linn. Family : Euphorbiaceae

Chief Characters :

1. Shrub, latex yeilding.
2. Alternate phyllotaxy.
3. Cymose inflorescence, yellow coloured flowers.
4. Fruit - capsule.

Synonyms : Sehunda, Simhatunda, Vajri, Vajradruma, Sudha, Guda, Samanta dugdha.

Properties : Rasa - Katu; Guna - Snigdha, Laghu (Latex), Guru; Virya - Ushna and Vipaka - Katu.

Pharmacological Actions : Kaphavatahara, Rechana, Deepana.

Indications : Shoola, Ashthila, Udara, Adhmana, Kushta, Arshas, Vrana, Shotha, Unmada, Jwara, Pleeha, Pandu, Dushivisha.

Therapeutic Uses :

1. Piles : Haridra powder mixed with snuhi latex should be applied. (S.S., C.S., R.M.)
2. Udara : One suffering from udararoga should use the course of pippali (upto 1000) impregnated with snuhi latex and on milk diet. (V.M.)

Parts Used : Tuber, Root, Leaf, Latex, Stem.

Preparations & Dosage : Juice 5-10 ml.; Powder ½-1 gm.; Latex 125-250 ml.

Specific Formulations : Vajrakshara, Snuhyadi taila.

विरेचनानां सर्वेषां सुधा तीक्ष्णतमा मता ।
सङ्घातं हि भिनत्त्याशु दोषाणां कष्टविभ्रमा ॥
तस्मान्नैषा मृदौ कोष्ठे प्रयोक्तव्या कदाचन ।
न दोषनिचये चाल्पे सति मार्गपरिक्रमे ॥
पाण्डुरोगोदरे गुल्मे कुष्ठे दूषीविषार्दिते ।
श्वयथौ मधुमेहे च दोषविभ्रान्तचेतसि ॥
रोगैरेवंविधैर्ग्रस्तं ज्ञात्वा सप्राणमातुरम् ।
प्रयोजयेन्महावृक्षं सम्यक् स ह्यवचारितः ॥
सद्यो हरति दोषाणां महान्तमपि सञ्चयम् । च०क०

183
KAMPILLAKA

Mallotus philippensis Lamk. Family : Euphorbiaceae

Chief Characters :

1. Tree grows upto 10m. height.
2. Oval shaped simple leaf, alternate phyllotaxy.
3. Small male and female flowers, whitish yellow in colour, spike inflorescence.
4. Fruit - capsule.

Synonyms : Karkasha, Chandra, Raktanga, Rochana, Rechana.

Properties : Rasa - Katu; Guna - Laghu, Ruksha, Tikshna; Virya - Ushna and Vipaka - Katu.

Pharmacological Actions : Kaphapittahara (B.P.), Rechana, Kaphahara (D.N.)

Indications : Krimi, Gulma, Udara, Ashmari, Prameha, Vrana, Visha, Adhmana.

Therapeutic Uses :

1. Krimi : The powder (1½ tola) mixed with jaggery expels worms from abdomen. (B.P.)
2. Vrana : The oil prepared with kampillaka on external application heals the wound. (C.S.)

Parts Used : Fruit hairs, Flowers.

Preparations & Dosage : 1-3 gm.

Specific Formulations : Krimighatini vati.

कम्पिल्ल: कफपित्तास्रकृमिगुल्मोदरव्रणान् ।
हन्ति रेची कटूष्णश्च मेहानाहविषाश्मनुत् ।। भा०प्र०

184
PUTRAJĪVAKA

Putranjiva roxburghii Family : Euphorbiaceae

Chief Characters :

1. Tree grows upto 10 m. height.
2. Simple leaf, alternate phyllotaxy.
3. Yellow coloured flowers.
4. Fruit - round cherry shaped wit white hairs.

Synonyms : Garbhakara, Yashtipushpa, Garbhadha, Sleepadapaha, Arthasadaka.

Properties : Rasa - Madhura, Lavana, Katu; Guna - Guru, Ruksha; Virya - Sheeta and Vipaka - Madhura.

Pharmacological Actions : Kaphavatahara (B.P.), Vrishya, Garbhada, Chakshushya, Pittahara (R.N.), Kaphakara (R.N.).

Indications : Daha, Trishna, Mutrakricchra, Shleepada, Vandhyatva.

Therapeutic Uses :

1. The fresh juice relieves shleepada. (S.Ch. 19)
2. The external application of seed relieves vispota. (B.P.)
3. Root of putranjivaka with vishnukranta and sivalingi should be taken during pregnancy for eight days. It provides male child. (B.P.)

Parts Used : Seed, Leaf.

Preparations & Dosage : Leaf powder 3-6 gm.; Leaf juice 10-20 ml.

पिबेत् सर्षपतैलं वा श्लीपदानां निवृत्तये ।
पूतीकरञ्जपत्राणां रसं वापि यथाबलम् ॥
अनेनैव विधानेन पुत्रञ्जीवकजं रसम् ॥ सु०चि०

185
BHŪMYĀMALAKĪ

Phyllanthus urinaria Family : Euphorbiaceae

Chief Characters :

1. Annual herb.
2. Simple leaf, alternate phyllotaxy.
3. Flowers are green or white coloured.
4. Fruit - echinate.

Synonyms : Shiva, Tamalaki, Bahupatra, Bhudatri, Bahuphala, Bahuvirya, Ajata.

Gana :

Charaka : Kasahara, Shwasahara.

Properties : Rasa - Tikta, Kasaya, Madhura; Guna - Guru, Ruksha; Virya - Sheeta and Vipaka - Madhura.

Pharmacological Actions : Kaphapittakara, Vatakara, Rechana.

Indications : Daha, Trishna, Shwasa, Kasa, Kandu, Raktapitta, Pandu, Kamala, Amlapitta, Prameha.

Therapeutic Uses :

1. Janndice : Paste of bhumyamalaki made with butter milk relieves jaundice.
2. Haemorrhage : Seeds of bhumyamalaki taken with rice water alleviate in two or three days metrorrhagia, haematuria and diarrhoea with blood. (B.S.)

Parts Used : Whole plant.

Preparations & Dosage : Powder 3-6 gm.; Juice 10-20 ml.

तामलकी हिमा तिक्ता कषाया मधुरा लघुः ।
रोचनी पाण्डुपित्तास्रकफकुष्ठविषापहा ॥
जयेच्छ्वासतृषादाहहिध्माकासक्षतक्षयान् ॥ कै०नि०

186
SWARṆĀKṢĪRĪ

Euphorbia thomsoniana Family : Euphorbiaceae

Chief Characters :

1. Perennial herb.
2. Simple leaf, alternate phyllotaxy.
3. Yellow coloured flowers.
4. Fruit - capsule.

Synonyms : Katuparni, Peetadugdha, Kanchanaksheeri.

Gana :

Charaka : Bhedaniya.

Properties : Rasa - Tikta; Guna - Laghu, Ruksha; Virya - Sheeta and Vipaka - Katu.

Pharmacological Actions : Kaphapittahara, Bhedana, Vishahara.

Indications : Krimi, Kandu, Anaha, Kushta.

Therapeutic Uses :

1. Skin diseases : Juice of swarnakshiri removes ringworm. (S.B.)
2. Rabies : Bakuchi and swarnakshiri root mixed with jaggery are made into sweet boluses. They destroy the poisoning by dog bite if taken for three days keeping on wholesome diet. (S.B.)

Parts Used : Seed, Root, Latex, Oil.

Preparations & Dosage : Powder 1-3 gm.; Latex 5-10 drops; Oil 10-20 drops; Juice 5-10 ml.

हेमाह्वा रेचनी तिक्ता भेदन्युत्क्लेशकारिणी ।
कृमिकण्डूविषानाहकफपित्तास्त्रकुष्ठनुत् ॥ भा०प्र०

187
KAṄKUṢṬHA

Garcinia morella Desr. Family : Guttiferae

Chief Characters :

1. Tree, grows upto 15 m height.
2. Simple leaf, alternate phyllotaxy.
3. Male and female flowers occur at the leaf bases.
4. Fruit - berry.

Synonyms : Kakakushta, Viranga, Kolakakula, Tamala, Tapiccha.

Properties : Rasa - Tikta, Katu; Guna - Laghu, Ruksha; Virya - Ushna and Vipaka - Katu.

Pharmacological Actions : Kaphahara, Rechana, Varnya.

Indications : Krimi, Shotha, Udara, Adhmana, Gulma, Anaha, Udavarta, Shoola, Vrana.

Therapeutic Uses :

1. Shwasapradhan jwara (Pneumonia) : It is given for inducing vomiting to alleviate the condition by removing kapha.
2. Constipation : It is taken along with rock salt, ela in a smaller dose.

Parts Used : Gum.

Preparations & Dosage : 50-125 mg.

कङ्कुष्ठं तिक्तकटुकं वीर्ये चोष्णं प्रकीर्तितम् ।
गुल्मोदावर्तशूलघ्नं रसरङ्गव्रणापहम् ।। ध०नि०

188
JAYAPĀLA

Croton tiglium Family : Euphorbiaceae

Chief Characters :

1. Decidious tree.
2. Simple leaf.
3. Recemose inflorescence.
4. Fruit - capsule.
5. Consists of white coloured flowers.

Synonyms : Dantibeeja, Tintidi phala, Jaypala, Dravanti.

Properties : Rasa - Katu; Guna - Guru, Snigdha; Virya - Ushna and Vipaka - Katu.

Pharmacological Actions : Pittakaphahara, Rechana, Deepana, Vishahara (B.P.), Kaphavatahara (R.N.).

Indications : Jalodara, Kushta, Krimi, Shotha.

Therapeutic Uses :

1. Udararoga : In severe condition oil of danti and dravanti seeds should be given internally. (A.H.)
2. Wound : Paste of dravanti and cirabilva cleans the wounds. (S.S.)
3. Snake poison : Use of jayapala as collyrium in eyes.

Parts Used : Seed, Seed oil.

Preparations & Dosage : Seed powder 25-50 mg.; Oil ½ drop.

Specific Formulations : Ecchabhedi, Jalodarari.

जैपालः कटुरुष्णश्च कृमिहारी विरेचनः ।
दीपनः कफवातघ्नो जलोदरविनाशनः ॥ रा०नि०

189

NĀGADANTĪ

Croton oblongifolius Roxb. Family : Euphorbiaceae

Chief Characters :

1. The tree grows upto a height of 5-6 m.
2. Simple leaf, alternate phyllotaxy.
3. Recemose inflorescence.
4. Flowers are green in colour.
5. Fruit - capsule, lepidote.

Synonyms : Hastidanti.

Gana :

Susruta : Arkadi.

Properties : Rasa - Katu; Guna - Guru, Tikshna; Virya - Ushna and Vipaka - Katu.

Pharmacological Actions : Kaphapittahara.

Indications : Udara, Krimi, Gulma, Anaha, Kushta.

Parts Used : Seed, Root.

Preparations & Dosage : Powder 25-50 mg.

नागदन्ती कटुस्तिक्ता रूक्षा वातकफापहा ।
मेधाकृद्विषदोषघ्नी पाचनी शोथनाशिनी ॥
गुल्मशूलोदरव्याधिकुष्ठदोषनिकृन्तनी ॥ रा०नि०

190
VAṬA

Ficus bengalensis Family : Moraceae

Chief Characters :

1. Tree.
2. Simple leaf, alternate phyllotaxy.
3. Hypanthodium inflorescence.

Synonyms : Raktaphala, Sringi, Nyagrodha, Dhurva, Skandhaja, Kshiri, Vysravana, Vasa, Bahupada, Vanaspati.

Properties : Rasa - Kashaya; Guna - Guru, Ruksha; Virya - Sheeta and Vipaka - Katu.

Pharmacological Actions : Kaphapittahara, Grahi, Varnya, Mutra sangrahaniya, Stambhana.

Indications : Visarpa, Daha, Yonidosha, Vrana, Trishna, Chardi, Ra-ktapitta, Yoniroga, Vandhya, Vyanga.

Therapeutic Uses :

1. Sringa churned in water relieves vandhyatwa. (Shodhala)
2. The tender leaves of vata on external application is used in vyanga. (B.P.)
3. Latex of vata should be applied. It destroys maggots in wound. (V.D.)

Parts Used : Bark, Latex, Leaf, Fruit, Tender leaf and tender aerial roots.

Preparations & Dosage : Decoction 50-100 ml.; Powder 3-6 gm.

Specific Formulations : Nyagrodhadi churna, Nyagrodhadi ghrita.

वटः शीतो गुरुग्राही कफपित्तव्रणावहः ।
वर्ण्यो विसर्पदाहघ्नः कषायो योनिदोषहृत् ॥
वटाङ्कुरा मसूराश्च प्रलेपाद् व्यङ्गनाशनम् । भा०प्र०

191
AŚWATTHA

Ficus religiosa Linn. Family : Moraceae

Chief Characters :

1. Tree grows upto 20 m. height.
2. Heart shaped leaves with long petiole, alternate phyllotaxy.
3. Hypanthodium inflorescence, violet colour.

Synonyms : Bodhidru, Pipala, Chalapatra.

Properties : Rasa - Kashaya, Madhura; Guna - Guru, Ruksha; Virya - Sheeta and Vipaka - Katu.

Pharmacological Actions : Pittakaphahara, Varnya, Vrishya, Yonivishodhana, Vranasodhana-ropana.

Indications : Vrana, Raktavikara, Yoniroga, Daha, Prameha, Vatarakta, Kushta, Dustavrana.

Therapeutic Uses :

1. Vatarakta : The bark decoction relieves even severe vatarakta. (C.S.)
2. Vomiting : The supernantent portion of water mixed with charred bark powder checks even severe vomiting. (C.D.)
3. Aphrodisiac : The milk boiled with the fruits, root, bark and tender leaves act as an aphrodisiac in combination with sugar & honey. (S.S.)

Parts Used : Bark, Fruit, Latex, Tender leaf.

Preparations & Dosage : Decoction 50-100 ml.

Specific Formulations : Udumbaradi lehya, Chandanadya ghrita.

पिप्पलो दुर्जरः शीतः पित्तश्लेष्मव्रणास्रजित् ।
गुरुस्तुवरको रूक्षो वर्ण्यो योनिविशोधनः ॥ भा०प्र०

192
PLAKṢA

Ficus lacor Buch. Family : Moraceae

Chief Characters :

1. It is a deciduous tree.
2. Simple leaf, alternate phyllotaxy.
3. Hypanthodium inflorescence.
4. Fruit - white with red spots.

Synonyms : Jati, Parkati, Pakadi.

Gana :

Charaka : Mutrasangrahaniya.
Sushruta : Nyagrodhadi.

Properties : Rasa - Kashaya; Guna - Guru, Ruksha; Virya - Sheeta and Vipaka - Katu.

Pharmacological Actions : Kaphapittahara, Mutrasangrahaniya.

Indications : Vrana, Yoniroga, Daha, Shotha, Raktapitta.

Therapeutic Uses :

1. Menorrhagia & metrorrhagia : Lump of the powdered bark of plaksha mixed with honey should be kept in lubricated vagina. (C.S.)
2. Diarrhoea with blood : Barks of plaksha, sallaki and tinisha are pounded with milk and mixed with honey . Its intake checks blood. (S.S.)
3. Eyesipelas : Cold paste of the tender leaves and bark mixed with profuse ghee should be applied. (C.S.)

Parts Used : Bark.

Preparations & Dosage : Decoction 50-100 ml.

प्लक्षः कषायः शिशिरो व्रणयोनिगदापहः ।
दाहपित्तकफास्रघ्नं शोथहा रक्तपित्तहृत् ॥
रक्तदोषहरो मूर्च्छाप्रलापभ्रमनाशनः ॥ भा०प्र०

193
TŪDA

Morus alba Family : Moraceae

Chief Characters :

1. It is tree and grows upto a height of 15 m.
2. Simple leaf, alternate phyllotaxy.
3. Spike inflorescence.
4. Cosists of green coloured flowers.
5. Fruit - achene.

Synonyms : Tula, Puga, Kramuka, Brahmadaru.

Properties : Rasa - Madhura, Amla (Amaphala); Guna - Guru; Virya - Sheeta, Ushna (Amaphala) and Vipaka - Madhura.

Pharmacological Actions : Pittavatahara.

Indications : Jwara, Daha, Trishna, Krimi, Swarabhanga.

Therapeutic Uses :

Swarabheda : Decoction of the leaves is useful for gargling.

Parts Used : Fruit, Leaf, Bark.

Preparations & Dosage : Decoction 50-100 ml.

तूदस्तूलश्च पूगश्च क्रमुको ब्रह्मदारु च ।
तूतं पक्वं गुडस्वादु हिमं पित्तानिलापहम् ।
तदेवामं गुरु सरमम्लोष्णं रक्तपित्तकृत् ॥ भा०प्र०

194
KĀKODUMBARA

Ficus hispida Linn. Family : Moraceae

Chief Characters :

1. Tree, grows upto 5 m. height.
2. Oval shaped simple leaf, opposite phyllotaxy.
3. Hypanthodium inflorescence.

Synonyms : Malaya, Phalgu, Jaghanephala.

Properties : Rasa - Kashaya, Tikta; Guna - Ruksha, Laghu; Virya - Sheeta and Vipaka - Katu.

Pharmacological Actions : Kaphapittahara, Grahi, Shukrala, Brimhana, Stambhana.

Indications : Switrakushta, Pandu, Kamala, Arshas, Vrana.

Therapeutic Uses :

1. Alarkavisha : The root of kakodumbara and seeds of dhattura are pounded together on internal administration relieves toxic effect of dog bite. (V.S.)
2. Switra : The decoction of vibhitaka bark and malapu root mixed with avalguja seed powder relieves leucoderma. (Chikitsa Kalika)
3. Raktapradara : The intake of fruit juice mixed with honey relieves pradara. (Y.R.)

Parts Used : Root, Fruit, Latex, Bark.

Preparations & Dosage : Bark powder 1-3 gm.

Specific Forumulations : Kanchana gutika.

काकोदुम्बरिका फल्गुर्मलयूर्जघनेफला ।
मलयू: स्तम्भकृत्तिक्ता शीतला तुवरा जयेत् ॥
कफपित्तव्रणश्वित्रकुष्ठपाण्ड्वर्शकामला: ॥ भा०प्र०

195
CIRABILWA

Holoptelea integrifolia Family : Ulmaceae

Chief Characters :

1. Tree.
2. Simple leaf, alternate phyllotaxy.
3. Green coloured flowers.
4. Fruit - samara.

Synonyms : Karanji, Udakirya, Karabhanjika.

Gana :

Charaka : Lekhaniya, Bhedaniya.
Sushruta : Sleshmasamshamana.

Properties : Rasa - Tikta, Kashaya; Guna - Laghu, Ruksha; Virya - Ushna and Vipaka - Katu.

Pharmacological Actions : Kaphapittashamaka.

Indications : Krimi, Kushta, Prameha, Chardi, Arsha.

Therapeutic Uses :

1. Worms : The juice of chirabilwa should be taken with honey. (S.S.)
2. Piles : Paste of citraka, putika and sunthi is mixed with alkali of putika should be used. (S.S.)
3. Colic : Leaf buds of cirabilwa fried in oil should be taken. (S.S.)

Parts Used : Bark.

Preparations & Dosage : Decoction 50-100 ml.

करञ्जी स्तम्भनी तिक्ता तुवरा कटुपाकिनी ।
वीर्योष्णा वमिपित्तार्शःकृमिकुष्ठप्रमेहजित् ॥ भा०प्र०

196
PANASA

Artocarpus integrifolia Linn. f Family : Moraceae

Chief Characters :

1. It is an evergreen tree.
2. Simple leaf, alternate phyllotaxy.
3. Hypanthodium inflorescence.
4. Fruit - large.

Synonyms :Kantakiphala, Palasa, Brihatphala, Amasayaphala.

Properties : Rasa - Madhura, Kashaya; Guna - Guru, Snigdha; Virya - Sheeta and Vipaka - Madhura.

Pharmacological Actions : Pittavatahara, Balya, Brimhana, Tarpana, Shukrala, Mamsala, Medokara, Vistambhi (Unripe fruit), Vatala, Mutral (Seed), Vrishya (Seed).

Indications : Raktapitta, Vrana, Kshaya, Krishata, Gulma.

Therapeutic Uses :

1. Skin disorders : Decoction made from its root is useful.
2. Poisoning : Decoction made from its leaves is useful.
3. Diarrhoea : Decoction of the bark is useful.

Parts Used : Fruit, Leaf, Latex, Bark, Root.

Preparations & Dosage : Decoction 50-100 ml.

पनसः कण्टकिफलः पनसोऽतिबृहत्फलः ।
पनसं शीतलं पक्वं स्निग्धं पित्तानिलापहम् ॥
तर्पणं बृंहणं स्वादु मांसलं श्लेष्मलं भृशम् ।
बल्यं शुक्रप्रदं हन्ति रक्तपित्तक्षतव्रणान् ॥
आमं तदेव विष्टम्भि वातलं तुवरं गुरु ।
दाहकृन्मधुरं बल्यं कफमेदोविवर्धनम् ॥
पनसोद्भूतबीजानि वृष्याणि मधुराणि च ।
गुरूणि बद्धविट्कानि सृष्टमूत्राणि संवदेत् ॥
मज्जा पनसजो वृष्यो वातपित्तकफापहः ।
विशेषात् पनसो वर्ज्यो गुल्मभिर्मन्दवह्निभिः ॥ भा०प्र०

197
AKṢOṬA

Juglans regia Linn. Family : Juglandaceae

Chief Characters :

1. Deciduous tree grows upto 30m. in height.
2. Paripinnate compound leaf, alternate phyllotaxy.
3. Spike inflorescence, with greenish coloured, male and female flowers on separate spikes.
4. Fruit - nut.

Synonyms : Sailabhavapeelu, Karparala.

Properties : Rasa - Madhura; Guna - Guru, Snigdha; Virya - Ushna and Vipaka - Madhura.

Pharmacological Actions : Vatahara, Kaphapittahara, Shukrala.

Indications : Amavata, Vatarakta, Krimi, Shotha, Kushta, Gandamala, Prameha, Katishoola, Vataroga, Sirashoola, Sweta pradara.

Therapeutic Uses :

1. Sandhivata : The fruit is very useful in osteo-arthritis and can be considered as a good nervine tonic. (Indian Medicinal Plants, Kirtikar & Basu).
2. Impotency : The kernels are supposed to possess aphrodisiac properties. (Khory)

Parts Used : Juice, Leaf, Bark.

Preparations & Dosage : Powder 1-2 gm.; Decoction 40-80 ml.

Specific Formulations : Amritprasha ghrita.

पीलुः शैलभवोऽक्षोटः कर्पूरालश्च कीर्तितः ।
अक्षोटकोऽपि वातात् सदृशः कफपित्तकृत् ॥ भा०प्र०

198
KAṬPHALA

Myrica nagi Thumb. Family : Myricaceae

Chief Characters :

1. Evergreen tree grows upto 20 m. height.
2. Oval shaped simple leaf, alternate phyllotaxy.
3. Male and female flowers arranged in spike inflorescence.
4. Consists of red aromatic flowers.
5. Fruit - drupe.

Synonyms : Somavalka, Kaitarya, Kumbhika, Sriparnika, Kumudika, Bhadra, Bhadravati, Mahavalkala.

Gana :

Charaka : Sandhaniya, Sukrashodhana, Vedhana sthapana, Kashayaskandha.

Sushrut : Lodhradi, Surasadi, Lakshadi, Parushakadi.

Properties : Rasa - Kashaya, Tikta, Katu; Guna - Laghu, Tikshan; Virya - Ushna and Vipaka - Katu.

Pharmacological Actions : Vatakaphahara, Vedanasthapana, Shukrasodhana, Sandhaniya.

Indications : Aruchi, Jwara, Udara, Raktapitta, Shwasa, Kasa, Pratishyaya, Kandu, Arshas, Prameha, Kantha roga.

Therapeutic Uses :

1. Fever : In fever caused by kapha, the formulation consisting of katphala, puskaramula, karkatashringi and pippali mixed with honey is efficacious. It alleviates kapha and its associated symptoms. (V.M.)
2. Head diseases : In head disease caused by kapha katphala powder should be taken as snuff or as gargles for alleviating kapha. (S.S.)
3. Conjuctivitis : In conjuctivitis caused by pitta, acqueous solution of katphala should be used as eye-drops. (S.S.)

Parts Used : Bark.

Preparations & Dosage : Powder 3-5 gm.

Specific Formulations : Katphaladi churna.

कट्फलस्तुवरस्तिक्तः कटुर्वातकफज्वरान् ।
हन्ति श्वासप्रमेहार्शः कासकण्ड्वामयारुचिः ॥ भा०प्र०

199
MĀYĀPHALA

Quercus incana Family : Cupiliferae

Chief Characters :

1. Evergreen tree.
2. Simple leaf, alternate phyllotaxy.
3. Spike inflorescence.
4. Involucre of bracts form a cup.
5. Fruit - nut.

Synonyms :Mayaka, Majjaphala.

Properties : Rasa - Kashaya; Guna - Laghu, Ruksha; Virya - Sheeta and Vipaka - Katu.

Pharmacological Actions : Kaphapittahara, Grahi, Deepana.

Indications : Atisara, Grahani, Pravahika, Shwetapradara, Arshas, Mukha-danta roga, Yonisrava.

Therapeutic Uses :

1. Dental disorders : It is useful for gargling.
2. Piles : It is useful as dusting powder in rectal prolapse, piles and wounds.
3. Menorrhagia : Wicks (varti) made of it should be kept in vagina.

Parts Used : Gall.

Preparations & Dosage : Powder 1-3 gm.

Specific Formulations : Vajradanta manjana, Mayaphaladi lepa.

An insect by the name Adleria gallae tinctoriae Oliv. forms a gall and it is known as mayaphala which means not a true fruit.

मायूकं शीतलं रूक्षं कषायं लघु दीपनम् ।
विपाके कटुकं ग्राहि कफपित्तहरं परम् ॥ शो०

200
BHŪRJAPATRA

Betula utilis Family : Betulaceae

Chief Characters :

1. Tree.
2. Simple leaf, alternate phyllotaxy.
3. Spike inflorescence.
4. Fruit - nut.

Synonyms : Bhurja, Charmi, Bahulavalkala, Sucharma, Bhojapatra.

Properties : Rasa - Kashaya; Guna - Laghu; Virya - Ushna and Vipaka - Katu.

Pharmacological Actions : Sleshmapittahara, Vishahara, Bhutagrahakara, Rakshasoghna, Medhohara.

Indications : Karnaruja, Graharoga, Raktavikruti, Medoroga, Apasmara, Unmada, Vrana, Raktapitta.

Therapeutic Uses :

1. Garbhasomga : The dhupa of bark is used in garbhasanga. (A.H.)
2. Kushta : Bhurja, lasuna, sirisha, kasisa, guggulu and shigru soaked in cow's bile and then powdered is applied as dushing powder and anointment. (C.S.)
3. Wound : In wound caused by vata, covering is provided with the leaves of eranda, bhurja, putika and haridra.

Parts Used : Bark.

Preparations & Dosage : Powder 3-6 gm.; Decoction 5-10 ml.

भूर्जपत्रः स्मृतो भूर्जश्चर्मी बहुलवल्कलः ।
भूर्जो भूतग्रहश्लेष्मकर्णरुक्पित्तरक्तजित् ।।
कषायो राक्षसघ्नश्च मेदोविषहरः परः ।। भा०प्र०

201
SOMA

Ephedra gerardiana Family : Gnetaceae

Chief Characters :

1. Perennial plant.
2. Spike inflorescence.
3. Simple leaf, opposite phyllotaxy.

Synonyms : Somalata, Somavalli, Somaksheeri, Dwijapriya.

Properties : Rasa - Kashaya, Tikta, Katu; Guna - Laghu, Ruksha; Virya - Ushna and Vipaka - Katu.

Pharmacological Actions : Tridoshahara, Rasayana, Hridya. (B.P.)

Indications : Shwasa, Mutrakricchra, Hridroga, Pratishyaya.

Therapeutic Uses :

1. Rasa sindoora-1 part, soma churna-20 parts together taken in the dosage of 5-10 ratti with madhu relieves kasa and shwasa. (S.Y.S.)
2. In inflammation associated with severe pain it is used as anointment.

Parts Used : Stem.

Preparations & Dosage : Powder 1-3 gm.

Specific Formulations : Soma yoga.

सोमवल्ली सोमलता सोमक्षीरि द्विजप्रिया ।
सोमवल्ली त्रिदोषघ्नी कटुस्तिक्ता रसायनी ॥

202
SARALA

Pinus longifolia Roxb. Family : Pinaceae

Chief Characters :

1. Evergreen tree.
2. Monocieous plant and consists of female and male cones. Turpentine oil is extracted from the sap wood of pinus excelsa.

Synonyms : Surabhidaruka, Peetavriksha, Gandhabiroja (Niryasa).

Gana :

Charaka : Purishavirajaneeya.
Sushrut : Eladi.

Properties : Rasa - Kashaya, Tikta, Katu; Guna - Laghu, Snigdha, Tikshana; Virya - Ushna and Vipaka - Katu.

Pharmacological Actions : Kaphavata shamaka, Vrana sodhana.

Indications : Dustavrana, Kushta, Krimi, Shotha.

Therapeutic Uses :

1. Wound : Wounds should be fumigated with sriveshtaka, sarjarasa, sarala, devadaru and other heart woods. (S.S.)
2. Urustambha : Paste of pippali, pippalimula, sarala and devadaru should be taken with honey. (C.S.)

Parts Used : Gum, Oil, Wood.

Preparations & Dosage : Oil 1-3 drops; Powder 1-3 gm.

सरलः पीतवृक्षः स्यात्तथा सुरभिदारुकः ।
सरलो मधुरस्तिक्तो कटुपाकरसो लघुः ॥
स्निग्धोष्णा कर्णकण्ठाक्षिरोगरक्षोहरः स्मृतः ।
कफानिलस्वेददाहकासमूर्च्छाव्रणापहः ॥

203
HAPUṢĀ

Juniperus communis Family : Cupressaceae

Chief Characters :

1. Gymnosperm, perennial herb.
2. Whorled phyllotaxy.
3. Flowers are arranged like cones.
4. Blue and black coloured fruit.

Synonyms : Havusha, Visra.

Properties : Rasa - Tikta, Katu, Kashaya; Guna - Guru, Mridu; Virya - Ushna and Vipaka - Katu.

Pharmacological Actions : Vatakaphahara, Deepana.

Indications : Udara, Arshas, Grahani, Gulma, Shoola.

Therapeutic Uses :

1. Udara roga : In case of intestinal obstruction, butter milk should be taken with hapusa, yavani, jiraka and rock salt. (C.S.)
2. Piles : Citraka, Hapusa and hingu should be given with butter milk. (C.S.)

Parts Used : Fruit, Oil.

Preparations & Dosage : Powder 3-5 gm.; Oil 1-2 drops.

हपुषा दीपनी तिक्ता कटूष्णा तुवरा गुरुः ।
पित्तोदरसमीरार्शोग्रहणीगुल्मशूलहृत् ॥ भा०प्र०

204
ŚAṬĪ

Hedychium spicatum Family : Zingiberaceae

Chief Characters :

1. Perennial herb.
2. White coloured flowers, spike inflorescence.
3. Simple leaves.
4. Fruit - capsule.

Synonyms : Palasi, Sadagrantha, Gandha moolika, Gandharika, Gandhavadhu, Vadhu, Prithupalasika, Gandhapalasi.

Gana :

Charaka : Hikka nigrahana, Shwasahara.

Properties : Rasa - Katu, Tikta, Kashaya; Guna - Laghu, Tikshna; Virya - Anushna and Vipaka - Katu.

Pharmacological Actions : Kaphavatashamaka, Grahi.

Indications : Shotha, Kasa, Shwasa, Shoola, Vrana, Asyamala, Sidhma, Hikka, Jwara.

Therapeutic Uses :

1. Hricchoola : Trikatu, bhumyamalaki and shati churna relieve all kinds of vasti and hricchsoola. (Y.R.)
2. Semen disorder : In case of grathita shukra, ghee cooked with shati should be used. (S.S.)
3. Amavata : Paste of shati and shunthi mixed with decoction of punarnava should be taken for a week. (V.M., B.P.)

Parts Used : Tuber.

Preparations & Dosage : Powder 1-3 gm.

Specific Formulations : Shatyadi churna, Shatyadi kwatha.

शटी पलाशी षड्ग्रन्था सुव्रता गन्धमूलिका ।
गन्धकारिका गन्धवपुर्वधूः पृथुपलाशिका ।।
भवेद्गन्धपलाशी तु कषाया ग्राहिणी लघुः ।
तिक्ता तीक्ष्णा च कटुकानुष्णास्यमलनाशिनी ।।
शोथकासव्रणश्वासशूलहिध्मग्रहापहा ।। भा०प्र०

205
TAVAKṢĪRA

Curcuma angustifolia Family : Zingiberaceae

Chief Characters :

1. Perennial having root stack.
2. Leaves - barrel shaped, big in size.
3. Yellow coloured flowers, spike inflorescence.

Synonyms : Tugakseeri, Tavaksheera.

Gana :

Sushruta : Kakolyadi.

Properties : Rasa - Madhura; Guna - Laghu, Snigdha; Virya - Sheeta and Vipaka - Madhura.

Pharmacological Actions : Vatapittashamaka, Brimhana, Vrishya.

Indications : Swasa, Kasa, Kshaya, Mutrakricchra.

Parts Used : Tuber.

Preparations & Dosage : Powder 3-6 gm.

तवक्षीरी क्षयश्वासकासघ्नी मधुरा हिमा ॥ अ०स०सू०

206
ĀMRAGANDHĪ HARIDRĀ

Curcuma amada Roxb. Family : Zingiberaceae

Chief Characters :

1. Perennial herb grows upto 1½ m. height.
2. Big leaves with long petiole.
3. Light yellow coloured flowers.
4. Spike inflorescence.

Synonyms : Darvibheda, Amragandha, Surabhidaru, Daru, Karpoor, Padmapatra, Surimata, Surataraka.

Properties : Rasa - Katu, Tikta, Madhura; Guna - Laghu, Ruksha; Virya - Sheeta and Vipaka - Katu.

Pharmacological Actions : Kaphapittashamaka, Vatala.

Indications : Kandu, Prameha, Kushta, Shwitra, Krimi, Vrana.

Therapeutic Uses :

Shwitra : The powder is administered internally in the treatment of shwitra. (N.A.)

Parts Used : Rhizome.

Preparations & Dosage : Juice 5-10 ml.; Powder 1-2 gm.

आम्रगन्धि हरिद्रा सा या शीता वातला मता ।
पित्तहृन्मधुरा तिक्ता सर्वकण्डुविनाशनी ।। भा०प्र०

207
NĀGADAMANĪ

Crinum asiaticum Linn. Family : Amaryllidaceae

Chief Characters :

1. It is a perennial plant.
2. Radicle leaves.
3. White coloured big flowers, umbel inflorescence.
4. Fruit - capsule.

Synonyms : Sukhadarshana.

Properties : Rasa - Madhura, Tikta; Guna - Snigdha, Picchila; Virya - Sheeta and Vipaka - Madhura.

Pharmacological Actions : Vatapittahara, Balya.

Indications : Kasa, Shwasa, Mutrakricchra, Daurbalya, Jwara, Kushta, Shotha.

Therapeutic Uses :

The nasya of the tuberpaste relieves snake poison. (R.R.S.)

Parts Used : Root, Leaf.

Preparations & Dosage : Juice 10-20 ml.; Root powder 1-2 gm.

बलामोटा कटुस्तिक्ता लघुः पित्तकफापहा ।
मूत्रकृच्छ्रव्रणान् रक्षो नाशयेज्जालगर्दभम् ॥
सर्वग्रहप्रशमनी निःशेषविषनाशिनी ।
जयं सर्वत्र कुरुते धनदा सुमतिप्रदा ॥

208
MAHĀBHARĪ VACĀ

Alpinia galanga Family : Zingiberaceae

Chief Characters :

1. Perennial herb consists of root stalk.
2. Leaves - barrel shaped with acute tip.
3. White coloured big flowers, panicle inflorescence.
4. Indehiscent capsule.

Synonyms : Kulanjana, Gandhamoola, Sthulagranthi, Malaya vacha.

Properties : Rasa - Katu; Guna - Laghu, Tikshna, Ruksha; Virya - Ushna and Vipaka - Katu.

Pharmacological Actions : Kaphavatashamaka, Deepana, Swarya, Hridya.

Indications : Shwasa, Kasa, Hridroga, Kushta, Mukharoga, Kantharoga.

Parts Used : Rhizome.

Preparations & Dosage : Powder 1-3 gm.

Specific Formulations : Kulinjanadyavaleha.

सुगन्धाऽप्युग्रगन्धा च विशेषात् कफवातनुत् ।
सुस्वरत्वकरी रुच्या हृत्कण्ठमुखशोधिनी ॥ भा०प्र०

209
KEBUKA

Costus speciosus Koen. Family : Zingiberaceae

Chief Characters :

1. Herb consists of tuberous root.
2. Simple leaf, alternate phyllotaxy.
3. Spike inflorescence.
4. White coloured big flowers.
5. Fruit - capsule.

Synonyms : Kembuka.

Gana :

Charaka : Krimighna, Tiktaskandha.

Properties : Rasa - Tikta, Kashaya; Guna - Laghu, Ruksha; Virya - Sheeta and Vipaka - Katu.

Pharmacological Actions : Kaphapittahara, Deepana, Pachana, Hridya, Vatala, Grahi, Garbhashaya sankochana.

Indications : Kushta, Prameha, Kasa, Raktavikara.

Therapeutic Uses :

1. Wound : Juice of kebuka should be taken keeping on pungent diet. (S.S.)
2. Filaria : Juice of kebuka rhizome mixed with bida salt should be taken as remedy. (S.S.)

Parts Used : Tuber.

Preparations & Dosage : Powder 3-6 gm.; Juice 10-20 ml.

केबुकं कटुकं पाके तिक्तं ग्राहि हिमं लघु ।
दीपनं पाचनं हृद्यं कफपित्तज्वरापहम् ॥
कुष्ठकासप्रमेहास्रनाशनं वातलं कटु ॥ भा०प्र०

210
KADALĪ

Musa paradisiaca Linn. Family : Musaceae

Chief Characters :

1. Tree like herb grows upto 3-6 m.
2. Pseudostem, leaves rectangular shaped.
3. Spadix inflorescence.
4. Red or violet coloured flowers.
5. Fruit - berry.

Synonyms : Varana, Mocha, Ambusara, Amsumatephala.

Properties : Rasa - Madhura; Guna - Guru, Snigdha; Virya - Sheeta and Vipaka - Madhura.

Pharmacological Actions : Pittavatahara, Vrishya, Brimhana, Kaphakrita, Vishtambhi.

Indications : Trishna, Daha, Kshaya, Prameha, Netraroga, Amalapitta (Kadalikanda).

Therapeutic Uses :

1. Prameha : The fruits are to be administered with ghee (Shodhala).
2. Vrana : The leaf paste is applied externally for healing the infected wounds. (V.M.)
3. Shwasa-kasa : Fruit boiled in gomutra or heated on live charcoal relieves kasa-shwasa. (V.M.)

Parts Used : Tuber, Flower, Fruit.

Preparations & Dosage : Juice 10-20 ml.; Powder 1-2 gm.

Specific Formulations : Shankha vati.

कदली वारणा मोचाऽम्बुसारांऽशुमती फला ।
मोचाफलं स्वादुशीतं विष्टम्भि कफकृद्गुरु ॥
स्निग्धं पित्तास्रतृड्दाहक्षतक्षयसमीरजित् ।
पक्वं स्वादु हिमं पाके स्वादु वृष्यञ्च बृंहणम् ।
क्षुत्तृष्णानेत्रगदहृन्मेहघ्नं रुचिमांसकृत् ॥ भा०प्र०

211
ANĀNĀSA

Ananas comosus Merr. Family : Bromeliaceae

Chief Characters :

1. Annul herb.
2. Simple leaf, radical leaves.
3. Red coloured flowers.
4. Racemose inflorescence.
5. Fruit - berry.

Synonyms : Bahunetra, Ananna, Anarasa, Kautukasamjnaka.

Properties : Rasa - Madhura (Ripen fruit), Amla (Unripen fruit); Guna - Guru, Snigdha; Virya - Sheeta and Vipaka - Madhura.

Pharmacological Actions : Vatapittashamaka, Balya, Artavajanana, Mutrala, Shleshmala, Tarpana, Garbhapatakara (Unripen fruit juice).

Indications : Krimi, Shoola, Kamala, Ashmari, Kashtartava, Rajorodha, Mutrakriccha, Koshtagata vata.

Therapeutic Uses :

1. Krimi : The leafy juice (20 ml.) with honey is useful in worm infestation.
2. Kamala : The intake of fruit juice (50-100 ml.) is useful in relieving jaundice.
3. Hikka : The intake of leafy juice mixed with sugar controls Hiccup.

Parts Used : Fruit.

Preparations & Dosage : Juice 25-50 ml.

बहुनेत्रफलं चाम्लं कृमिघ्नं मधुरं सरम् ।
बल्यं वातहरं रुच्यं श्लेष्मलं तर्पणं गुरु ॥ राजनिघण्टु

212
SUDARŚANA

Crinum latifolium Family : Amaryllidaceae

Chief Characters :

1. Perennial shrub with bulb.
2. Leaves - barrel shaped, wavy margin.
3. White flowers, umbel inflorescence.
4. Fruit - capsule.

Synonyms : Somavalli, Chakrangi, Madhuparnika.

Properties : Rasa - Madhura, Tikta; Guna - Ruksha, Tikshna; Virya - Ushna and Vipaka - Madhura.

Pharmacological Actions : Kaphahara.

Indications : Shotha, Raktavata, Kushta.

Therapeutic Uses :

1. Pradara : Fine paste of the root of sudarshana taken with milk checks the disease. (R.M.)
2. Kushta : Cakramarda seeds and jeeraka in equal parts with a piece root of sundarshana destroy ringworm and kushta. (C.D.)

Parts Used : Tuber, Leaf.

Preparations & Dosage : Leaf juice 5-10 ml.; Powder 1-2 gm.

सुदर्शना सोमवल्ली चक्राङ्गी मधुपर्णिका ।
वत्सादनी च दध्याली मेचका मेचका तथा ॥
दध्याली स्वादु तिक्तोष्णा कफशोफास्रवातजित् ॥ कै०नि०

213
KUṄKUMA

Crocus sativus Linn. Family : Iridaceae

Chief Characters :

1. A herb consisting of tuberous root.
2. Radical leaves occur.
3. Light violet coloured flowers.
4. Fruit - loculicidal capsule.

Synonyms : Ghusruna, Rakta, Kashmira, Peetaka, Vara, Sankocha, Pisuna, Dheera, Bahlika, Sonitabhidha.

Properties : Rasa - Katu, Tikta; Guna - Snigdha; Virya - Ushna and Vipaka - Katu.

Pharmacological Actions : Tridoshahara, Varnya, Shonita sthapana.

Indications : Chardi, Shiroruja, Vyanga, Vrana, Krimi, Netraroga.

Therapeutic Uses :

1. Suryavarta/Ardhavabhedaka : Kesara mixed with sugar is fried in ghee and ghee is administered as nasya to relieve suryavarta and ardhavabhedaka shiroroga. (Sodhala)
2. Mutrarodha/Udavarta : The decoction of kumkuma is administered. (Sushruta)

Parts Used : Stamens of the flower.

Preparations & Dosage : Stamens ½-1 gm.

Specific Formulations : Kumkumadi ghrita, Kumkumadhya taila.

कुङ्कुमं घुसृणं रक्तं काश्मीरं पीतकं वरम् ।
सङ्कोचं पिशुनं धीरं बाह्लीकं शोणिताभिधम् ॥
काश्मीरदेशजे क्षेत्रे कुङ्कुमं यद्भवेद्धि तत् ।
सूक्ष्मकेसरमारक्तं पद्मगन्धि तदुत्तमम् ॥
बाह्लीकदेशसञ्जातं कुङ्कुमं पाण्डुरं मतम् ।
केतकीगन्धयुक्तं तन्मध्यमं सूक्ष्मकेशरम् ॥
कुङ्कुमं पारसीकं यन्मधुगन्धि तदीरितम् ।
ईषत्पाण्डूरवर्णं तत् ह्यधमं स्थूलकेशरम् ॥
कुङ्कुमं कटुकं स्निग्धं शिरोरुग्व्रणजन्तुजित् ।
तिक्तं वमीहरं वर्ण्यं व्यङ्गदोषत्रयापहम् ॥ भा०प्र०

214
TĀLAMŪLĪ

Curculigo orchioides Gaertn. Family : Hypoxidaceae

Chief Characters :

1. It is a perennial plant.
2. Leaves - barrel shaped.
3. Yellow coloured flowers.
4. Fruit - capsule.

Synonyms : Talapatri.

Properties : Rasa - Madhura, Tikta; Guna - Guru, Snigdha, Picchila; Virya - Ushna and Vipaka - Madhura.

Pharmacological Actions : Vatapitta shamaka, Brimhana, Rasayana, Vrishya.

Indications : Arshas, Kleebatwa, Grahani, Mutrakricchra, Kushta, Kasa.

Therapeutic Uses :

1. Retention of urine : Decoction of talapatri should be used. (B.S., A.H.)
2. Aphrodisiac : Regular use of the powder of krishna musali mixed with ghee acts as aphrodisiac. (V.V.)

Parts Used : Tuberous root.

Preparations & Dosage : Powder 3-6 gm.-

मुशली मेधुरा वृष्या वीर्योष्णा बृंहणी गुरुः ।
तिक्ता रसायनी हन्ति गुदजान्यनिलं तथा ॥ भा०प्र०

215
VĀRĀHĪKANDA

Dioscorea bulbifera Linn. Var. sativa Family : Dioscoriaceae

Chief Characters :

1. Climber.
2. Simple leaves, alternate and opposite phyllotaxy.
3. Light green or violet coloured flowers, spike inflorescence.
4. Fruit - capsule.

Synonyms : Varahi, Sukari, Krodhakanya, Grishti, Charmakaraluka, Varahavadana, Varada.

Properties : Rasa - Madhura, Tikta, Katu; Guna - Laghu, Snigdha; Virya - Ushna and Vipaka - Katu.

Pharmacological Actions : Kaphavatahara, Pittakara, Rasayana, Shukrala, Balya, Varnya, Deepana.

Indications : Prameha, Kushta, Krimi.

Therapeutic Uses :

1. The powder of varahi and oil on external application relieves nadivrana. (S.Ch. 17)
2. Rasayana : Powder of varahi tuber mixed with honey is taken with milk. After it is digested, milk, ghee and boiled rice should be taken as diet. (S.S.)
   Fresh varahi tuber should be taken with milk keeping on milk diet without cereals for a month and then for the next month on milk and cereals. (A.H.)

Parts Used : Tuber.

Preparations & Dosage : Powder 3-6 gm.

शौकरो मधुरस्तिक्तः कटुको रसपाकयोः ।
शुक्रायुः स्वरवर्णाग्निबलपित्तविवर्धनः ॥
कफकुष्ठमरुन्मेहकृमीन् हन्ति रसायनम् ॥ कै०नि०

216
VANAPALĀṆḌU

Urginea indica Family : Liliaceae

Chief Characters :

1. Herb with bulb.
2. Leaves - long with sharp acute tip.
3. Light green coloured flowers, racemose inflorescence.
4. Fruit - loculicidal capsule.

Synonyms : Kolakanda.

Properties : Rasa - Tikta, Katu; Guna - Laghu, Tikshana; Virya - Ushna and Vipaka - Katu.

Pharmacological Actions : Kaphavatashamaka, Hridya, Mutrala.

Indications : Hridroga, Kushta, Krimi, Mutrakricchra.

Therapeutic Uses :

Skin disorders : The paste is useful as anointment.

Parts Used : Bulb.

Preparations & Dosage : Powder 120-200 gm.

पलाण्डुर्यवनेष्टश्च दुर्गन्धो मुखदूषकः ।
पलाण्डुस्तु गुणैर्ज्ञेयो रसोनसदृशो बुधैः ॥
स्वादुः पाकैः रसेऽनुष्णः कफकृन्नातिपित्तलः ।
हरते केवलं वातं बलवीर्यकरो गुरुः ॥ भा०प्र०

Vanapalāṇḍu

कोलकन्दः कटुश्चोष्णः कृमिकुष्ठविनाशनः ।
वान्तिहृच्च परं हृद्यो मूत्रलो विषवारणः ॥ द्र०गु०वि०

217

DWIPĀNTARA VACĀ

Smilax glabra Roxb. & Family : Liliaceae
Smilax feron Wall. Family : Liliaceae

Chief Characters :

1. Perennial creeper.
2. Simple leaves, alternate phyllotaxy.
3. White coloured small flowers, umbel inflorescence.
4. Fruit - berry.

Synonyms : Chopchini, Madhusnuhi.

Properties : Rasa - Tikta; Guna - Laghu, Ruksha; Virya - Ushna and Vipaka - Katu.

Pharmacological Actions : Vatahara, Deepana, Sakrut-mutra vishodhana.

Indications : Phiranga, Vatavyadhi, Apasmara, Tanuvedana, Vibandha, Adhmana, Shoola, Unmada.

Therapeutic Uses :

Phiranga : The powder of tuber with honey relieves phiranga. (B.P.)

Parts Used : Tuber.

Preparations & Dosage : Powder 3-6 gm.

Specific Formulations : Chopachinipaka.

द्वीपान्तरवचा किञ्चित्तिक्तोष्णा वह्निदीप्तिकृत् ।
विबन्धाध्मानशूलघ्नी शकृन्मूत्रविशोधिनी ॥
वातव्याधीनपस्मारमुन्मादं तनुवेदनाम् ।
व्यपोहति विशेषेण फिरङ्गामयनाशिनी ॥

218
UŚAVA

Smilax zeylanica Linn. Family : Liliaceae

Chief Characters :

1. Perennial climber.
2. Simple leaves, alternate phyllotaxy.
3. White coloured small unisexual flowers.
4. Umbel inflorescence.
5. Fruit - berry.

Properties : Rasa - Madhura, Tikta; Guna - Laghu, Ruksha, Tikshna; Virya - Ushna and Vipaka - Katu.

Pharmacological Actions : Tridoshahara, Deepana.

Indications : Adhamana, Shoola, Vibandha, Kushta, Vatavyadi, Apasmara, Unmada.

Parts Used : Tuber.

Preparations & Dosage : Powder 3-6 gm.

219
LĀṄGALĪ

Gloriosa superba Linn. Family : Liliaceae

Chief Characters :

1. Perennial creeper.
2. Simple leaves, alternate phyllotaxy.
3. Corymb inflorescence, red coloured flowers.
4. Fruit - septicidal capsule.

Synonyms : Halini, Kalihari, Sakrapushpi, Visalya, Agnisikha, Ananta, Vahni vaktra, Garbhanuta.

Properties : Rasa - Kashaya, Tikta, Katu; Guna - Laghu, Tikshna; Virya - Ushna and Vipaka - Katu.

Pharmacological Actions : Sleshmahara, Pittala, Garbhapataka, Sara.

Indications : Krimi, Kushta, Shotha, Arsas, Vrana, Shoola.

Therapeutic Uses :

1. For removal of placenta, the root paste should be applied to limbs. (S.Sa. 10)
2. External application of root paste to umbilicus, vagina etc. induces labour.

Parts Used : Tuber.

Preparations & Dosage : Powder 250-500 mg.; 3-6 gm. for abortion.

Specific Formulations : Kasisadi taila, Langali rasayana, Langalyadi vati.

कलिहारी सरा कुष्ठशोषार्शोव्रणशूलजित् ।
सक्षारा श्लेष्मजित्तिक्ता कटुका तुवरापि च ॥
तीक्ष्णोष्णा कृमिहृल्लघ्वी पित्तला गर्भपातिनी ॥ भा०प्र०

220
SURAÑJĀNA

Colchicum luteum Family : Liliaceae

Chief Characters :

1. Perennial plant.
2. Simple leaves, radicle.
3. Funnel shaped flowers.
4. Fruit - septicidal capsule.

Properties : Rasa - Tikta, Katu; Guna - Laghu, Ruksha; Virya - Ushna and Vipaka - Katu.

Pharmacological Actions : Kaphavata shamaka, Vedana sthapana, Rakta shodhaka.

Indications : Vatarakta, Shotha, Amavata, Gridhrasi.

Therapeutic Uses :

1. Amavata : The paste made up of nagakesara and egg yolk is externally applied to reduce inflammation.
2. Wound : The powder is useful for dusting the wounds.

Parts Used : Tuber.

Preparations & Dosage : Powder 125-375 mg.

Specific Formulations : Suranjanavalehya.

सुरञ्जानं तु कटुकं तिक्तं वीर्योष्णमेव च ।
कफवातहरं रक्तशोधनमामनाशनम् ॥ द्र०गु०वि०

221
MŪSALĪ

Asparagus adscendens Family : Liliaceae

Chief Characters :

1. Perennial herb.
2. White coloured branches and stem covered with thorns.
3. Fruit - berry.

Properties : Rasa - Madhura, Tikta; Guna - Guru (B.P.), Snigdha; Virya - Ushna (B.P.), Sheeta (R.N.) and Vipaka - Katu.

Pharmacological Actions : Vatahara (B.P.), Vrishya, Brimhana, Rasayana, Kaphakara (R.N.), Vatapittahara (S.N.), Pittahara (R.N.).

Indications : Arshas, Daha, Mutrakricchra, Shukrakshaya, Klaibyata.

Therapeutic Uses :

1. Freckles : The root of musali pounded with goat's milk and mixed with honey is applied on face. (A.H.)
2. Deafness : One should take powder of musali and bakuchi in order to alleviate deafness. (B.S.)
3. Aphrodisiac : Powder of musali root combined with guduchi sattva, kapikacchu gokshura, shalmali, sharkara, amalaki and suspended in milk added with ghee should be taken. It arouses sex urge and increases libido. (S.G.; B.P.)

मुशली मधुरा शीता वृष्या पुष्टिबलप्रदा ।
पिच्छिला कफदा पित्तदाहश्रमहरा परा ॥ रा०नि०

222
NĀRIKELA

Cocos nucifera Linn Family : Arecaceae

Chief Characters :

1. It is a tree grows upto 30 mts.
2. Compound leaves.
3. Light green coloured flowers, spadix inflorescence.
4. Fruit - drupe.

Synonyms : Dridhaphala, Langali, Kurchashirshaka, Tunga, Skandhapala, Trinaraja, Sadaphala.

Properties : Rasa - Madhura; Guna - Guru, Snigdha, Laghu (Coconut water); Virya - Sheeta and Vipaka - Madhura.

Pharmacological Actions : Vatapittahara, Brimhana, Balya, Vasti sodhana, Vishtambhi, Hridya, Shukrala (Coconut water).

Indications : Dahajwara, Gulma, Shoola, Raktatisara (Flower) Mutrakricchra (Coconut water).

Therapeutic Uses :

1. Flower paste taken with curd relieves mutra sharkara. (B.P.)
2. Coconut water relieves suryavarta and ardhavabedhaka (C.D.)

Parts Used : Fruit, Flower, Oil, Root, Alkali etc.

Preparations & Dosage : Fruit 10-20gm.; Alkali 1-2gm.; Oil 10-20 drops.

Specific Formulations : Narikela kanda, Narikela lavana, Narikelamirta.

नारिकेलफलं शीतं दुर्जरं बस्तिशोधनम् ।
विष्टम्भि बृंहणं बल्यं वातपित्तास्रदाहनुत् ॥
विशेषत: कोमलनारिकेलं निहन्ति पित्तज्वरपित्तदोषान् ।
तदेव जीर्णं गुरुपित्तकारि विदाहि विष्टम्भिमतं भिषग्भि: ॥
तस्याम्भ: शीतलं हृद्यं दीपनं शुक्रलं लघु ।
पिपासापित्तजित् स्वादु बस्तिशुद्धिकरं परम् ॥ भा०प्र०

223
PŪGA

Areca catechu Family : Arecaceae

Chief Characters :

1. It is a tree and grows upto a height of 30 mts.
2. Spadix inflorescence.
3. Compound leaves.
4. Fruit - berry.

Synonyms : Kramuka, Guvaka, Gokshata, Puga, Pugi, Udwega.

Gana :

Sushruta : Salasaradi, Shyamadi.

Properties : Rasa - Kashaya, Madhura; Guna - Ruksha, Guru (Half fruit); Virya - Sheeta and Vipaka - Katu.

Pharmacological Actions : Kaphapittahara, Deepana, Mohajanaka, Abhisyandi (Ardha phala), Tridoshahara (Boiled fruit).

Indications : Krimi, Atisara, Asyavairasya, Prameha, Pravahika.

Therapeutic Uses :

1. Decoction of pugiphala and khadira used in kshudrameha. (Sushruta)
2. Pugiphala rasa with jambira is taken in purishaja krimi. (Y.R.)

Parts Used : Fruit.

Preparations & Dosage : Powder 1-3 gm.

Specific Formulations : Pugakhanda.

पूगं गुरु हिमं रूक्षं कषायं कफपित्तजित् ।
मोहनं दीपनं रुच्यमास्यवैरस्यनाशनम् ॥
आर्द्रं तद् गुर्वभिष्यन्दि वह्निदृष्टिहरं स्मृतम् ।
स्विन्नं दोषत्रयच्छेदि दृढमध्यं तदुत्तमम् ॥ भा०प्र०

224
TĀLA

Borassus flabellifer Linn Family : Arecaceae

Chief Characters :

1. The tree grows upto 50 mts. height.
2. Spadix inflorescence.
3. Dioceious plant. Consists of white coloured flowers.
4. Fruits - drupe with stony endocarp.
5. A separate stony endocarp is present for the 3 seeds.

Synonyms : Lekhyapatra, Trinaraja, Mahonnata.

Properties : Rasa - Madhura; Guna - Laghu, Snigdha; Virya - Sheeta and Vipaka - Madhura.

Pharmacological Actions : Pittasleshmakara/Mutrala (Fruit), Vatapittaghna/Sleshmala (Talamajja), Pittala (Talarasa), Madakari (Rasa).

Indications : Amlapitta, Vishama jwara, Mutrakricchra.

Therapeutic Uses :

1. The decoction of root relieves mutrakricchra & mutravaivarnya. (C.S.)
2. The decoction of root with tandulodaka relieves mutraghata.
3. Ash of tala flowers mixed with jaggery alleviates spleenomegaly. (C.D.)

Parts Used : Fruit.

तालस्तु लेख्यपत्रः स्यात्तृणराजो महोन्नतः ॥
पक्वं तालफलं पित्तरक्तश्लेष्मविवर्धनम् ।
दुर्जरं बहुमूत्रञ्च तन्द्राऽभिष्यन्दशुक्रदम् ॥
तालमज्जा तु तरुणः किञ्चिन्मदकरो लघुः ।
श्लेष्मलो वातपित्तघ्नः सस्नेहो मधुरः सरः ॥
तालजं तरुणं तोयमतीव मदकृन्मतम् ।
अम्लीभूतं तदा तु स्यात्पित्तकृद्वातदोषहृत् ॥ भा०प्र०

225
KHARJŪRA

Phoenin sylvestris Family : Arecaceae

Chief Characters :

1. Tree.
2. Paripinnate compound leaf.
3. Spadix inflorescence.
4. Male flowers - white coloured and female flowers - green coloured.
5. Fruit - berry.

Synonyms : Bhumi kharjuika, Swadari, Duraroha, Mriducchada, Skandaphala.

Properties : Rasa - Madhura; Guna - Guru, Snigdha; Virya - Sheeta and Vipaka - Madhura.

Pharmacological Actions : Vatakaphahara, Hridya, Tarpana, Balya, Shukrala, Vistambhi, Vrishya, Brimhana.

Indications : Raktapitta, Kshaya, Jwara, Atisara, Trishna, Kasa, Shwasa, Mada, Murccha.

Therapeutic Uses :

The leaf decoction and honey relieve krimi. (B.R.)

Parts Used : Fruit, Juice, Leaf.

Preparations & Dosage : Decoction 50-100ml.

खर्जूरीत्रितयं शीतं मधुरं रसपाकयो: ।
स्निग्धं रुचिकरं हृद्यं क्षतक्षयहरं गुरु ।
तर्पणं रक्तपित्तघ्नं पुष्टिविष्टम्भशुक्रदम् ॥
कोष्ठमारुतहृद् बल्यं वान्तिवातकफापहम् ।
ज्वरातिसारक्षुत्तृष्णाकासश्वासनिवारकम् ॥
मदमूर्च्छामरुत्पित्तमद्योद्भूतगदान्तकृत् ।
महतीभ्यां गुणैरल्पा स्वल्पखर्जूरिका स्मृता ॥ भा०प्र०

226
RAKTANIRYĀSA

Daemonorops propingues Family : Palmae

Chief Characters :

1. Tree.
2. Compond leaf - alternate phyllotaxy.
3. Spadix inflorescence.
4. Red coloured fruit exudation is known as raktaniryasa.

Properties : Rasa - Kashaya; Guna - Laghu, Ruksha; Virya - Sheeta and Vipaka - Katu.

Pharmacological Actions : Kaphapitta shamaka, Raktastambhana, Vranaropana.

Indications : Raktapitta, Rakta pradara, Raktarshas, Atisara, Pravahika.

Therapeutic Uses :

Accidental wounds and chronic ulcers : Its powder is useful for dusting the wounds.

Parts Used : Fruits exudation.

Preparations & Dosage : Powder 1-3gm.

ज्ञेयस्तु रक्तनिर्यासः कषायः रूक्षशीतलः ।
कफपित्तहरो रक्तस्तम्भनो व्रणरोपणः ॥ द्र०गु०वि०

227
KETAKĪ

Pandanus tectorius Soland Family : Pandanaceae

Chief Characters :

1. Perennial shrub grows upto 5 m. height.
2. Long leaves with serrate margin.
3. Male and female flowers occur on different plants and consists of white aromatic flowers.
4. Fruit - drupe.

Synonyms : Suchika pushpa, Jambuka, Krakacacchada.

Properties : Rasa - Tikta, Madhura, Katu; Guna - Laghu, Snigdha; Virya - Ushna and Vipaka - Katu.

Pharmacological Actions : Pittakaphahara, Varnya, Balya, Rasayana, Chakshushya.

Indications : Jwara, Prameha, Kushta, Masurika.

Therapeutic Uses :

1. Vataja gulma *:* Kshara is made from its root and administered internally along with oil. (Vrinda)
2. Mutrakricchra *:* Its root juice and root paste should be given orally along with ghee. (Vaidya Manorama)

Parts Used : Flower, Root.

Preparations & Dosage : Arka 40-60ml.; Sharbat 20-40ml.; Powder 1-3 gm.

Specific Formulations : Chandrakala rasa.

केतकी कुसुमं वर्ण्यं केशदौर्गन्ध्यनाशनम् ।
हेमाभं मदनोन्मादवर्धनं सौख्यकारि च ॥
तस्यास्तनोऽतिशिशिरः कटुः पित्तकफापहः ।
रसायनकरो बल्यो देहदार्ढ्यकरः परः ॥ रा०नि०

228
SŪRAṆA

Amorphophallus companulatus Family : Araceae

Chief Characters :

1. Pereinnial plant.
2. Compound leaves.
3. Spadix inflorescence; consists of light green or violet coloured flowers.
4. Fruit - berry.

Synonyms : Arshoghna, Kandula.

Properties : Rasa - Kashya; Guna - Laghu, Ruksha; Virya - Ushna and Vipaka - Katu.

Pharmacological Actions : Kaphavatahara, Deepana, Pachana.

Indications : Arshas, Pleeha roga, Gulma, Shoola, Krimi, Kasa

Contraindications : Shwasa, Dadrukushta, Raktapitta.

Therapeutic Uses :

1. Piles : The tuber of surana pasted with mud should be cooked by closed heating. Then it should be taken with oil and salt. It destroys haemorrhoids. (A. H.; V. M.; S.G.).
   Intake of buttermilk mixed with surana powder and kutaja bark destroys haemorrhoids. (R.M.)
2. Valmika and Sleepada : The paste of surana tuber mixed with honey and ghee is applied to alleviate valmika and sleepada. (H.S.)

Parts Used : Tuber.

Preparations & Dosage : Powedr 3-6gm.

Specific Formulations : Surana modaka.

सूरणो दीपनो रूक्षः कषायः कण्डुकृत् कटुः ॥
विष्टम्भी विशदो रुच्यः कफार्शःकृन्तनो लघुः ।
विशेषादर्शसे पथ्यः प्लीहगुल्मविनाशनः ॥
सर्वेषां कन्दशाकानां सूरणः श्रेष्ठ उच्यते ।
दद्रूणां कुष्ठिनां रक्तपित्तिनां न हितो हि सः ।
सन्धानयोगं सम्प्राप्तः सूरणो गुणवत्तरः ॥ भा०प्र०

229
MĀNAKANDA

Alocasia indica Family : Araceae

Chief Characters :

1. Herb.
2. Spadix inflorescence with light yellow or green coloured flowers.
3. Fruit - berry.

Synonyms : Manaka, Mahapatra.

Properties : Rasa - Madhura; Guna - Guru, Snigdha; Virya - Sheeta and Vipaka - Madhura.

Pharmacological Actions : Vatapittahara.

Indications : Shotha, Raktapitta, Arshas, Mutrakricchra, Vibandha, Shoola.

Therapeutic Uses :

Stiffness or palsy of tongue : Ash of manaka mixed with salt and oil should be rubbed on the tongue. (C.D.)

Parts Used : Tuber, Leaf, Stem.

Preparations & Dosage : Tuber powder 5-10gm.; Juice 10-20ml.

Specific Formulations : Manakadi vati, Manakadi gutika.

मानकः स्यान्महापत्रः कथ्यन्ते तद्गुणा अथ ।
मानकः शोथहृच्छीतो रक्तपित्तहरोऽलघुः ।। भा०प्र०

230
KUMBHIKĀ

Careya arborea Roxb Family : Barringtoniaceae

Chief Characters :

1. Tree grows upto the height of 20 m.
2. Simple leaf alternate phyllotaxy.
3. Spike inflorescence.
4. White coloured big flower.
5. Fruit - oval shaped.

Synonyms : Katabhi, Katambhara, Swadupushpa, Madhuranu.

Properties : Rasa - Katu; Guna - Ruksha, Laghu; Virya - Ushna and Vipaka - Katu.

Pharmacological Actions : Kaphahara, Vishahara, Shukrahrut (Fruit).

Indications : Prameha, Arshas, Krimi, Kushta, Nadivrana.

Therapeutic Uses :

Vrana : The external application of pounded leaf heals the infected wound without fail. (Nighantu Adarsha)

Parts Used : Bark, Leaf, Fruit.

Preparations & Dosage : Powder 1-3gm.; Decoction 50-100ml.

वारिपर्णी कुम्भिका स्याद्वारिमूली खमूलिका ।
शैवालं जलनीली स्याच्छैवलं जलजश्च तत् ॥
वारिपर्णी हिमा तिक्ता लघ्वी स्वाद्वी सरा कटुः ।
दोषत्रयहरी रूक्षा शोणितज्वरशोषकृत् ॥
शैवालं तुवरं तिक्तं मधुरं शीतलं लघु ।
स्निग्धदाहतृषापित्तरक्तज्वरहरं परम् ॥

231
KAŚERUKA

Scirpus grossus **Linn** Family : Cyperaceae

Chief Characters :

1. Shrub grows upto 3 m. height.
2. Large leaves, consists of brown coloured flowers.
3. Spike inflorescence.
4. Fruit - drupe.

Synonyms : Chichoda.

Gana :

Charaka : Madhuraskandha, Kashayaskandha.

Properties : Rasa - Madhura, Kashaya; Guna - Ruksha, Guru (K.N.) Laghu (B.P.); Virya - Sheeta and Vipaka - Madhura.

Pharmacological Actions : Pittahara, Grahi, Shukrala, Stanyajanana.

Indications : Daha, Trishna, Prameha, Raktapitta, Kamala, Shukrakshaya, Netra roga.

Therapeutic Uses :

1. Eye disease : Powder of kaseru and madhuka is put in cloth pouch which is kept in water. The liquid so prepared is useful as eyedrop (S.S.; V.M.)
2. Miscarriage : Paste of kasheru, shringataka and lotus root should be used with boiled milk. (S.S.)

Parts Used : Tuber.

Preparations & Dosage : 5-10 gm.

Specific Formulations : Kashervadi peya, Kashervadi lepa.

कशेरुकं हिमरूक्षं मधुरं तुवरं गुरु ।
संग्राहि शुक्रलं स्तन्यकफमारुतवर्धनम् ॥
पित्तशोणितदाहघ्नं नयनामयनाशनम् ।
वृष्यं मेहं तृषां हन्याद्विष्टम्भि कृमिकारि च ॥
कशेरुकस्य पुष्पं तु पित्तघ्नं कामलापहम् ॥ के०नि०

232
VAṀŚA

Bambusa arundinaceae Family : Poaceae

Chief Characters :

1. Perennial shrub.
2. Bisexual flowers, spike inflorescence.
3. Small spikelet arranged in panicle inflorescence.
4. Consists of white coloured flowers.
5. Fruit - caryopsis.

Synonyms : Twaksara, Karmara, Trinadwaja, Shataparva, Venu, Maskara, Tejana, Trinadwaja.

Properties : Rasa - Madhura, Kashaya; Guna - Laghu, Ruksha; Virya - Sheeta and Vipaka - Katu, Madhura.

Pharmacological Actions : Kaphapittahara, Sara, Chedana, Vasti shodhana.

Indications : Koshta, Vrana, Shotha, Prameha, Mutrakricchra.

Therapeutic Uses :

1. Prameha : Barley shaped fruits of vamsha should be given as dietary preparation like that of yava. (C.S.)
2. Menorrhagia : Decoction of bamboo nodes 20 gm and shatapushpa 40 gm. mixed with jaggery induces menses. (S.R.)
3. Rabies : Root of ankota and vamsha pounded with milk should be taken. It alleviates rabies. (B.P.)

Parts Used : Root, Leaf, Fruit, Vanshalochana.

Preparations & Dosage : Decoction 50-100 ml.; Vanshalochana 1-3 gm.

Specific Formulations : Sitopaladi churna, Talishadi churna.

वंशः सरो हिमः स्वादुः कषायो बस्तिशोधनः ।
छेदनः कफपित्तघ्नः कुष्ठास्त्रव्रणशोथजित् ॥
तत्करीरः कटुः पाके रसे रूक्षो गुरुः सरः ।
कषायः कफहृत् स्वादुर्विदाही वातपित्तलः ॥
तद्यवास्तु सरा रूक्षाः कषायाः कटुपाकिनः ।
वातपित्तकरा उष्णा बद्धमूत्रा कफापहाः ॥ भा०प्र०
वंशजा बृंहणी वृष्या बल्या स्वाद्वी च शीतला ।
तृष्णाकासज्वरश्वासक्षयपित्तास्त्रकामलाः ॥
हरेत् कुष्ठं व्रणं पाण्डुं कषाया वातकृच्छ्रजित् ॥ भा०प्र०

233
KUŚA

Desmostachya bipinnata stapf. Family : Poaceae

Chief Characters :

1. Perennial herb grows upto 90 cm. height.
2. Long leaves with a hairy tip.
3. Light brown coloured flowers, panicle inflorescence.
4. Fruit - caryopsis.

Synonyms : Darbha, Barhi, Suchyagra, Yajnabhushana.

Gana :

Charaka : Stanyajanana, Mutravirechaniya.
Sushruta : Trunapanchamuladi.

Properties : Rasa - Madhura, Kashaya; Guna - Laghu, Snigdha; Virya - Sheeta and Vipaka - Madhura.

Pharmacological Actions : Tridoshahara, Mutravirechaniya, Stanyajanana.

Indications : Ashmari, Mutrakricchra, Trishna, Pradara, Vastishoola, Visarpa.

Therapeutic Uses :

1. Rakta pradara : Its root is grinded along with rice water and orally administered for 3 days. (Vrinda)
2. Dysuria : One suffering from paittika dysuria should take cold decoction of shatavari, kasa, kusha, gokshura, vidari, shali, ikhsu and kasheruka added with honey and sugar. (C.S.)
3. Piles : Kusha root mixed with bala root is taken with rice water for arresting bleeding from piles, menorrhagia and metrorrhagia. (B.S.)

Parts Used : Root.

Preparations & Dosage : Decoction 50-100 ml.

Specific Formulations : Trinapanchamula kwatha, Kushavaleha, Kushadya ghrita.

दर्भद्वयं त्रिदोषघ्नं मधुरं तुवरं हिमम् ।
मूत्रकृच्छ्राश्मरीतृष्णाबस्तिरुक् प्रदरास्रजित् ॥ भा०प्र०

234
ŚARA

Saccharam munja Family : Poaceae

Chief Characters :

1. Perennial grass.
2. Pale violet or green coloured - spikelete arranged in panicle inflorescence.
3. Fruit - Rectangular.

Synonyms : Bhadramunja, Bana, Tejana, Ikshuveshtana, Morja, Munjataka, Sthuladarbha, Sumekhala.

Properties : Rasa - Madhura, Tikta, Kashaya; Guna - Laghu, Snigdha; Virya - Sheeta and Vipaka - Madhura.

Pharmacological Actions : Tridoshahara, Vrishya.

Indications : Daha, Trishna, Visarpa, Mutrakricchra, Akshiroga.

Therapeutic Uses :

1. Calculus : Ghee cooked with kusha, kasa, sara etc. breaks calculus caused by pitta.
2. Thirst : Water processed with saradi panchamula and cooked and added with sugarcandy should be taken. (C.S.)
3. Cough : In case of cough goat's milk processed with sara root etc. should be given (C.S.)

Parts Used : Root.

Preparations & Dosage : Decoction 50-100 ml.

Specific Formulations : Trinapanchamula kwatha.

मुञ्जद्वयं तु मधुरं तुवरं शिशिरं तथा ।
दाहतृष्णाविसर्पास्रमूत्रकृच्छ्राक्षिरोगजित् ॥
दोषत्रयहरं वृष्यं मेखलासूपयुज्यते ॥ भा०प्र०

235
KĀŚA

Saccharum spontaneum Linn Family : Poaceae

Chief Characters :

1. Perennial herb grows upto 3 m. height.
2. Consists of long leaves.
3. Spike inflorescence.
4. Consists of white colored flowers.

Synonyms : Kaseksha, Ikshurasa, Ikswalika, Potagala, Ikshugandha.

Gana :

Charaka : Stanyajanana, Mutravirechaniya, Madhuraskandha, Kashayaskandha.
Sushruta : Trunapanchamuladi, Viratarvadi.

Properties : Rasa - Madhura, Kashaya; Guna - Laghu, Snigdha; Virya - Sheeta and Vipaka - Madhura.

Pharmacological Actions : Vatapittahara, Mutrala, Stanyajanana.

Indications : Mutrakricchra, Ashmari, Raktapitta, Pittajaroga, Kshaya, Daha.

Therapeutic Uses :

1. Pradara : Root pounded in tandulodaka cures pradara (Yogatarangni).
2. Ajeerna : The root decoction relieves the indigestion caused due to ingestion of flesh of birds like kapota, paravata etc. (B.P.)

Parts Used : Root.

Preparations & Dosage : Decoction 50-100 ml.

Specific Formulations : Trinapanchamula kwatha, Kushavaleha, Kushadya ghrita.

काशः स्यान्मधुरस्तिक्तः स्वादुपाको हिमः सरः ।
मूत्रकृच्छ्राश्मदाहस्रक्षयपित्ताक्षिरोगजित् ॥ भा०प्र०

236
NALA

Arundo donax Linn. Family : Poaceae

Lobelia nicotianaeefolia Companulaceae is also considered as one of the sources of Nala.

Chief Characters :

1. It is a perennial plant.
2. Leaves - long with acute tip.
3. Light greenish yellow flowers are arrangd in panicle inflorescence.
3. Fruit - caryopsis.

Synonyms : Shunyamadhya, Dhamana, Vibhishana, Potagala.

Properties : Rasa - Madhura, Tikta, Kashaya; Guna - Laghu, Snigdha; Virya - Ushna (B.P.) / Sheeta (D.N.) and Vipaka - Madhura.

Pharmacological Actions : Kapharaktahara, Pittahara, Vrishya, Mutrala.

Indications : Hricchula, Vastishoola, Yonishoola, Daha, Visarpa, Raktapitta, Mutrakricchra.

Therapeutic Uses :

1. Retention of urine : By taking cooled decoction of nala, kusha, kasa, ikshu and bala added with sugar, retention of urine is relieved. (B.P.)
2. Rabies : Nala root pounded with water is useful as intake and paste. (A.S.)

Parts Used : Root.

Preparations & Dosage : Decoction 50-100 ml.

Specific Formulations : Trinapanchamula kwatha, Pancha trinaksheera.

नलस्तु मधुरस्तिक्तः कषायः कफरक्तजित् ॥ भा०प्र०

237
DŪRVĀ

Cynodon dactylon Family : Poaceae

Chief Characters :

1. Perennial creeper.
2. Spike inflorescence with violet coloured flowers.
3. Fruit - caryopsis.

Synonyms : Shweta durva - Golomi, Shatavirya;
Neela durva - Sahasravirya, Shatavalli, Bhargavi, Ruha, Shataparva.

Properties : Rasa - Tikta, Madhura, Kashaya; Guna - Laghu; Virya - Sheeta and Vipaka - Madhura.

Pharmacological Actions : Kaphapittahara, Varnya, Praja sthapana.

Indications : Trishna, Daha, Kushta, Raktapitta, Pradara, Mutrakricchra.

Therapeutic Uses :

1. The paste of durva relieves dysmenorrhoea. (C.D.)
2. The root paste along with haridra relieves all skin disorders. (G.N.)
3. Oil cooked with durva juice and paste of darvi bark is an excellent remedy for wound healing.
4. One should take durva, tender leaves of vata and white girikarnika with honey to relieve haemorrhage. (S.S.)

Parts Used : Whole plant.

Preparations & Dosage : Juice 10-20 ml.

Specific Formulations : Durvadi kwatha, Durvadhya gritha and Durvadya taila.

दूर्वाः कषाया मधुराश्च शीताः पित्ततृषारोचकवान्तिहन्त्र्यः ।
सदाहमूर्च्छाग्रहभूतशान्तिश्लेष्मश्रमध्वंसनतृप्तिदश्च ॥ रा०नि०

238
ROHIṢA

Cymbopogan martini Family : Poaceae

Chief Characters :

1. Herb growing upto 2 mts. height.
2. Leaves - barrel shaped.
3. Spike inflorescence.
4. Consists of red coloured flowers.

Synonyms : Kattruna, Devajagdha, Sougandhika, Bhutika, Dhyamapoura, Dhupagandhika.

Properties : Rasa - Tikta, Kashaya, Katu (B.P.); Guna - Laghu, Ruksha, Tikshna; Virya - Ushna and Vipaka - Katu.

Pharmacological Actions : Pittlakapha hara, Stanyajanana, Kaphavata shamaka.

Indications : Hridroga, Kantharoga, Raktapitta, Shoola, Kasa, Jwara.

Therapeutic Uses :

1. Chronic coryza : Rohisha, jiraka, vacha, tarkari and chanaka should be inhaled.
2. Headache : Paste of trivrt, kushta, sarngeshta, devadaru and rohisa pounded with yavakshara and salt and slightly heated should be applied on head. (S.S.)
3. Scropion sting : Mushroom growing on elephant faeces and rohisa root should be pounded with shleshmataka juice and made into a pill which is rubbed and pasted on the spot. (A.H.)

Parts Used : Stem, Leaf, Flower, Oil.

Preparations & Dosage : Decoction 50-100 ml.; Oil 1-3 drops.

रौहिषं तुवरं तिक्तं कटुपाकं व्यपोहति ।
हृत्कण्ठव्याधिवातास्रशूलकासकफज्वरान् ॥ भा०प्र०

239
HAṀSARĀJA

Adiantum lunulatum Family : Polypodiaceae

Chief Characters :

1. Perennial herb having root stock
2. Fern shaped leaves or cuniate shaped leaves.

Synonyms : Hamsapadi, Keetamala, Tripadika, Raktapadi.

Properties : Rasa - Kashaya; Guna - Guru; Virya - Sheeta and Vipaka - Madhura.

Pharmacological Actions : Kaphapittahara, Vishahara.

Indications : Visarpa, Daha, Atisara, Luta visha, Agnirohini, Vrana.

Therapeutic Uses :

It is useful for external application in visarpa, plague, luta visha and in pitta predominant inflammatory conditions.

Parts Used : Whole plant.

Preparations & Dosage : Juice 50-100 ml.; Powder 1-3 gm.

Specific Formulations : Hamsapadi panaka.

हंसपादी गुरुः शीता हन्ति रक्तविषव्रणान् ।
विसर्पदाहातीसारलूताभूताग्निरोहिणीः ॥ भा०प्र०

240
MAYŪRAŚIKHĀ

Adiantum caudatum Family : Polypodiaceae

Actinopteris radiata is also considered as one of the sources for Mayurasikha.

Chief Characters :

1. Perennial fern (maiden hair fern).
2. Compound leaf.

Synonyms : Sahasrahi, Madhucchada, Neelakantha sikha.

Properties : Rasa - Madhura, Tikta, Kashaya; Guna - Laghu, Ruksha; Virya - Sheeta and Vipaka - Katu.

Pharmacological Actions : Kaphapittahara, Vishahara.

Indications : Atisara, Pravahika, Prameha.

Therapeutic Uses :

1. Sterility : The root paste along with milk taken in ritukala facilitates conception. (G.N.)
2. Calculus : Root of mayurashikha is taken with rice water to relieve caliculi. (A.H.)
3. Snake poison : Mayurashikha mixed with ghee and taken with rice water destroys all types of snake poison. (G.N.)

Parts Used : Whole plant.

Preparations & Dosage : Juice 10-20 ml.

मयूराह्वा शिखा शीता कषाया कटुपाकिनी।
लघ्वी पित्तकफौ रक्तमतिसारं विनाशयेत् ॥ कै०नि०

241
ŚAILEYA

Parmelia perlata Family : Parmeliaceae

Synonyms : Shilapushpa, Vriddha, Kalanusaryaka.
It is a lichen.

Properties : Rasa - Tikta, Kashaya; Guna - Laghu, Snigdha; Virya - Sheeta and Vipaka - Katu.

Pharmacological Actions : Kaphapittahara, Hridya, Vishahara.

Indications : Kandu, Kushta, Ashmari, Daha, Raktasrava.

Therapeutic Uses :

1. Oedema : In oedema caused by vata, oil processed with shaileya, kusha, aguru and devadaru etc. is useful. (C.S.)
2. Wound : Powder consisting of sarjaka, tuttha, kasisa shaileya, rasanjana and manahshila alleviates wound and its spread. (S.S.)

Parts Used : Whole plant.

Preparations & Dosage : Powder 1-3 gm.

शैलेयं तु शिलापुष्पं वृद्धं कालानुसार्यकम् ।
शैलेयं शीतलं हृद्यं कफपित्तहरं लघु ॥
कण्डूकुष्ठाश्मरीदाहविषहृल्लासरक्तहृत् ॥ भा०प्र०

242
ŚAIVĀLA

Ceratophyllum demersum Family : Ceratophyllaceae

Chief Characters :

1. Hydrophyte.
2. Whorled phyllotaxy.
3. Fruit - drupe.

Synonyms : Shaivala, Jalaneeti.

Properties : Rasa - Madhura, Tikta, Kashaya; Guna - Laghu, Snigdha; Virya - Sheeta and Vipaka - Katu.

Pharmacological Actions : Pittahara.

Indications : Daha, Trishna, Jwara.

Therapeutic Uses :

1. Erysipelas : Shaivala, nalaroot, gojihva and vrshakarni are used as paste. (C.S.)
2. Thirst : Paste of shaivala, lotus, mud and also of parched flour mixed with sours and ghee is applied. (C.S.)
3. Scorpion poisoning : Shaivala mixed with camel tooth counteracts scorpion sting. (A.H.)

Parts Used : Whole plant.

Preparations & Dosage : Fresh juice 10-20 ml.

243
CHATRAKA

Agaricus campestris Family : Agaricaceae

Chief Characters :

1. Fungus hairy fruiting body consisting of light violet coloured spores.
2. Basidio carp - fruit.

Synonyms : Silindhraka, Bhumi chatra.

Properties : Rasa - Madhura; Guna - Guru, Snigdha, Picchila; Virya - Sheeta and Vipaka - Madhura.

Pharmacological Actions : Vatapitta shamaka, Kaphakara.

Indications : Shopha, Daha, Amlapitta, Chardi, Atisara, Jwara.

Therapeutic Uses :

Kshaya and shosha : Its ksheerapaka should be given. It alleviates the condition.

Parts Used : Whole plant.

सर्पच्छत्रकवर्ज्यास्तु वह्व्योऽन्याश्छत्रजातय: ।
शीता: पीनसकर्त्र्यश्च मधुरा गुर्व्य एव च ॥ च०सू०
सर्वे संस्वेदजा: शीता दोषता पिच्छिलाश्च ते ।
गुरवश्छर्द्यतीसारज्वरश्लेष्मामयप्रदा: ॥ भा०प्र०

244
ŚAṆAPUṢPĪ

Crotalaria verrucosa Family : Fabaceae

Chief Characters :

1. Shrub grows upto 1 mt. height.
2. Simple leaves, alternate phyllotaxy.
3. yellow coloured flowers, racemose inflorescence.
4. Fruit - legume.

Synonyms : Ghanta, Sanapushpa samakriti, Ghantarava.

Gana :

Charka : Vamanopaga, Udardaprashamana.

Properties : Rasa - Katu, Tikta, Kashaya; Guna - Laghu, Ruksha, Tikshna; Virya - Ushna and Vipaka - Katu.

Pharmacological Actions : Kaphapittahara, Vamaka.

Indications : Kantha roga, Hridroga, Mukha roga, Kushta.

Therapeutic Uses :

1. For ripening of abscess : Seeds of shana, mulaka and shigru ripen the abscess.
2. Rasayana : One who takes fruits of shana cooked with milk followed by intake of milk does not suffer from senility. (S.S.)

Parts Used : Root, Leaf.

Preparations & Dosage : Root powder 3-6 gm.; Leaf juice 50-100 ml.

शणपुष्पी स्मृता घ्रष्टा शणपुष्पसमाकृतिः ।
शणपुष्पी कटुस्तिक्ता वामिनी कफपित्तजित् ॥ भा०प्र०

245
SŪCĪ

Atropa belladonna Family : Solanaceae

Chief Characters :

1. Simple leaves, alternate phyllotaxy.
2. Yellow or red coloured flowers, funnel shaped.
3. Fruit - berry.

Synonyms : Madani, Deerghamula, Karmarda phala.

Properties : Rasa - Katu, Tikta; Guna - Laghu, Ruksha; Virya - Ushna and Vipaka - Katu.

Pharmacological Actions : Kaphavatahara, Shula prashamana, Vedanasthapana.

Indications : Kasa, Shwasa, Vrana, Shotha, Hridroga, Shoola, Agnimandhya.

Therapeutic Uses :

In inflammatory disorders it is useful for anointing or can be used for massaging the part.

Parts Used : Root & Leaf.

Preparations & Dosage : Powder 30-60 mg.

सूची तिक्ता कटुर्लघ्वी रुदोष्णा मदकारिणी ।
कफवातहरा पित्तकरा धातुप्रशोषणी ॥
लालाप्रसेकशमनी शूलप्रशमनी भृशम् ।
प्रलापजननी हृद्या वेदनाश्नापनी तथा ॥
कासे श्वासे व्रणे शोथे वातव्याधो हृदामये ।
अग्निमान्द्ये विषे शूले प्रस्वेदे च प्रशस्यते ॥ द्र०वि०

246
DUGDHIKĀ

Euphorbia hirta Linn Family : Euphorbiaceae

Euphorbia thymifolia Burm is also considered as one of the sources for dugdhika.

Chief Characters :

1. Annual plant.
2. Opposite phyllotaxy, simple leaves with serrated margins.
3. Consists of green or rose coloured flowers.
4. Fruit - capsule.

Synonyms : Nagarjuni, Swaduparni, Vikshirini, Ksheerini.

Properties : Rasa - Katu, Tikta, Madhura; Guna - Guru, Ruksha, Tikshna; Virya - Ushna and Vipaka - Katu.

Pharmacological Actions : Kaphahara, Vatala, Vrishya, Mutrala, Garbhakarini. (B.P.)

Indications : Krimi, Shwasa, Kasa, Udara,Mutrakricchra.

Therapeutic Uses :

1. The kalka of dhugdhika with pepper is used in snake poisoning.
2. Ghee cooked with kantakari and dugdhika alleviates bleeding piles with pain. (C.S.)
3. Dugdhika steamed with cooked rice and taken with the same after adding oil checks dysentry with blood. (V.S.)

Parts Used : Whole plant.

Preparations & Dosage : Juice 10-20 ml.; Powder 1-3 gm.; Paste 10-20 gm.

दुग्धिका स्वादुपर्णी स्यात्क्षीरा विक्षीरिणी ।
दुग्धिकोष्णा गुरु रुक्षा वातला गर्भकारिणी ॥
स्वादुक्षीरा कटुस्तिक्ता सृष्टमूत्रा मलापहा ।
स्वदुविष्टम्भिनी वृष्या कफकुष्ठक्रिमिप्रणुत् ॥ भा०प्र०

SECOND PAPER

Part - B

- Introduction of Jantava Dravyas
- Introduction of Vargokta Dravyas
- Pharmacognistical Study of Certain Dravyas
- Modern Pharmacology

1
AṄGARASA

Ayurvedic classics mentioned the usage of animate and inanimate substances alongwith vegetable drugs. The bile, blood, muscular tissue, urine, faeces, skin, horns, nails and hairs of different animals are utilised in Ayurvedic therapeutics to process different formulations. Charaka advocates in the management of loss of blood, to administer blood of animals like goat and birds etc. as a substitution. Similarly intake of semen of buffalo's is indicated in shukra kshaya. The bodily secretions of musk deer, civet cat etc. are also utilised in the process of different medicines. In the modern medical system different hormones like insulin, adrenalin, thyroxine, oxytocin and biliary secretions are indicated in the management of different diseases.

Thus angarasas (bodily secretions) of animals are having wider therapeutic applicability in the management of different disorders.

2
AGNIJĀRA

Ambra grasea (Sperm whale)

Synnonyms : Ambera, Tundamaya

Properties : Rasa - Katu; Guna - Laghu, Ruksha; Virya - Ushna and Vipaka - Katu.

Pharmacological Actions : Tridoshaghna, Deepana, Pachana, Anulomana, Hridya, Vajeekarana, Balya.

Indications : Dhanurvata, Shoola, Grahani, Pratishyaya.

Therapeutic Uses :

1. Pakshaghata : Agnijara, saindhava lavana mixed with vatahara tailas should be used for massage externally. (Anubhuta)
2. Vajeekarana : Pills made up ot jatiphala, ahiphena, agnijara processed in bhringaraja swarasa should be taken. (Anubhuta)

Preparations & Dosage : 1-3 gms.

Amber is the morbid exretion contained in the intestines or caelcum of the sperm-whale. It is in the form of a concrete mass found floating on the sea waters (Red sea or shores of Africa). A single whale's excretion has been found to weigh 750 lbs. It is opaque, dark brownish or pinkish in colour with a peculiar fragrance. It contains ambrein (85%) and acts as stimulant, antiseptic and antispasmodic. It is used in general weakness, epilepsy, spasms and nervous debility.

3
KASTŪRĪ

***Moschus moschiferus* (Musk-deer)**

Synonyms : Mruganabhi, Mrugamada, Sahasrabhita.

Properties : Rasa -Tikta, Katu; Guna - Laghu, Ruksha, Tikshna; Virya - Ushna and Vipaka - Katu.

Pharmacological Actions : Kaphavata shamaka, Vrishya.

Indications : Kasa, Shwasa, Chardi, Shosha, Dourgandhya.

Therapeutic Uses :

1. Akshepaka vata : Ahiphena and kasturi combindly should be used. (Anubhuta)
2. Shwasa hrichhula : Kasturi should be taken along with shrungi bhasma and paushkaramula. (Anubhuta)

Preparations & Dosage : 60-120 mg.

Specific Formulations : Kasturibhairava rasa, Mrugamadasava.

Musk proper is an inspissated and dried secretion (testicular extract) from the preputial follicles of the male musk deer (*Moschus moschiferus*). Musk is found in these animals only in the rutting season for the purpose of attracting the female. Musk contains ammonia, oleine, cholesterine fat, wax and yields by distillation a small percentage of viscid, colourless oil with a very powerful and agreeable odour of musk. Bhavamishra describes three varities of musk viz. Kamrupa, Nepala and Kashmira. Among these three, Kamarupa is considered superior to others.

4
GOROCANA

Fel Bovinum purifcatum

Synonyms : Rochana, Gouri, Mangalya.

Properties : Rasa - Tikta; Guna - Laghu, Ruksha; Virya - Ushna, Sheeta (B.P.) and Vipaka - Katu.

Pharmacological Actions : Kaphavatahara, Medhya, Lekhana, Sothahara.

Indications : Apasmara, Agnimandya, Pandu, Kamala, Shotha, Mutrakricchra.

Therapeutic Uses :

1. Shwitra kushta : Paste of manahsila, vidanga, karisa, gorochana, swarna pushpi should be used externally as an ointment. (C.S.)
2. Bhutonmada : The powder of pippali, marica, saindhava lavana, gorochana etc. along with honey should be used as collyrium. (B.P.)
3. Yonivyapada : Silk cloth soaked in bile of cow and fish for 21 times should be placed in vagina in acharana yoni vyapada. (B.P.)

Preparations & Dosage : 2-6 gms.

Specific Formulations : Balarka rasa.

6x-bile or 6x-gall is prepared by evaporating ox-gall to one-third, adding alcohol, filtering, distilling off and evaporating until it acquires a suitable consistence for making pills. It acts as anti-spasmodic, cholagogue and laxative.

5
PRAVĀLA

Corallium rubrum

Synonyms : Vidruma, Bhoumaratna.

Gana : Navaratna. (R.R.S.)

Properties : Rasa - Madhura, Kinchit amla; Guna - Laghu, Ruksha; Virya - Sheeta and Vipaka - Madhura.

Pharmacological Actions : Tridoshahara, Mainly kaphavata hara, Balya, Vishaghna, Deepana, Pachana.

Indications : Kshaya, Kasa, Raktapitta, Netra roga.

Therapeutic Uses :

1. Kasa/Shwasa : Powder of vamsalochana, rasa sindura, pravala bhasma and shukti bhasma should be taken. (Rasa Tarangini)

2. Mutrakricchra : Pravala bhsma or pishti should be taken along with decoction of shatavari and kokilaksha. (Rasa Tarangini)

   Pravala bhasma in the dosage of 2 rattis should be taken along with tandulodaka in kapha predominant mutra kricchra.

Preparations & Dosage : Pishti bhasma 120-360 mg.

Specific Formulations : Pravala panchamruta, Kamadudha rasa.

The skeleton of C. rubrum is called as coral. The animal dies when the calcium contents becomes very high. Coral is found in Red sea, Mediterranean sea adn Atlantic occean. It is made up of numerous minute pieces, each piece is minutely and longitudinally furrowed. The red colour of the coral is due to its iron content.

6
PŪTI (KHATTĀŚĪ)

***Viverra civetta* Linn.**

Gana : Susrutha : Parnamruga varga.

Properties : Rasa - Katu, Tikta; Guna - Laghu, Ruksha; Virya - Ushna and Vipaka - Katu.

Pharmacological Actions : Kaphavatahara, Chakshushya.

Indications : Kandu, Kushta, Shwasa, Hridroga, Netraroga.

Therapeutic Uses :

1. Sirahshoola : Gandha marjara virya should be used as nasya. (Anubhuta)
2. Swara : Intake of powder of pippali, bharngi, shunthi, pushkaramoola and puti gives relief. (Anubhuta)

Preparations & Dosage : 1-2 gm.

Specific Formulations : Dhanvantari vati.

V. civetta is a small animal resembling cat found in Malabar region of India. A pouch situated between the anus and genital organs contains semi-liquid, unctuous secretion of musky perfume. Civet is mainly used for perfumery and acts as aphrodisiac and anti-spasmodic. The empty pouch is filled with dry grass is being sold under the name of Khattashi for the purpose of perfumary.

7
MUKTĀ

Mytilus margaritiferus

Synonyms : Sashiratna, Muktaphala, Mouktika, Shuktija.

Gana : Navaratna (R.R.S.)

Properties : Rasa - Madhura; Guna - Laghu; Virya - Sheeta and Vipaka - Madhura.

Pharmacological Actions : Kaphapittahara, Deepana, Vishahara, Chakshushya, Vrishya.

Indications : Daha, Kasa, Shwasa, Netraroga, Raja yakshma, Jeerna jwara, Asthi sosha.

Therapeutic Uses :

1. Hikka : Mukta bhasma taken along with swarna gairika and katuka rohini cures the condition. (Rasa Tarangini)
2. Rajayakshma : Mukta bhasma and pravala bhasma mixed with kajjali should be pounded with the juice of beejapura and incenerated by laghu puta. The processed medicine is given for a period of one month in the dose of 2 ratti (250 mg.) to relieve rajayakshma. (Rasa Tarangini)

Preparations & Dosage : Bhasma. 120-150 mg.

Specific Formulations : Kamadudha rasa, Vasantakusumakara.

Pearl mussel has nearly a semi-circular shell with greenish colour externally and internally ornamented with the most beautiful nacre.

8
ŚAṄKHA

Turbinella rapa (Class : Mollusca)

Synonyms : Kambu, Trirekha, Sankhaka, Sunada.

Gana : Uparatna (B.P.)

Properties : Rasa - Katu; Guna - Laghu, Ruksha, Teekshna; Virya - Ushna and Vipaka - Katu.

Pharmacological Actions : Kaphavatahara, Deepana, Pachana, Grahi.

Indications : Grahani, Amlapitta, Netraroga, Parinamashoola, Yuvanapidika.

Therapeutic Uses :

1. Atisara : Shankha bhasma should be taken along with lime juice in atisara and grahani. (Rasa Tarangini)
2. Amlapitta : Intake of shankha bhasma along with amalaki churna cures amlapitta. (R.S.)
3. Parinamashoola : Shankha bhasma should be taken along with trikatu powder or with pancha lavanas and jaggery. (Rasa Tarangini)
4. Netra roga : Collyrium made of suddha shankha and honey should be applied in netra roga by name arjuna.

Preparations & Dosage : 1/4-1/2 gm.

Specific Formulations : Shankha vati, Shankha dravaka, Chandrodaya varti.

Conch shell is often of an oblong form bulged in the middle and tepering at each end. The other variety i.e. conical variety consists of corkscrew type of upper portion with antapered end. The surface is hard, of a dull white colour and the interior is hollow. Conch is found in Indian ocean coasts.

9
ŚAMBŪKA

Achatina fulica

Synonyms : Kshudra shankha, Nakha shankha.

Properties : Rasa - Katu; Guna - Laghu, Ruksha; Virya - Ushna and Vipaka - Katu.

Pharmacological Actions : Deepana, Pachana, Anulomana.

Indications : Ajeerna, Parinama shoola, Gulma, Raktatisara, Netra roga.

Therapeutic Uses :

1. Parinama shoola : Shambuka bhasma should be taken with hot water (Cakradutta). The bhasma, marica and pancha lavana should be taken before and after the meals in parinama shoola (Rasa Tarangini).
2. Grahani : Equal quantities of shambuka bhasma and saindhava lavana should be taken with honey in vataja grahani. It gives faster relief (Rasa Tarangini).

Preparations & Dosage : 1-4 gm.

Specific Formulations : Shambukadi gutika.

The external shell is known as Shambhuka, which is brownish or dark brown in colour and the interior portion is white in colour. It consists of calcium carbonate, calcium phosphate, phosphate and sulphate of magnesium, iron, silica etc. Shell in the incinerated (bhasma) form used in the management of gastritis and peptic ulcer.

10

ŚUKTI

Ostrea edulis Linn.

Synonyms : Shuktika, Muktamata, Muktashukti.

Properties : Rasa - Madhura; Guna - Snigdha; Virya - Sheeta and Vipaka - Madhura.

Pharmacological Actions : Tridoshahara, Deepana, Vrishya, Balya, Chakshushya.

Indications : Shoola, Hridroga, Shwasa, Atisara, Grahani, Mutra sharkara, Pleeha vriddhi.

Therapeutic Uses :

1. Shoola : Intake of sukti bhasma with trikatu powder or with triphala and yashtimadhu powder gives immediate relief. (Rasa Tarangini)
2. Amlapitta : One should take shukti bhasma, swarnamakshika bhasma and yavakshara to get relief. (Rasa Tarangini)
3. Shwasa : One should take shukti bhasma, trikatu powder and honey with vasa juice for a period of one week. (Rasa Tarangini)

Preparations & Dosage : Bhasma 250 mg.

Common oyster shell is commonly found in the Atlantic and Indian ocean coasts. The shell has a sort of linage at one end and opens into two valves. The shell grey or dark brown in colour externally and white, smooth and shinning internally. It contains calcium carbonate (85-95%), calcium sulphate, calcium phosphate, phosphate and sulphate of magnesium alumina and silica.

11
VARĀṬIKĀ

Cypraea moneta Linn.

Synonyms : Kapardika, Charachara, Balakridanaka.

Gana : Sadharana rasa. (R.R.S.)

Properties : Rasa - Katu, Tikta; Guna - Laghu, Ruksha, Teekshna; Virya - Ushna and Vipaka - Katu.

Pharmacological Actions : Kaphavatahara, Deepana, Pachana, Bhedana, Grahi, Vrishya, Netrya.

Indications : Parinamashoola, Gulma, Vrana, Karnashoola.

Therapeutic Uses :

1. Grahani : The combination of varata bhasma, shankha bhasma and trikatu bhasma should be taken for a period of 1 week. (Rasa Tarangini)
2. Karnapuya : Fine powder of equal quantities of samudraphena and varata bhasma should be dropped into the ear. It stops puyasrava from the ear. (Rasa Tarangini)

Preparations & Dosage : 1-4 gm.

Specific Formulations : Bruhat lokanatha tasa, Kamadudha rasa.

Porcelaneous shells (marina shell) are smaller in size and upper surface is smooth, shining and covex. Base is compessed with a clef in the centre which runs longitudinally. The margin of the cleft is serrated on one side and depressed on the other. Three varieties of conries white, red and yellow are used in medicine.

12
MṚGAŚṚṄGA
(Stag's horn)

Cervus elephus

Synonyms : Enashringa, Harina shringa, Mrigavishanaka.

Properties : Rasa - Kashaya; Guna - Laghu; Virya - Ushna and Vipaka - Katu.

Pharmacological Actions : Vatakaphahara, Hridya.

Indications : Kasa, Hikka, Shwasa, Hridroga, Amavata.

Therapeutic Uses :

1. Hrichchula : Intake of shringi bhasma (1 ratti) mixed with honey relieves hrichchula and parshwa shoola (Rasa Tarangini). It can be administered with ghee (Bhaishajyaratnavali).
2. Shwasa : Intake of badara phala majja, pippali and apamarga beeja churna mixed with shringa bhasma mixed with honey relieves shwasa and hikka (Anuhuta).

Preparations & Dosage : 1-4 gm.

Stag's horn mainly consists of calcium phosphate.

1

IKṢU VARGA

Bhavamishra described 13 varieties of Ikshu with their identification, characteristics and also mentions various products prepared either from ikshu rasa or tastes as sweet like ikshu viz., guda, madhukhanda (sugar derived from honey), pushpasita (sugar derived from flowers), sitopala (sugar) etc.

Varieties of ikshu with their properties :

Varieties of ikshu	*Properties*
1. Paundrika 2. Bheeruka	Sheeta virya, madhura vipaka Brimhana, balya-vata-pitta, prashamana.
3. Koshakaraekshu	Raktapitta, kshayahara.
4. Kantaraekshu	Vrishya, brimhana, sara.
5. Vamshakaekshu	Kshara guna.
6. Shataporaka	Ushna virya, kshara guna and vatahara.
7. Tapasaekshu	Tarpaki, balya-vrishya and sleshma prakopaka.
8. Kandaekshu	Vataprakopaka and other gunas of tapasaekshu.
9. Suchipatra 10. Neelapora 11. Naipala 12. Deerghapatra	Vidahi, vata-kapha-pittahara.
13. Manogupta	Vatahara, trishnahara, raktapittahara.
Bala ikshu	Kapha, medoghna, pramehaghna
Taruna ikshu	Vata pittahara.
Vriddha ikshu	Raktapittahara, kshatahara, balya, vrishya.

Various preparations made out of ikshu rasa :

Preparations	*Properties*
1. Paryushita ikshu rasa	Kapha-pittakara, vatahara, mutrala.
2. Pakwa ikshu rasa	Kaphavatahara, gulmahara anahahara.
3. Danta nishapidita rasa	Pittaraktahara, avidahi.
4. Yantra nishpidita rasa	Vidahi, vishtambhi.
5. Phanita (Boiled sugarcane juice consisting of more liquid portion)	Brimhana, abhishyandi, sukrala, mutra-vasti shodhana.
6. Matsyandi (Molasses-boiled juice with less qualities of liquid portion)	Bhedanya, balya, brimhani, vrishya.
7. Guda (Jaggery)	Vrishya, mutra-shodhana, asrik-prasadhana (Jeerna gula); krimi, shwasa, kasakara (Nava guda).
8. Khanda (Sugarcandy)	Vrishya, chakshushya, brimhana, vatapittahara.
9. Sharkara (Pandery sugar)	Shukrala, vatapittahara, daha-murccha-jwara-chardihara.
10. Madhu-sharkara (Solidified honey)	Kaphapittahara, chardi-atisara-trishnahara. This will not come under ikshuvikara.

2
DUGDHA VARGA

Charaka attributes prime place to milk among jivaneeya drugs. Bhavamishra includes brimhana, balya, medhya, vajeekarana, ayushya, vayahsthapana and rasayana properties along with jivaneeya properties to it.

Indcations for drinking milk :

Jirna jwara, manoroga, shosha, murccha, bhrama, grahani, pandu, daha, trishna, hridroga, shoola, udavarta, gulma, vastiroga, arshas, atisara, yoni roga, garbhasrava.

Varieties of milk with their properties :

Source of milk	*Properties*
Gavya (Cow's)	Vatapitta sramshamana, kinchit kledakara.
Mahisha	Shukrakara, abhisyandikara, nidrakara, adhika kshudahara.
Aja (Goat's)	Grahi, raktapitta-atisarakara, kashaya, swasa-kasahara.
Mrigi (Deer's)	Having same properties of aja's milk.
Avika (Sheep's)	Ushna, ashmarihara, tarpaka, keshya, ahridya.
Badava (Mare's)	Ushna-balya-sosha-vatahara.
Ekasepha (animal's unsplit hoof)	Having same properties of badava milk.
Ushtra (Camel's)	Deepana, krimi-kushta-sothahara.
Hastini (Elephant's)	Vrishya, balya, chakshushya.
Nari (Woman's)	Deepana, vatapittahara, chakshushoolahara.

Properties of fresh milk :

1. *Gavya dharoshna ksheera* (warm milk drawn directly from the udder of the cow)—Deepana, tridoshahara.

2. *Dharasita* (Drawn directly from udder but cooled down)—Buffalow's milk is preferred to be taken in this form.

3. *Apakwa*—Woman's milk should be taken without boiling.

4. *Piyusha*—Piyusha is defined as the milk of the cow which has just delivered the calf.

5. *Santanika* (Cream on milk)—Vrishya, pittavatahara, tarpana, brimhana, shukrala.

6. *Kilataka*—Soild portion of the split milk.

7. *Morata*—Liquid portion of split.

All the varities of milk namely piyush, kilataka, morata are having properties like balya, vrishya, brimhana, hridya and vatapittahara.

8. *Boiled milk*—It acts as kapha-vatahara and boiled and cooled milk acts as pittahara. Milk added with khanda (sugarcandy) acts as vatahara and shukrala while milk taken with jaggery (guda) relieves mutrakricchra (dysuria) and increases pitta and kapha.

9. *Churned milk*—Milk of either of cow or goat should be boiled and churned before consumption. Phena (froth after churning) is balya, deepana and useul in jirna jwara, atisara and agnimandya.

Milk consumed during :

Forenoon	:	Vrishya, brimhana, deepaniya.
Midday	:	Deepana, balya, pitta-kaphahara.
Night	:	Chakshushya.

Milk alone should be consumed during night and should not be combined with rice as it causes indigestion.

3
MŪTRA VARGA

Varieties of mutra with their properties :

Source of mutra	*Property*
Gavya (Cow's)	Deepana, medhya, vata-kaphahara and pittakara. Indications include pleehodara, shwasa, kasa, shotha, shoola, gulma, kushta, kamala, pandu, karna shoola (local instillations).
Nara (Human)	Rasayana, Raktapamahara.

Female animal's urine is preferable in the case of cow, goat, sheep and buffalo and in the case of donkey, camel, elephant, man and horse, urine of male animal is said to be ideal. Bhavamishra gets the credit of investigating the therapeutic benefits of human urine and he may be regared as the father of "Auto urine therapy."

4
TAILA VARGA

Fatty material derived from oil of tila (sesamum), sarshapa (mustard) etc. are known as taila. Boiled ghee (medicated ghee) loses the potency after one year, while oil (cooked or uncooked—extracted through boiling or pressing) possess potency for a long time and Bhavamishra observes that older the oil better are its qualities, which was not mentioned by earlier acharyas who attributed such a property to asava and dhatu bhasmas.

Varieties of oil with their properties :

Name of the oil	*Property*
Tila tail (Oil of seíame seeds)	Lekhana, brimhana, grahi, chakshushya, medhya, keshya.
Sarshapa taila (Mustard oil)	Lekhana, arshoghna, kushta-kandu-krimihara.
Tuvari taila (Oil of tori)	Grahi, medodoshahara, vranasothahara.
Atasi taila (Lin seed oil)	Balya, grahi, vatahara.
Kusumbha taila (Safflower oil)	Vidahi, achakshushya, kaphakara.
Khasabija taila (Oil of khasa)	Balya, vrishya, vatakaphahara.
Eranda taila (Castcr oil)	Deepana, Vrishya, twachya, yoni-shukra visodhana. This oil is more specific remedy for amavata.
Sarjarasa taila (Oil of sal tree)	Vata-kaphahara and useful in visphot, vrana, kushta, pama, krimi.

According to Vagbhata all the oils possess similar properties attributed to their respective substances from which they are extracted.

5
MADYA VARGA

Bhavamishra describes different madyas (fermented beverages) under sandhana varga. Any drink/beverage which produces intoxination is defined as madya. All the varieties of madya are ushna virya, pittakara, vatahara, bhedana, deepana, pachana, and rochaka. Vyavayi and vikashi properties are specifically attributed to madya. Nava madya (fresh wine) acts as brimhana and ahridya whereas purana madya (old wine) is hridya. A person who takes madya in a regulated dosage judiciously acts as nector (amruta).

Varieties of madya with their properties :

Varieties of madya	*Properties*
Kanjika (Prepared from dhanya)	Vatahara, vastishothahara.
Tushodaka (Prepared from yava with husk)	Deepana, hridya, vasti, shothahara.
Aranala (Prepared from godhuma)	Deepana, kaphahara, bhedana.
Sauvira (From yava without husk)	Deepana, kaphahara, bhedana.
Dhanyamla (From flour of rice/kodrava)	Deepana and indicated in vata roga and in the preparation of asthapana vasti.
Shindaki (From rajika, mulaka patra)	Rochana, pitta-shleshmakara.
Shukta (From kandmula with sneha, lavana)	Pachana, bhedana, raktapittakara.
Asuta (From kandamula)	Pachana, vatahara.
Sura (From flour of shali)	Kaphakara, grahi and indica ted in shotha, gulma, arshas grahani.

Varieties of madya	*Properties*
Varuni (From punarnava & shali or juice of tala, kharjura)	Indicated in peenasa, adhmana, shoola etc.
Seedhu (From sugarcane juice boiled or unboiled)	Sadyosnehana, rochana, vibandha-medoroga, sopha,arshas, udara are the indications.

Madya prepared with drugs without boiling them is known as asava; an arista is defined as the madya prepared from decoctions by process of fermentation.

6
MADHU VARGA

The synonmys of madhu include makshika, madhvika, kshaudra, saragha, varativanta, bhringavranta and pushparasodbhava.

Grahi, lekhana, chakshushya, deepana, swarya, vrana shodhana, vrana ropana, srotovishodhana, prasada janaka, hladi, varnya, medhya, vrishya, rochana are some of the actions attributed by Bhavamishra. It is considered to be best among yogavahi substances. Generally, madhu is mentioned sheeta virya. Bhavamishra decribed eight varieties of madhu and details are given in the following table .

Variaties of madhu with their properties :

Varieties of madhu	*Properties*
1. Makshika (Best among all the varieties)	Netramayahara, kamala, arshas, kasa, shwasa, kshayaharana.
2. Bhramara	Abhisyandikara, rakta-pitta hara, sheeta virya.
3. Kshaudra	Pramehahara and all the indications of makshika are also given for kshaudra.
4. Pauttika	Ushnavirya, pittavatakara, vidahi, meha-mutra-kricchrahara.
5. Chatra	Tarpana, vishahara, krimi, shwitra, raktapitta, pramehahara, shita virya.
6. Arghya	Chakshushya, balya.
7. Auddalaka	Ruchya, swarya, vishaghna, ushna virya and pittakara.
8. Dala	This is not prepared by honey bee but the nector of flowers dropped as the leaves. Qualities are brimhana, deepana, chardi, pramehahara.

Purana madhu (old honey) is lekhaneeya and indicated in sthoulya (obesity). Honey should not be mixed with hot substances and contraindcated in pitta (ushna) prakriti fellow during summer season.

Mayana, madhucchishta, madhushesa, sikitha, madauaka are some of the synonyms given for bees-wax. Vranaropana (wound healing) is the important action and is indicated in fractures and skin diseases.

7
VĀRI VARGA

The synonyms for jala are—vari, paneeya, salila, neera, kilala, jala, ambu, kam, toya, paya, udaka, amba, jivana arna, amrita and ghanarasa.

- Jala
  - Divya (Atmospheric)
    - Dharaja (Torrential rain)
      - Ganga (Potable)
      - Samudra (Salty)
    - Karakabhava (Hail)
    - Taushara (Dew)
    - Haima (Snowfall)
  - Bhauma (Terrestrial)
    - Jangala vari
    - Anupa vari
    - Sadharana vari

Varieties of water with their properties :

Varieties of water	*Properties*
1. Dhara jala	Tridoshaghna, rasayana, balya, jeevaniya, tarpana.
2. Karaka jala	Pittahara, kaphavatakara.
3. Tusara jala	Vatala, Apathya, useful in urusthambha, prameha and galaganda.
4. Hima jala	Pittaghna, vatakara.
5. Nadeeya jala	Vatala, kaphapittahara, deepana, anabhishyandi. Godavari river water causes kushta (skin disorders).
6. Audbhida jala (Spring water)	Pittaghna, avidahi, balya, vatakara.
7. Nirjhara jala (Water fall)	Kaphahara, deepana, vatala.
8. Sarasa jala (Water of lakes)	Balya, baddha, mutra-mala-karaka.

Varieties of water	*Properties*
9. Tadaga jala (Water of ponds)	Vatala, baddha, mutra-purishkara.
10. Vapya jala (Tank with steps)	Pittakara, kapha-vatahara.
11. Kaupa jala (Deep well water)	Tridoshaghna (if sweet in taste), deepana, kapha-vatahara (alkaline in taste).
12. Chaunjaya jala (Rain from pits formed in rocks)	Deepana, pachana.
13. Palvala jala (Water of small pool)	Abhishyandi, tridoshakara.
14. Vikira jala (Water of burrows)	Pittaghna (sweet in taste), pittala (alkaline in taste).
15. Kaidar jala (Water of cultivable fields)	Abhishyandi, doshakrit.
16. Amshudaka (Water exposed to rays of sun and moon)	Tridoshahara, anabhishyandi balya, rasayana and medhya. During sharat ritu all varieties of water are healthy because of rise of agastya.

Regimen of drinking water :

Excessive intake of water or total avoidence of intake of water disturbs the digestion. So one is advised to drink water with frequent intervels.

8
MĀṀSA VARGA

Pisita, kravya, amisha, palala are the synonyms of mamsa. It is vatahara, brimhana, preenana and hridya.

Varieties of mamsa with their properties :

Variety of Mamsa	*Properties*
A. Jangala mamsa	
1. Jangala (Deer etc.)	Pitta-sleshmahara, balya.
2. Bilasaya (Snake etc.)	Brimhana, vatahara, baddhavitmutrata.
3. Guhashaya (Lion etc.)	Netra-guhyavikarahara.
4. Parnamriga (Wild cat, monkey etc.)	Vrishya, chakshushya, sristamutra-purushika.
5. Vishkira (Hen etc.)	Balya, vrishya, tridoshahara.
6. Pratuda (Pigion peacock etc.)	Pitta-kaphahara, baddhavarchas.
7. Prasaha (Crow, eagle ect.)	Unmadakara, bhasmaka, vyadhi janaka.
8. Gramya (Goat, horse etc.)	Deepana, brimhana, balya.
B. Anupa varga	
1. Kulechara	Vrishya, balya, mutrala.
2. Plava (Crane, swan etc.)	Balashukrakara.
3. Kosastha (Conch etc.)	Brihmana, balya, vrishya, bahuvarchaka.
4. Padina (Tortoise etc.)	Similar to that of koshastha.
5. Matsya (Fish)	Brimhana, vrishya, balya.

9
ŚŪKADHĀNYA VARGA

Bhavamishra enumerates five kinds of dhanyas namely—shali dhanya, vrihi dhanya, shuka dhanya, shimbi dhanya and kshudra dhanya. According to the harvesting period shali dhanya and vrihi dhanya are identified though they belong to species of rice. Paddy which is harvested in hemanta (dewy season) is identified as shali (paddy which yeilds white coloured rice) and paddy harvested in varsha ritu (rainy season) is called as vrihi dhanya.

Yava and godhuma are considered as shuka dhanya (grains with spikes, bristles or awns), mudga, masha etc. are called simbi dhanya (legumes/pulses) and kangu and other as kshudra/trina dhanya (inferior/coarse grains or grains from grass like plants).

Among shuka dhanya yava and godhuma are considered to be the most important varieties grown in India.

Yava

It consists of kashaya and madhura rasa, sheeta virya, katu vipaka and ruksha, guru and pichchila gunas. Yava possess deepana, medhya, swarya, balya, varnya, anabhisyandi and lekhana. In the cases of vrana it is also useful like tila (sesame). Yava produces more quantity of mala and flatus. It is indicated in peenasa, shwasa, kasa, urusthambha, trishna, kantha and twak rogas.

Charaka suggests yava as the principal diet for prameha vyadhi. Atiyava is inferior to yava dhanya.

Godhuma

Godhuma is otherwise known as sumana and is of three kinds—1. *Mahagodhuma* : which grows in western countries, 2. *Madhuli* : the grain of which is small and grows in madhyadesh (central parts) and 3. *Dirgha godhuma* : which is devoid of spike (nishulka). Godhuma consists of madhura rasa, sheeta virya and guru guna. Balya, shukrala, jivana, brimhana, varyna, vranya, ruchya and sandhanakara are some of the actions attributed to godhuma.

10
ŚIMBĪDHĀNYA VARGA

Samija, shimbibhava, supya and vaidala are the synonyms of shimbi dhanya. All the shimbi dhanya are generally consists of madhura rasa, sheeta virya, katu vipaka and ruksha guna, aggravate vata and cause distension of abdomen (flatulance) except mudga and masura.

Varieties of shimbi dhanya with their properties :

Variety of shimbi dhanya	*Properties*
1. Mudga (Green gram)	Netrya, jwaraghna.
2. Masha (Black gram)	Samsrana, tarpana, balya, shukrala, brimhana, bhinna mutramla, stanyajanana and indicated in arshas, shwasa and pakti shoola.
3. Rajamasha (Cowpea)	Tarpana, vataghna, stanyajanana, balya.
4. Nishpava (Flat bean)	Amlavipaka, ushna virya, stanyajanana, vibandhakara.
5. Makushtha (Kidney bean)	Grahi, vatala, jwaraghna, krimikara.
6. Masura (Lentil)	Grahi, jwarghna, vatala.
7. Adhaki (Red gram)	Grahi, varnya, vatala.
8. Chanaka (Bengal gram)	Vishtambhi, vatala, jwaraghna, balya (ardrabhrishta) shu-krahara.
9. Kalaya (Garden pea)	Grahi, vatala.
10. Triputa (Chickling vetch)	Grahi, khanjatwapangutwakari (gives rise to lameness of leg or legs), vatakopaka.
11. Kulutha (Horse gram)	Swedasangrahaka, pitta-raktakara, indicated in shwasa, kasa, hikka, ashmari, peenasa, daha, sthaulya, krimi.

12. Tila (Sesame)	Ushna virya, katu vipaka, kapha-pittahara, balya, keshya, stanyaja, vranya, dantya, grahi, vatahara.
13. Atasi (Linseed)	Achakshushya, shukraghna, vataghna
14. Sarshapa (Mustard)	Kapha-vatahara, indicated in kandu, kushta, kotha, krimi.
15. Rajika (Black mustard)	Similar to that of sarshapa.

11
LAVAṆA VARGA

Bhavamishra mentions the properties of different lavanas under Haritakyadi varga. Charaka renders the description in Sutrasthana under Aharopayogi varga while Sushruta gives the details about six lavanas in Lavana varga (Sut. 46).

Varieties of lavana with their properties :

Variety of Lavana	*Properties*
1. Saindhava (Rock salt)	Shita virya, tridoshahara, netraya, vrishya.
2. Shakambhariya (Sambhar salt) (Syn. Romaka)	Ushna, pittala, bhedi, abhisyandi.
3. Samudra (Common salt, sea salt)	Madhura vipaka, deepana, natyushna, bhedi, sleshmala.
4. Bida (Black salt)	This is artificially prepared by mixing rocksalt, amalaki, haritaki and sodium carbonate. The properites are—kapha-vatanulomana, deepana, vyavayi and indicated in vibandha, anaha, hrichchula.
5. Sauvarchala (Black salt, sonch salt) (artificially prepared from sodium chloride, sodium sulphide and sodium carbonate)	Deepana, bhedana, panchana, rochana, vatahara, udgara shuddhi, vibandha, anahahara
6. Audbhida (Salt from soil) (It is also known as panshulavana.)	Ksharaghna, vatahara.

12
ĀHĀROPAYOGĪ VARGA

Charaka, (Sutra sthana : 27th chapter) described aharopayogi varga among twelve vargas. In this varga details about different oils (tila, eranda, sarshapa, priyala, atasi, kusumbha etc.) were enumerated. Therapeutic utility of certain substances which are used in the preparation of food stuffs in day to day life were also described. The drugs namely shunthi, pippali, marica and hingu are having carminative property and aids the digestion of ingested food. Lavanas namely saindhava, sauvarchala, bida, kala, oudbhida, samudrika and pamshu alleiviate vata and enhances the tastes of deitetic substances. The drugs namely karavi (krishna jeeraka), kunchika (sthula jeeraka), ajaji (jeeraka), yavani and dhanyaka are used in the seasoning of diets to enhance the taste and these drugs also act as carminatives. In this varga Charaka has mentioned the pharmacological actions of kshara.

GUḌŪCĪ

History of the stem Tinospora cordifolia :

A transverse section of a mature stem about one cm. in diameter is circular with its outline broken up in one or more places by the openings of lenticels. The outermost tissue namely the cork or *phellem* can be differentiated into an outer zone of thin-walled wavy compressed cells with slightly brownish walls and an inner region of three or four rows of narrow tangentially elongated cells with colourless walls. The cork tissue is broken up in one or more places by the openings of lenticels. A single row of *phellogen* can be made out. A *phelloderm* consisting of five or more rows of cells is present next within of which the outmost rows are thinwalled and narrow, while the cells of the inner rows adjoining the cortex are larger. Scattered amidst the rows of phelloderm cells situated interior to or just within the lenticel openings are several groups of thickwalled cells, each group consisting of 2-10 cells that appear circular in T. S. These groups of *sclereids* are to be found only here.

The *cortex* is fairly wide and occupies a quarter of the radius of the stem. At the periphery of the cortex is a zone of chlorenchyma of three to five rows of regularly arranged thinwalled tangentially elongated cells. The bulk of the cortical cells situated inner to this layer are polygonal thinwalled and fully packed with simple rounded oblong or hemispherical starch grains measureing 9 to 22μ in length.

The centre of the stem is occupied by the *pith*. The vascular zone present between the pith and cortex is composed of ten to twelve or more wedge shaped radial strips of xylem (wood) crowned at their distal broader ends by semicircular strips of phloem the two together radially alternating with broad medullary rays that start from the pith and extend to the cortex. Ech vascular stand is bounded at its periphery by a crescent shaped group of thickwalled (pericyclic) fibres and the cortical cells just outside these groups are slightly elongate seeming to radiate out from the fibre groups. Within each patch of older phloem may be made out three or more tangential strips of collapsed cells which alternate with similar bands composed of few rows of large sized thinwalled cells containing starch grains. The more recently formed or functioning phloem which occupies only a smaller area is composed mostly of thinwalled polygonal to slightly tangentially elongated parenchyma cells some of which contain many small micro-crystals of calcium oxalate and a limited number of sieve tubes with their companion cells. Each strand of wood or xylem is wedgeshaped in T. S. and consists of several wide or large sized vessels, thickwalled xylem parenchyma and wood fibres. Most of the larger vessels appear occluded by several tyloses. The tyloses are comparatively narrow or longer than broad and have very thin walls or limiting membranes. In the primary xylem groups that are located at the innermost region of each xylem strand, the vessels are comparatively very narrow and are normally devoid of tyloses. The xylem parenchyma cells are nearly as thickwalled as the xylem fibres. Several of the parenchyma cells of the border rows on either side of each xylem strand situated adjacent to the medullary rays contain small rhomboidal crystals of calcium oxalate.

The medullary rays number 10 to 12 and most of them extend from the pith to the cortex. They are very broad being composed of 15 to 20 or more rows of cells. In each ray stretching radically along its middle up to the cortex is a strip of compressed collapsed cells region of the wood . The medullary rays are mostly multiseriate and composed of thinwalled radially elongated cells. These generally do not show the presence of starch grains in their cells as those of the stem. Radial strips of compressed and collapsed cells occur along the middle of the broader medullary rays as in those of the stem.

Stem and Root of Tinospora cordifolia
Different features

Morphological

The stem has characteristic lateral nodal swellings or tuberosites with two or three short downwardly pointed parrot-beak like projections. The roots do not show nodes or internodes and no such swellings are found. Other external features are nearly similar.

Anatomical

1. In T.S. of the stem, small groups of sclereids are found at the peripheral region of the cortex immediately below the complimentary tissue of the lenticels. These are not found in the aerial root sections.

2. Groups or patches of fibre groups occur just outside the phloem in stems. These are not found in roots.

3. The tyloses occluding the vessels of the stems are larger in number and possess thin cross septa whereas those in the root are fewer and appear simple.

4. Starch grains occur in abundance within the parenchymatous cells of the stem. These are scanty in roots.

MAÑJIṢṬHĀ

History of stem of Rubia cardifolia :

A very variable, prickly creeper or climber, up to 10 m. long, common throughout India, ascending to an altitude of 3,750 m. Rootstocks perennial, roots long, cylindric flexuose with thin, red bark; stems 4-angled; leaves very variable, cordate ovate to ovate-lanceolate; 2-8 in a whorl, normally 4, sometimes 1 pair larger; flowers small, white or greenish, or in shades of red and yellow, sweet-scented in many or few-flowered terminal panicles of cymes; fruits globose, or slightly 2-lobed, dark-purplish or black, fleshy with 2 small seeds.

R. cordifolia Linn. *sensu* Hook. f. is a complex group, exhibiting a wide range of morphological characters, and is distributed in Africa and Asia, extending into Australia. Indian madder of commerce consists of short stocks with numerous cylindrical, smooth and straight roots about the size of a quill. These are covered by a thin, brownish cork, which peels off in flakes exposing a red-brown bark marked by longitudinal furrows. The root is sweetish, followed by acrid and bitter taste. In West Bengal, the stem is preferred to root for extraction of dye, though both are used. A variety *R. cordifolia* var. *khasiana* Watt, commonly found throughout Assam and Manipur and extending westward to Nepal is reported to be far richer in the either *R. cordifolia* or *R. sikkimensis.*

Indian madder has long been employed in the country for dyeing coarse cotton fabrics, blankets and carpets The colour obtained from *R. cordifolia* though brighter is more fleeting than that from *R. tinctorum.*

The colouring matter present in roots of *R. cordifolia* is a mixture of purpurin (trihydroxy anthraquinone) munjistin (xanthopurpurin-2-carboxylic acid). Purpurin is the main colouring principle in the roots while manjistin an orange dye, occurs in the form of a glycoside accompanied by an isomeride ($C_{14}H_6O_6$ m.p. 2020). Besides purpurin and manjistin, the roots contains small amounts of xanthopurpurin or purpuroxanthin and pseudopurpurin (purpurin-3-carboxylic acid).

Roots are credited with tonic, astringent, antidysenteric, antiseptic and deobstruent properties. They are used in rheumatism and form an ingredient of several Ayurvedic preparations. Roots are said to be active against *Staphylococcus aureus* and are made into a paste for application into ulcers, inflammations and skin troubles. It is reported that after oral administration of the root decoction, the urine and bones of the patient show a red tinge. Roots are used also for colouring medicinal oils. A decoction of leaves and stems is used as a vermifuge.

Extract of *R. cordifolia* enters into the drug, Septilin, which is employed in the treatment of rhinosinal infections. Ethanolic extract of the aerial parts of the plant shows hypoglycaemic activity in albino rats, and maximum tolerated oral dose is 1.0 g/kg. of body weight. The plant gives positive tests for sterol, terpene and saponin (Mehta & Naik, *J. Indian med. Ass.* 1965, **45**,38; Dhar *et al., Indian J. exp. Biol.* 1968, **6**, 232. Maiti, *Bull. Bot. Surv. India,* 1968, **10**, 119).

The climber is much esteemed as *lalab*, a side dish with rice, by the Javanese, and is sometimes used as fodder (Laurie, *Indian For. Leafl.*, No. 82, 1945, 10; Uphof, 457).

KUṬAJA

History of stem bark of Holarrhena antidysenterica

The outer most tissue present in the stem bark of *Holarrhena antidysenterica* namely the outer bark has a thickness of about 1 mm. in barks about 12 mm. thick. The *cork* consists of 5 to 10 rows of almost rectangular cells having brown walls and yellowish contents. Inner to this there are two rows of narrow rectangular clear or colourless cells representing the *phellogen.* The *phelloderm* cells which are slightly smaller than the cortical cells are thinwalled and rectangular. Most of them contain rhomboidal crystals of calcium oxalate and some others contain small rounded starch grains. The cortical cells are large polygonal or tangentially elongated. They also contain rounded starch grains. Scattered in the cortex are a number of large stone cell groups. These form an almost continuous band at the inner region of the middle bark. Here the stone cells are arranged tangentially. The parenchymatous cells near the stone cell groups contain rhomboidal crystals of calcium oxalate. The inner bark which forms the major portion of the bark consists of several tangential rows of stone cells, the phloem elements and medullary rays. The stone cell groups are arranged in tangential rows separated by the medullary rays. The stone cells comprising the groups are large but not uniform in shape and size. They are generally long and are arranged radially. In some of the small sized stone cells rhomboidal crystals of calcium oxalate are present. The cells of the phloem parenchyma in between the rows of stone cell groups though not uniform in size, are small thinwalled and almost polygonal with very small intercellular spaces. Most of them are packed with starch grains and a few cells contain small rhomboidal crystals. The cut ends of several laticiferous ducts with brownish contents can be made out in this tissue. In the most recently formed phloem which forms the inner most part of the bark the cells are slightly smaller than those in middle bark and thin walled. Small sized crystals occur in a very few cells. Sieve tubes and companion cells are distinctly made out in the phloem. No mechanical elements are formed in this region but cut ends of laticiferous ducts are present.

Medullary rays : many, long. They are one to three-seriate and extend from innermost part of the bark upto the cortex. Most of them are straight, while a few are slightly wavy. All the ray cells are thin walled radially elongated and contain starch grains. The ray cells in the phloem region are smaller in size. The cells gradually enlarge towards the distal end of the rays and their starch grain content also increases.

DHATTŪRA

Microscopic characters of Datura fastuosa Linn. Solanaceae :

In a transverse section of a root of one cm. in diameter, the *phellem* or *cork* is the outermost tissue which is appreciably thin. It is composed of five to eight or occasionally ten rows of fairly large rectangular slightly tangentially elongate thinwalled cells devoid of contents. The outermost two to four rows appear in a crushed up or flattened condition.

A single row of *phellogen* is evident in fresh root but often not as a continuous layer. A distinct *phelloderm* is also not evident in most roots. When present it is seen to be composed of a few (two to four or five) rows of thinwalled cells somewhat similar in form but slightly larger (in size) than those of the cork.Inner to this is a wide zone composed of several rows of comparatively large thin walled parenchymatous cells extending as far as the phloem with the intercellular spaces distinct only at certain places. In certain roots (but not in all cases) the peripheral four to six rows here are different in form from those situated inner. These appear larger and appreciably tangentially elongated, the tangential length being three or four times the breadth. Most of the parenchyma cells are heavily loaded with starch grains. The starch grains are comparatively large though occasionally in some cells smaller grains are met with. A majority of the grains appear to be compound grains composed of two components and a lesser number with three or rarely with four components. A large number of simple and nearly spherical grains are also present. They vary in diameter from 10 to 21μ. The grains with two components are oblong in shape and vary in length from 16 to 34μ and those with three components are nearly spherical having a diameter varying from 15 to 36μ. The seperated components have one or more flat faces and a curved or convex face. In most cases a hilum is seen at one end of the grain or its component as a tiny dot and the striations are feebly pereeptible around the hilum.

A number of cells in this parenchymatous zone contain numerous micro-crystals of calcium oxalate similar to but larger than those present in *Withania somnifera* and spices of *Solanum.* The crystals appear mostly conical and arrowhead shaped.

Scattered amidst the *parenchyma* cells are present a few isolated or solitary thickwalled sclereids that appear square, some what circular or shortly rectangular oblong or polygonal in transverse section. The walls of these sclereids appear sparsely pitted the pits being not clear but distantly situated.

Phloem occurs in the form of short narrow radial, triangular or wedge shaped to rectangular strips separated by the vascular (phloem) rays. In addition to the usual thinwalled cells phloem elements it contains sections of a limited number of thickwalled cells that occur in scattered at ray either solitary of in groups of two or three. These fibre cells appear much smaller than the sclereds in the parenchymatous layer as seen in transverse section. In macerated material they are mostly long and narrow with the sides nearly parallel and only slightly tapering towards the ends which are not quite pointed but appear blunt or occasionally very truncate. The phloem fibres are much shorter than the wood fibres. Their walls are appreciably thick and sparsely pitted, the pits being oblique, and silt like. The parenchyma cells of the phloem are comparatively small. They do not generally contain starch grains. Several vascular (phloem) rays traverse radically across the phloem. They are mostly biseriate and several others form to six seriate. Uniseriate rays are also occasionally present as seen in tangential section. The ray cells are tangentially elongated at the distal ends of the rays where the rays appear wider. All the ray cells appear fully loaded with starch grains. A few of the ray cells contain micro-crystals similar to those found in the parenchyma cells. A narrow *cambial zone* of two or three rows of cells is evident outside the xylem.

The *xylem* occupies the bulk part of the root and shows both lignified and unlignified cells. The proportion to these xylem elements vary in roots of different plants or plants from different localities. In all cases however the centre of the root is occupied by a core of lignified xylem which may be small and nearly circular or larger and irregular in outline. Here can be made out the primary xylem which may be di-tri-or tetrarch the protoxylem appearing as thin wedge shaped strips outside the metaxylem which may consists of one or two vessels only as is the case in the di- and tri-arch roots or of more cells as in the tetrarch roots. The primary xylem is always found surrounded by lignified secondary xylem whose extent differs in different roots. The rest of the secondary xylem is composed of patches of unlignified parenchyma and lignified elements. The wood parenchyma occur as broad radial strands separated by xylem rays and interrupted by patches of various sizes of lignified elements.

VĀSĀ

History of the leaf of Adhatoda vasica :

A transverse section of the leaf shows the upper and lower epidermis with the mesophyll in between differentiated into palisade and spongy tissues and the section of the vascular bundle. Both the epidermal layers are covered with a thin cuticle and show the presence of stomata and hairs. The stomata present are of the cruciferous type : The hairs (trichomes) are of two types namely glandular and non-glandular the latter being two to six celled with the basal cell shorter than the others. The glandular trichomes are more frequently met within the upper epidermis. They are small and club shaped with one celled stalks. Their glandular heads are multicellular and brownish in colour. The epidermal cells are cubical to rectangular and thin walled in the transverse section. The walls of the lower epidermis as seen in peeled off tissues appear more wavy than those of the upper. On surface view the epidermal cells are polygonal. Some of the epidermal cells contain cluster crystals of calcium oxalate. There is a single row of vertically elongated palisade cells just inner to the upper epidermis. The spongy tissue in between the palisade layer and lower epidermis is composed of rounded or oblong thin walled cells. Most of these cells adjoining or nearer the palisade layer contain cluster crystals. At the midrib region adjoining and inner to the upper and lower epidermis are wide zones of collenchyma cells. The parenchymatous layer situated between the upper and lower zones of collenchyma and the vascular strand at the middle, is composed of fairly large sized rounded thinwalled (colourless) parenchyma cells with large inter cellular spaces. Some of these cells contain microcrystals and a few others prismatic crystals of calcium oxalate. The vascular strand present in the midrib region appears as a cresent or up wardly directed arc with the elements of xylem in the form of many short and narrow, wedge shaped up right strips separated by or alternating with narrow strips of parenchyma and with many small groups of phloem on the dorsal and ventral sides of the xylem. There is no sclerenchymatous bundle sheath encircling the vascular strand.

Diagnostic characters :

Leaves are simple, petiolate with light green colour. Flowers are found in short, dense axillary pedunceld spikes, each accompanied by one big bract and two small bracteoles. The young stem bears numerous glandular and non-glandular haris. The glandular hairs have a uni-cellular stalk and a quadricellular head. The pericycle in mature stem is thick-walled. The stele of the petiole consists of three vascular bundles of which the centre is the largest and fan shaped. The lamina represents a dorsiventral structure. The epidermal cells being sinuous. Trichomes, both glandular and non glandular, are present on both the surfaces. Cystolithos elongated and cigar shaped are of wide occurence and are found in the cortical and pith regions of the stem, cortex of the petiole and the midrib and spongy tissue. Oil globules are present mainly in the mesophyll of the leaf precentage of alkaloids determined is 0.5408-1.1050.

PIPPALĪ

Histology of the root of Piper longum

A transverse section of a root about 4 mm. in diameter is almost circular and the outline regular. *Cork* is the outermost tissue and appears as a narrow strip slightly brown in colour. It consists of only a few (3 to 5) rows of cells. The cork cells are all thinwalled and rectangular to slightly tangentially elongated. The *phellogen* is not evident in many specimens.

The *cortex* within is fairly wide and parenchymatous except for a few small thickwalled cells.The cortical cells are large sized thinwalled and rounded to oblong with large intercellular spaces. The cell walls of the peripheral rows are slightly thickened but not lignified. The rounded cortical cells measure 40 to 60µ in diameter and the oblong cells 60 to 90µ x 50 to 75µ. Most of these cells are heavily loaded with starch. The starch grains appear spherical or oval and are compound consisting usually of 2 to 6 components or rarely more. They measure up to 15µ in length. Separated components of the grains also occur in abundance. A few cortical cells contain minute prismatic crystals of calcium oxalate. Many secretory cells are found scattered in the cortex. Most of them appear nearly filled with large globules of a light yellow colour. A number of thick walled cells are found scattered in the cortex. They are smaller than the other cells and appear circular in the transverse section and their diameter varies from 30 to 48µ. A wavy ring (endodermis) composed of one row of rectangular cells with their side walls slightly thickened can be distinctly made out.

The centre of the root is occupied by pith, 180µ in diameter and it is surrounded by 4 to 6 wedge-shaped radiating strips of vascular tissue having their wider ends towards the periphery. The cells composing the pith are polygonal and thinwalled and contain starch grains similar to those present in the cortical cells. Six groups of primary xylem bundles are present outside the pith. They are evenly spaced. In each vascular strip the xylem is about 1 mm. in length appears wedge-shaped and is composed of xylem vessels, xylem parenchyma and wood fibres and its wider end is crowned with a hemispherical strip of phloem 60µ in thickness. There are many xylem vessels and these appear arranged in 3 or 4 radial rows. Their diameters vary from 18 to 60µ. The xylem parenchyma cells when compared to the wood fibers are fewer but are nearly as thickwalled as the firbers. A strip of cambium composed of one or two rows of narrow thinwalled rectangular cells is present between the xylem and phloem. The phloem is composed of many sieve tubes with their companion cells that can be distinctly made out towards the inner region of the phloem and small thinwalled polygonal phloem parenchyma cells. The cells at the outer convex side are slightly compressed and appears tangentially elongated. One or two groups of small stone cells composed of 2 or 3 cells about 15µ in diameter are present at the peripheral region of the phloem. The outer border of phloem is limited by a row of pericyclic cells found just inner to the endodermis.

Medullary rays : There are four to six broad wedgeshaped medullary rays with their wider ends at the periphery and alternating with the radiating bands of vascular tissue. Each ray is ten to fifteen or more cell rows wide towards the outer region and extends from the pith up to the endodermis. The ray cells are all thinwalled cubical to slightly radially elongated and arranged in regular radial rows. Most of the cells are heavily loaded with starch grains similar to those present in the cortex. Some cells contain minute crystals of calcium oxalate and a few cells have oil globules. In some specimens narrow strips of interfascicular cambial cells are found connecting the fascicular cambia present in vascular strips. The presence of large quantity of compound starch grain is peculiar to *Piper longum.*

ARJUNA

Histology of the root of Terminalia arjuna

Leaves are dorsiventral, single layered, cuticularised. Upper and lower dermis bear unicellular glandular and non-glandular trichomes and the lower dermis is provided with ranunculaccous stomata. In the midrib region, the epideımis several layers of thick-walled collenchymatous and thinwalled parenchymatous tissues surround the central vascular cylinders. Vascular wall is open, bicollateral i.e. xylem surrounded by phloem. Few secretory ducts are observed in the parenchymatous tissue and in the central regions.

Abundant cluster crystals of calcium oxalate are noted in the phloem and parenchymatous tissues. Mesophyll is composed of palisade and spongy cells. Inside is double layered. Stomatal index is 14.0—15.5. Vein-islet numbers cells—19 sq. mm. and palisade ratio varies from 7-12.

Stem bark :

The young stem shows typical combretaceous type of hair having swollen and tapering apex. Transverse section of the bark shows cork, thin-walled parenchymatous ground tissue with embedded cells of calcium crystals and secondary phloem with patches of selerencyma fibres, mucilage, secreting ducts, seleranchyma of fibres and tanniniferous cells.

Mature bark shows a broad zone of phloem consisting of ceratencyma, phloem parenchyma, phloem fibres and crystal fibres. The latter contains rosette crystals of calcium oxalate.

Fruit :

Transverse section shows epidermis and hypodermis. Secretary canals, ducts and vascular supply are present. The seeds are composed of stone cells, fibres and vascular supply.

SĀRIBĀ

Microscopic characters of the root of H. indicus :

The young root shows a single layer of epidermis followed by 4-8 layers of isodiametric cortical parenchyma arranged more of less in radial rows. The endodermis is distinct. The pericycle encloses a diarch to hexarch stele, the tri- and tetrarch conditions being more common. The phellogen arises in the pericycle and soon the tissues outside the pericycle are ruptured.

In a mature root, 6-8 mm. diameter thick, the cork consists of 4-14 layers of narrow, rectangular, tangentially elongated cells which gets mostly compressed excepting the inner 2-3 layers of cells. The cork cells are polyhedral in surface view and filled with brown contents. The phellogen is single layered; the phelloderm is represented by 8-16 layers of polyhedral cells, some of which show secondary radial wall formation. The secondary phloem consists of sieve tubes, companion cells, phloem parenchyma and medullary rays. Sieve tubes are collapsed in the outer phloem but remain intact in the inner region. The cells of the parenchyma are bigger in the outer phloem and become smaller in the inner region. Medullary rays are 4-20 cells high and 1-3 cells wide, but uniseriate rays 5-8 cells high are very common. The ray cells in the outer phloem are somewhat tangentially elongated and bigger. Laticiferous vessels of non-articulated, but unbranched type are present both in the phelloderm and the phloem.

The wood shows 2 to 3 growth rings and is composed of vessels, parenchyma, tracheids, fibres tracheids and medullary rays; all the elements being lignified. The vessels occure singly or in the group of 2-3. They are usually cylindrical, drum-shaped, some being greatly bordered pits and transverse to oblique pits and are moderately thick-walled, elongated with wide lumen and tapering extremities which possess peg-like outgrowth in some cases. The xylem parenchyma are rectangular or elongated at one end and pitted. The rays are 1-3 cells wide and 6-10-15-25 cells high, uni-seriate rays being more common, the cells are oblong to radially elongated and simple pitted. Pith is absent.

AŚVAGANDHĀ

Histology of the root of Withania somnifera (Linn.) Dunal Solanaceae :

A transverse section of the root shows only a narrow cork and cortex enclosing a wide central woody region which is parenchymatous for the most part and storage in function. A T.S. of a fresh root 2 cms. in diameter shows a *cork* light brown in colour, at the outside, of 320μ width. Cork is composed of 12 to 16 rows of thinwalled cubical to slightly tangentially elongated cells. Inner to the cork is the *phellogen* composed of one row of narrow thinwalled tangentially elongated cells. One or two rows of cork cells just outer to the phellogen have a yellow colour. This ring of yellow colour is quite distinct even in the specimen, brought from the bazaar, but this colour fades away by the action of microscopical reagents. The *cortex* is fairly wide, from 2 to 3 mm. in thickness and composed of fairly large, thinwalled, slightly tangentially elongated cells. Most of the cortical cells are fully packed with moderately large starch grains. The starch grains are compound having 2 to 5 components and almost rounded with a diameter of 15 to 30μ. The different components are also found separately. There are many smaller starch grains of diameter 9μ. So there is considerable variation in the size of the starch grains. Striations are fairly visible in the larger grains. Several of the cortical cells are completely filled with micro-crystals of calcium oxalate. These very minute crystals are mostly triangular in shape. Inner to the cortex is the *phloem* in the form of a narrow ring enclosing the wood and intercepted by the medullary rays. It is composed of small sized thinwalled polygonal cells. Sieve tubes and the companion cells are not very prominent and comparatively few in number. Some of the cells of this tissue are found to be filled with microcrystals as in the cortex. A distinct *cambium* is present composed of one or two rows of narrow thinwalled cells appearing broadly rectangular in T.S.

The *wood* which forms the major part of the root is 12 to 14 mm. in diameter. It is composed almost entirely of secondary xylem and wood rays. The peripheral part of the wood is composed of thickwalled fibres, in which are small patches of thinwalled parenchyma as well as scattered or radially arranged rows of small groups of vessels and tracheids all together forming a circular zone or band of thickwalled tissue. The rest of the root namely the wide central portion is composed almost entirely of thinwalled parenchyma in which occur scattered several small groups of vessels and tracheids. In each group the number of vessels varies from 4 to 8. They vary in length from 80 to 400μ and their diameter varies from 16 to 108μ. The vessels may be short and wide tailed at both ends or long and thickwalled with ends tapering. Their length varies from 50 to 800μ and width from 16 to 20μ. The parenchyma cells are all thin walled, fairly large, rectangular and most of them fully loaded with starch grains similar to those in the cortical cells. Others are full of micro-crystals of calcium oxalate. A few larger groups of vessels are found towards the centre of the wood and the centre of the root shows a diarch primary xylem.

Medullary rays : There are many long uni-to-bi-seriate medullary rays most of which extend from the centre of the wood up to the cortex. The ray cells are radially elongated and completely packed with starch grains. The ray cells within the wood in the thinwalled parenchymatous region are thinwalled radially elongated and heavily loaded with starch grains. The ray cells at the peripheral region of the wood are also radially elongated, but some of the cells are slightly thickwalled. The ray cells at the region of phloem are thinwalled and mostly rectangular while those at the distal ends of the medullary rays are larger and tangentially elongated.

ŚATĀVARĪ

Histology of the root of Asparagus racemosus Willd. (Asparagaceae):

A transverse section of the root is nearly circular. It shows an outer exodermis which is light yellow in colour within which is a wide cortex surrounding a ring or cirelet of vascular bundles and a central pith. The outermost tissue is formed of 6 to 10 rows of compactly arranged polygonal to slightly radially elongated slightly thickwalled cells whose walls are suberised as well as lignified. These cells measure 54 to 135μ x 25 to 60μ in T.S. The length of these cells in L.S. varies from 800 to 1050μ. The number of rows of cells of this zone varies slightly at different levels of the root. Towards the distal or apical narrower end of the root in addition to the exodermis, the outer piliferous layer is present at certain regions which is seen to be composed of small thinwalled mostly rectangular cells many of which are modified into root hairs. At certain portions of this region this layer is seen ruptured and replaced by a dark pigmented mass of broken down cells.

The cortex which forms 3/4ths the diameter of the T.S. of the root is composed of 20 to 25 rows of cells in the basal, 30 to 45 rows in the middle and 25 to 30 rows at the distal regions of the tuberous root. The cortical cells are thinwalled and circular or oval with distinct intercellular spaces. The cells of the outer region are smaller in size than those of the inner region. The diameter of the cells of the cortex varies from 45 to 120μ. Scattered within the cortex are a number of cells which contain raphide bundles of calcium oxalate. The raphide containing cells are found to be smaller in size than the adjacent of surrounding cells in a longitudinal section of the root. Each raphide bundle consists of a large number of acicular crystals. These vary in length in different cells but crystals belonging to the same bundle (cell) are of equal length. The length of the crystals varies from 45 to 75μ. Scattered amidst the cortical cells are a limited number of narrow comparatively thickwalled lignified cells with numerous circular or oval pits on their walls the thickness of the walls varying in different cells. Their length also varies from 350 to 400μ. The innermost three or four rows of cortical cells immediately outside the endodermis are modified into elongate very thick-walled lignified cells with numerous circular or oval pits on their walls. The thickness of the walls varies in different cells. Their length varies from 190 to 370μ. The *endodermis* consists of a single row of narrow rectangular thinwalled cells. The central stele shows the typical monocotyledonous type of structure. Just within the endodermis is the *pericycle* consisting of a single row of thinwalled rectangular cells. The xylem and phloem groups number from twenty to twentyfive and are arranged along alternate radii in a circle surrounding a large central pith. The xylem vessels have spiral and pitted thickenings. The proto xylem elements have a diameter of 12-20 to 50μ and the later formed mentaxylem vessels a diameter of 60 to 100μ. Their length varries from 500 to 2500μ. Tracheids with pitted thickening on the walls are also present. They are however shorter and much narrower than the vessels. The phloem parenchyma cells are polygonal and thinwalled. There is a zone of thickwalled tissue at the periphery of pith within which the metaxylem elements appear embedded. Their cells are considerably long as seen in L. S. with numerous oblique pits on the walls and have one or two fairly distantly spaced thin transverse speta.

The centre of the root is occupied by the pith which is composed of small rounded mostly thinwalled cells with large intercellular spaces. The diameter of the pith cells varies from 21 to 48μ. Scattered within the pith are a few cells whose walls are slightly thickened (similar to those in the cortex). These cells are however narrower and nearly three to four times longer than those occuring in the cortex.

MODERN PHARMACOLOGY

1. Antimicrobials & Antibiotics :

Cotrimoxozole : A fixed dose combination of

Trimethoprim and sulfamenthoxazole - 50 mg + 400 mg B.D. 2 B.D. for 2 days then 1 B.D.	All adverse effects of sulphonamides can be produced nausea, vomiting, stomatitis headache and rashes.
Occinolones :	
Nalidixic acid - 0.5-1.0 gm. TDS	Gastrointestinal upset and rashes, headache, drowsiness, vertigo, visual, disturbances, occasionally seizures in children.
Fluroquinolones :	
Ciproflaxam - 250 mg.	Nausea, vomiting, bad taste, anorexia, dizziness, headache, restlessness, anxiety, insomnia, confusion, tremor, tendoniter, tendon, rupture etc.
Pencillin G (Benzyl pencillin) - 60 g	Pain at I.M. injection site, nausea on oral ingestion, thrombophlebitis of injected vein, mental confusion, muscular twitching, convulsions & coma.
Extended spectrum pencillins :	
Aminopecillin - Ampicillin 0.5-2 g oral/I.M./I.V.	Diarrhoea on oral ingestion. Marked alternation of bacterial flora, rashes etc.
Amoxicillin - 0.5-1 g TDS oral	Incidence of diarrhoea is less.
Carboxypencillin - Carbenicillin - 1-2 g I.M. or 1-5 g I.V. every 4-6 hrs.	Higher doses may cause bleeding by interfering with platelet function.

Cephalosporins : are bactericidal.

Adverse effects : Pain after I.M. injection, diarrhoea, thrombophlebitis, nephrotoxicity, bleeding, hypersensitivity reactions caused by cephalosporins are similar to pencillin.

Tetracyclines : Primarily bacteriostatic.

Dose : 250, 500 mg cap.

Adverse effects : Epigastric pain, nausea, vomiting, diarrhoea, esophageal ulceration, thrombophlebitis, of the injected vein, pain at the injection site. Kidney damage is prominent in existing kidney disease, phototoxicity, antianobolic, liver damage etc.

Chloramphenicol : Primarily bacteriostatic.

Dose : 250-500 mg 6 hrly	Bone marrow depression, aplastic anaemia, agranulocytosis, thrombocytopenia, non dose related indiosyncratic reaction. Gray baby syndrome etc.

Aminoglycoside antibiotics : Drugs effective against gram negative bacteria.

1. Streptomycin - 0.75, 1 g	Vestibular disturbances, rashes, eosinophilia, fever, exfoliative dermatitis have been reported. Pain at injection site is common.
2. Gentamycin - 1-1.5 ml/kg/ I.V. 8 hrly	More nephrotoxic.
3. Neomycin - 0.25-1 g Q.D. oral	Highly toxic to inernal ear and to kidney.

Macrolide antibiotics :

Erythromycin - 250-500 mg 6 hrly	Mild to severe epigastric pain, diarrhoea—occasional. High doses may cause reversible hearing impairment.
Clarithromycin - 250 mg B.D. for 7 days	Similar to erythromycins, Pseudomembranous enterocolitis is reported.

Miscellaneous antibiotics :

Clindamycin - 150-300 mg Q.D. oral	Rashes urticaria, abdominal pain, diarrhoea & pseudomembranous enterocolitis.

Antitubercular drugs :

Firstline drugs : These drugs have high antitubercular efficacy as well as low toxicity are used routinely.

1. Isoniazid - 5 mg/kg 300 mg>50 kg	Peripheral neuritis, paresthesias, numbness, mental disturbances are most important dose dependent toxic effects & hepatitis.
2. Rifampcin - 10 mg/kg 600 mg>50 kg	Hepatitis - major adverse effect, breathlessness which may be associated with shock & collapse, purpura, haemolysis, shock & renal failure.
3. Pyrazinamide - 25-30 mg/kg 1500 mg>50 kg.	Hepatotoxicity, hyperuricemia, gout may occur, arthralgia, flushing, rashes, fever & loss of diabetic control.
4. Ethambutol - 15 mg/kg 100 mg above 50 kg	Loss of visual acuty or colour vision, field defects due to optic neuritis are most importnat dose & duration dependant toxicity, hyperuricemia etc.
5. Streptomycin - 15 mg/kg 1000 mg>50 kg.	Ototoxicity & nephrotoxicity.

Antileprotic drugs :

1. **Sulfones :**

Dapsone - 100 mg/day	Mild haemolytic anaemia, nausea & anorexia, methaemoglobinaemia, headache, paresthesias, mental symptoms, drug fever etc.

2. **Phenazine derivative :** Clofazimine - 50-100 mg	Reddish black discolouration of skin, discolouration of hair and body secretions may occur. Drying of skin & itching etc. Enteritis with intermittent loose stools, nausea, abdominal pain, anorexia & weight loss may occur.
3. **Rifampcin** - 600 mg monthly dose	Relativily nontoxic
4. **Other antibiotics :** Ofloxacin - 400 mg/day Clarithromycin - 500 mg/day	

Antifungal drugs : These are drugs used for superficial & deep fungal infections.

I. Antibiotics :

(a) **Polyenes :**	
1. Amphotericin B - 50-100 mg Q.D.	Toxicity is high, acute reaction occurs with each infusion and consists of chills, fever, aches and pain allover, nausea, vomiting and dyspnoea.
2. Nystatin - 5 lac U TDS	Nausea and bad taste in mouth.
(b) Heterocyclic benzofuran Griscofulvin - 125-250 mg Q.D.	Headache followed by G.I.T. disturbances, CNS symptoms & peripheral neuritis are occasional.
(c) Clotrimazole - 1% lotion Topical treatment	Local irritation with stinging and burning sensation.
(d) Ketaconazole	Nausea, vomiting, loss of appetite, headache, paresthesia, rashes, hair loss, menstrual irregularities in women, g ynaecomastia, lose of hair & libido and oligospermia may be the mainfestations.

Antiviral drugs :

1. Anti herpes virus :

Idoxuridine - 1% solution -	Ocular irritation, edema of lids & photophobia.
Acyclovir - 200 mg/vial for inj.	Topical - Stinging & burning sensation. Oral - Headache, nausea, malaise & CNS effects. I.V. - Rashes swealing, emesis & fall in B.P. may occur.
Zidovudine - - 500 mg/day - Adults	Anaemia & neutropenia.
- 150 mg/m^2 - Children	Nausea, anorexia, abdominal pain, headache, insomnia & myalgia are common at the start of therapy.
Amantadine - 100 mg B.D. - 5 mg/m^2 - Children	Insomnia, dizziness, nightmares, lack of mental concentration. Hallucination postural hypotension, ankle oedema.

Antimalarial drugs :

1. 4-Aminoquinolines - Chloroquine - 250 mg	Nausea, vomiting, anorexia, epigastric pain, uncontrolled itching, uneasiness, headache. Parenteal - Hypotension, cardiac depression, arrhythmias & CNS toxicity including convulsions.
2. Quinine - 300 mg	Cinchonism consisting of ringin in ears, nausea, vomiting, headache, mental confusion, vertigo, difficulty in hearing, visual defects etc.
3. Primaquine - 15 mg daily for 2 wks 0.2 mg/kg - Children	Abdominal pain, G.I.T. upset, weakness/uneasiness in chest, haemolysis, methaemoglobinaemia and cyanosis.

Antiamoebic drugs : These are drugs useful in infection caused by protozoa entamoeba histolytica.

1. Tissue amoebicides :

(a) for both intestinal & extraintestinal amoebiasis :

1. Nitroimidazoles - Metronidazole - 200 mg	Anorexia, nausea, metallic taste, abdominal cramps, headache, glossitis, dryness of mouth etc.
Tinidazole - 2 gm OD for 3 days	Metallic taste, nausea, rash.
2. Alkaloids - Emetine 60 mg/2 ml inj.	Highly toxic

(b) For extraintestinal amoebiasis only

1. Chloroquine - 600 mg for 2 days followed by 300 mg daily for 2-3 wks.

Luminal amoebicides :

Diloxanide furoate 500 mg TDS	Flatulence occasional, nausea, itching and rarely urticaria.
8-Hydroxy Quinolines 250-500 mg TDS	Nausea, transient loose & green stools, pruritus, goitre on prolonged medication.

Antihelminthics : These are drugs that either kill (vermicide) or expel (vermifuge) infesting helminthes.

1. Mebendazole - 100 mg	Diarrhoea, nausea, abdominal pain, allergic reactions, loss of hair and granulocytopenia have been reported with higher doses.
2. Albendazole - 400 mg	Gastrointestinal side effects, dizziness in few etc.
3. Piperazine - 4.5 g OD	Nausea, vomiting, abdominal discomfort, urticaria are occasional.

Anticancer drugs : These either kill cancer cells or modify their growth.

1. Alkylating agent - Cyclophosphamide 2-3 mg/kg/day oral	Alopecia and cystitis are prominent.
2. Antimetaboliter - Methotrexate - 2.5 mg tab	Major toxicity on bone marrow megaloblastic anaemia, high doses produce pancytopenia etc.
3. Vinca alkaloids - - Vincristene - 1.5 mg/m^2 BSA I.V. wkly	Peripheral neuropathy and alopecia.
Vinblastine - 0.1-0.15 mg/kg I.V.	Bone marrow depression is more prominant while neurotoxicity & alopecia are less marked.

Miscellaneous cytotoxic drug :

4. Cisplastin - 50-100 mg/m^2 I.V. BSA every 3-4 wks.	Renal impairment, deafness, neuropathy, hyperuricaemia.

2. Harmones :

Insulin :

Insulin zincsuspension 40U/80U/ml/strength	Hypoglycaemia, local reaction, swelling, erythema, stinging, lipodystrophy after long usage edema.

Oral hypoglycemic drugs : These drugs lower blood glucose levels and are effective orally.

I. Sulphonyl ureas :

	Adverse effects
First generation : Tolbutamide - 0.5-3 g - 2-3 times **Second generation :** Gilbenclamide 5-15 mg - OD/BD Glipizide - 5-20 mg/OD/BD	Hypoglycaemia, nausea, vomiting, flatulence, diarrhoea, constipation, headache, weight gain, paresthesias, rarely hypersensitivity reaction occur.

II. **Biguanides :**

1. Phenformin - 25-150 mg OD/TDS 2. Metformin - 0.5-2 g BD/QID	Abdominal discomfort, anorexia, nausea, metallic taste, mild diarrhoea & tiredness, lacticacidosis, vit B_{12} deficiency.

Corticosteroids :

I. **Glucocorticoids :**

	Adverse effects
1. Short acting : Hydrocortisone - 20 mg (Cortisol) Cortisone - 25 mg	Cushing's habitus, fragile skin, purple striae, hyperglycemia. Delayed healing, peptic ulceration, gloucoma.
2. Intermediate acting : Prednisolone - 5 mg Methyl prednisolone - 4 mg 3. Long acting : Paramethasone - 2 mg Dexomethasone - 0.75 mg Betamethasone - 0.75 mg	Muscular weakness, growth lretardation, Psychiatric disturbances, suppression of hypothalamo pituitary adrenal axis osteoporosis, susceptibility to infection etc.

Mineral Corticoids :

1. Desoxycorticosterone acetate - 2.5 mg sublingual	Sodium & water retention, edema, hypokalaemic alkalosis.
2. Fludrocortisone - 0.2 mg	Progressive rise in B.P.

Antiestrogens :

1. Clomiphene citrate - 50 mg OD for 5 days, starting from 5th day of cycle in sterility	Polycystic ovaries, multiple pregnancy, hot flushes, gastric upset, vertigo, allergic dermatites. Risk of ovarian tumour.
2. Tamoxifen citrate 10-20 mg BD	Hot flushes, vomiting, vaginal bleeding, menstrual irregularities, dermatites, anorexia, depression, mild leucopenia & ocular changes.

3. Vitamins :

Vitamins are nonenergy producing organic compounds, essential for normal human metabolism that must be supplied in small quantities in the diet.

Vitamins are traditionally divided into two parts :

1. Fat soluble vitamins - A, D, E & K.
2. Water soluble vitamins - B complex & C.

Fat soluble vitamins :

Vitamins	Deficiency symptoms	Therapeutic dosage	Adverse effects
1. Vitamin A (Retinol)	Xerosis of eye, bitot spots, keratomalacia, corneal opacities, night blindness phrynoderma hyperkeratinization, tendency to urinary stone formation, sterility. Abortions, fetal malformations, growth retardation, impairment of senses.	50,000-100,000 I.V./I.M. or orally for 1-3 days followed by intermittent supplement doses. **Prophylaxis :** 3000-5000 I.V./ day **Daily requirement :** 5000 U in adult 3000 U in children below 5 yrs.	Nausea, vomiting, itching, erythema, dermatitis, exfoliation, hair loss, bone & joint pains, loss of appetite, irritability, bleeding, increased intracranial tensions & chronic liver disease.
2. Vitamin D (Calciferol)	Rickets in children, osteomalacia in adults, fall of plasma calcium & phosphate levels	3000-4000 IU/ day. Prophylaxis : 400 IU/day.	Hyperkalaemia, weakness, fatigue, vomiting, diarrhoea, sluggishness, polyuria, albuminuria, nephrocalcinosis, hypertension, growth retard-

			ation in children, ectopic, calcium deposition.
3. Vitamin E Tocopherol	Sterility in male & recurrent abortion in female rats, degenerative changes in spinal cord & nucleus gracilis degenerative lesion in skeletal muscles & heart haemolytic & hypoplastic anaemia.	10-30 mg/day Daily requirement : 3-15 mg	Creatinuria & impaired wound healing.
4. Vitamin K	Bleeding tendency. Haematuria first to occur other common sites of bleeding are G.I.T., nose & under the skin ecchymosis.	5-10 mg/day oral or parenteral.	Rapid I.V. inj. of emulsified Vit K produces flushing, breathlessness, a sense of constriction in the chest fall in B.P.

Water soluble vitamins :

Vitamin B complex group :

1. Thiamine Aneurine B_1	Dry Beriberi- Neurological symptoms are prominent. Wet Beriberi - Cardiovascular system is primarily effected.	100 mg/day Prophylactic 2-10 mg/day Daily requirement : 1-2 mg	Nontoxic, sensitivity reaction, sometimes occur on parenteral injection.

2. Niacin B_3	Pellagra - cardinal manifestation are- dermatitis, diarrhoea, dementia anaemia & hypoproteinemia	200-500 mg/day Prophylactic : 20-30 mg/day Daily requirement : 15-20 mg	
3. Pyridoxin Vitamin B_6	Seborrhic dermatitis, glossitis, growth retardation, mental confusion, lowered seizure threshold or convulsions, anaemia, peripheral neuritis	10-50 mg/day Prophylactic 2-5 mg/day Daily requirement : 1-2 mg	
4. Riboflavin Vitamin B_2	Angular stomatitis, magenta pigmentation of tongue, glossitis, cheliosis, burning feet blepharospasm, photophobia, burning, lacrimation, seborrheic follicular keratosis of nasolabial folds etc.	2-10 mg Daily requirement : Adult : 1.5-3 mg Child 0.6-2 mg/ day.	Excess riboflavine may impart fluorescense to urine during its excretion.
5. Pantothenic acid (Vit B_1)	Deficiency in human beings not known. In animals resulted in keratitis, dermatitis, ar-	10-50 mg Daily requirement : below 5 mg	

	rest of growth, depigmentation of hair, neuro-muscular degeneration, fatal bilateral adrenal haemorrhage.		
6. Biotin	Usually not encountered in human beings. But deficiency may produce seborrheic dermatitis, lassitude, anorexia & paraesthesia.		
7. Ascorbic acid (Vit C)	Scurvy - characterised by perifollicular haemorrhages, petechiae, ecchymoses, swollen, inflammed, bleeding & spongy gums, amaemia.	200-500 mg/day. Prophylactic : 50 mg/day. Dialy requirement : 30 mg for adults, 5 mg/kg in children.	Increased excretion of oxalate with stone formation & kidney damage.

Index of Latin Names of Drugs

Abbies webbiana	TĀLĪŚAPATRA	327
Abroma augusta	PIŚĀCA KĀRPĀSA	388
Abrus precatorius	GUÑJĀ	419
Acacia arabica	BABBŪLA	445
Acacia catechu	KHADIRA	213
Acacia farnesiana	IRIMEDA	442
Achatina fulica	ŚAMBŪKA	607
Achyranthes aspera	APĀMĀRGA	305
Aconitum ferox	VATSANĀBHA	151
Aconitum heterophyllum	ATIVIṢĀ	152
Acorus calamus	VACĀ	340
Adathoda vasica	VĀSĀ	291
Adiantum caudatum	MAYŪRAŚIKHĀ	590
Adiantum lunulatum	HAṀSARĀJA	589
Adina cordifolia	HARIDRĀ	471
Aegle marmelos	BILVA	172
Aerva lanata	GORAKṢAGUÑJĀ	522
Agaricus campestris	CHATRAKA	593
Ailanthus excelsa	ARALU	401
Alangium salvifolium	AṄKOṬA	417
Albizzia lebbeck	ŚIRĪṢA	209
Alhagi camelorum	YAVĀSA	191
Allium cepa	PALĀṆḌU	346
Allium sativum	RASONA	334
Alocasia indica	MĀNAKANDA	579
Aloe barbadensis	KUMĀRĪ	336
Alpinia galanga	MAHĀBHARĪ VACĀ	558
Alstonia scholaris	SAPTAPARṆA	260
Althoea officinalis	KHATMĪ	385
Altingia excelsa	SILHAKA	452
Ambra grasea	AGNIJĀRA	600
Amorphophallus companulatus	SŪRAṆA	578
Anacyclus pyrethrum	ĀKĀRAKARABHA	477
Ananas comosus	ANĀNĀSA	561
Andrographis paniculata	KĀLAMEGHA	514
Anethum sowa	ŚATAPUṢPĀ	235

Angelica glauca	CORAKA	468
Annona squamosa	SĪTĀPHALA	355
Anogeissus latifolia	DHAVA	453
Anthocephalus indicusa	KADAMBA	470
Apium graveolens	AJAMODĀ	239
Aquilaria agallocha	AGURU	313
Areca catechu	PŪGA	573
Argemone mexicana	SATYĀNĀŚĪ	362
Argyreia nervosa	VṚDDHADĀRUKA	502
Aristolochia bracteolata	KĪṬAMĀRĪ	526
Aristolochia indica	ĪŚWARĪ	525
Artemisia maritima	CAUHĀRA	474
Artemisia vulgaris	DAMANAKA	473
Artocarpus integrifolia	PANASA	546
Arundo donax	NALA	586
Asparagus adscendens	MŪSALĪ	571
Asparagus racemosus	ŚATĀVARĪ	338
Asteracantha longifolia	KOKILĀKṢA	513
Atropa belladonna	SŪCĪ	595
Averrhoa carambola	KARMARAṄGA	396
Azadirachta indica	NIMBA	177
Bacopa monnieri	BRĀHMĪ	285
Balanites aegyptiaca	IṄGUDĪ	402
Baliospermum axillare	DANTĪ	318
Balsamodendron mukul	GUGGULU	173
Bambusa arundinaceae	VAṀŚA	582
Barleria prionitis	SAIREYAKA	512
Barringtonia acutangula	HIJJALA	455
Bauhinia purpurea	KĀÑCANĀRA	205
Benincasa hispida	KŪṢMĀṆḌA	229
Berberis aristata	DĀRUHARIDRĀ	156
Bergenia lingulata	PĀṢĀṆABHEDA	450
Betula utilis	BHŪRJAPATRA	550
Blepharis edulis	UṬAṄGANA	515
Blumea lacera	KUKUNDARA	479
Boerhaavia diffusa	PUNARNAVĀ	303
Bombax ceiba	ŚĀLMALĪ	167
Borassus flabellifer	TĀLA	574
Boswellia serrata	ŞALLAKĪ	404
Boswellia serrata	KUṄDURU (ŚALLAKĪ)	405

Brassica campestris	SARṢAPA	365
Brassica juncea	RĀJIKĀ	366
Bryophyllum calycinum	PARṆABĪJA	451
Buchanania latifolia	PRIYĀLA	416
Butea monosperma	PALĀŚA	186
Caesalpinia bonduc	LATĀKARAÑJA	197
Caesalpinia sappan	PATRĀṄGA	433
Callicarpa macrophylla	PRIYAṄGU	517
Calotropis gigantea	ARKA	266
Cannabis sativa	BHAṄGĀ	323
Caplophyllum inophyllum	PUNNĀGA	377
Capparis decidua	KARĪRA	374
Capparis sepiaria	HIṀSRĀ	372
Capparis zeylanica	VYĀGHRANAKHĪ	373
Capsicum annum	KAṬUVĪRA	507
Careya arborea	KUMBHIKĀ	580
Carica papaya	ERAṆḌAKARKAṬĪ	459
Carissa carandas	KARAMARDA	493
Carum carvi	KṚṢṆAJĪRAKA	244
Carum copticum	YAVĀNĪ	240
Cassia absus	CAKṢUṢYA	439
Cassia angustifolia	MĀRKAṆḌIKĀ	443
Cassia auriculata	ĀVARTAKĪ	444
Cassia fistula	ĀRAGWADHA	211
Cassia occidentalis	KĀSAMARDA	435
Cassia tora	CAKRAMARDA	434
Cedrus deodara	DEVADĀRU	325
Celastrus paniculatus	JYOTIṢMATĪ	179
Centella asiatica	MAṆḌŪKAPARṆĪ	231
Centipeda minima	CHIKKIKĀ	483
Centratherum anthelminticum	ARAṆYAJĪRAKA	478
Ceratophyllum demersum	ŚAIVĀLA	592
Cervus elephus	MṚGAŚṚṄGA	610
Chenopodium ambrosiodes	SUGANDHAVĀSTUKA	527
Cichorium intybus	KĀSANĪ	484
Cinnamomum camphora	KARPŪRA	312
Cinnamomum tamala	PATRAKA (TEJAPATRA)	529
Cinnamonum zeylanicum	TWAK	311
Cissampelos pariera	PĀṬHĀ	155
Cissus quadrangularis	ASTHISAṀHĀRAKA	410

Citrullus colocynthis	INDRAVĀRUṆĪ	227
Citrus medica	BĪJAPŪRA	397
Citrus medica	NIMBŪKA	171
Cleome gynandra	TILAPARṆĪ	371
Clerodendron phlomidis	AGNIMANTHA	295
Clerodendrum serratum	BHĀRṄGĪ	297
Clerodendurm infortunatum	BHĀṆḌĪRA	516
Clitoria ternatea	APARĀJITĀ	188
Coccinia grandis	BIMBĪ	465
Cocculus hirsutus	PĀTĀLAGARUḌĪ	357
Cocos nucifera	NĀRIKELA	572
Colchicum luteum	SURAÑJĀNA	570
Coleus amboinicus	PARṆAYAVĀNĪ	520
Commiphora myrrha	BOLA	403
Convolvulus pluricaulis	ŚAṄKHAPUṢPĪ	274
Corallium rubrum	PRAVĀLA	603
Corchorus fascicularis	CAÑCU	395
Cordia dichotoma	SLEṢMĀTAKA	499
Coriandrum sativum	DHĀNYAKA	237
Costus speciosus	KEBUKA	559
Crataeva religiosa	VARUṆA	159
Crinum asiaticum	NĀGADAMANĪ	557
Crinum latifolium	SUDARŚANA	562
Crocus sativus	KUṄKUMA	563
Crotalaria verrucosa	ŚAṆAPUṢPĪ	594
Croton oblongifolius	NĀGADANTĪ	539
Croton tiglium	JAYAPĀLA	538
Cucumis sativus	TRAPUṢA	460
Cuminum cyminum	JĪRAKA	242
Curculigo orchioides	TĀLAMŪLĪ	564
Curcuma amada	ĀMRAGANDHĪ HARIDRĀ	556
Curcuma angustifolia	TAVAKṢĪRA	555
Curcuma longa	HARIDRĀ	328
Cuscuta reflexa	AMARAVALLĪ	505
Cymbopogan martini	ROHIṢA	588
Cynodon dactylon	DŪRVĀ	587
Cyperus rotundus	MUSTĀ	342
Cypraea moneta	VARĀṬIKĀ	609
Daemonorops propingues	RAKTANIRYĀSA	576
Dalbergia lanceolaria	GORAKṢA	424

Dalbergia sissoo	ŚIṀŚAPĀ	428
Datura metel	DHATTŪRĀ	281
Daucus carota	GARJARA	467
Delphinium denudatum	NIRVIṢĀ	350
Dendrophthoe falcata	BANDĀKA	531
Desmodium gangeticum	ŚĀLAPARṆĪ	192
Desmostachya bipinnata	KUŚA	583
Dichrostachys cinerea	VĪRATARU	430
Digitalis purpurea	HṚTPATRĪ	509
Dioscorea bulbifera	VĀRĀHĪKANDA	565
Diospyros tomentosa	TINDUKA	491
Dipterocarpus turbinatus	AŚWAKARṆA	382
Dolichos biflorus	KULATTHA	440
Eclipta alba	BHṚṄGARĀJA	252
Elattaria cardamomum	ELĀ	332
Embelia ribes	VIḌAṄGA	258
Ephedra gerardiana	SOMA	551
Erythrina indica	PĀRIBHADRA	429
Eucalyptus globulus	TILAPARṆA	454
Eupatorium triplinerve	ĀYĀPĀNA	481
Euphorbia hirta	DUGDHIKĀ	596
Euphorbia neriifolia	SNUHĪ	532
Euphorbia thomsoniana	SWARṆĀKṢĪRĪ	536
Euryale ferox	MAKHĀNNA	363
Fel Bovinum purifcatum	GOROCANA	602
Ferula foetida	HIṄGU	234
Ficus bengalensis	VAṬA	540
Ficus hispida	KĀKODUMBARA	544
Ficus lacor	PLAKṢA	542
Ficus racemosa	UDUMBARA	322
Ficus religiosa	AŚWATTHA	541
Ficus rumphii	AŚMANTAKA	423
Flacourtia ramontchi	VIKAṄKATA	376
Foeniculum vulgare	MIŚREYA	236
Fumaria parviflora	PARPAṬAKA	364
Garcinia indica	VṚKṢĀMLA	381
Garcinia morella	KAṄKUṢṬHA	537
Garcinia morella	TAMĀLA	379
Garcinia pedunculata	AMLAVETASA	400
Gardenia gummifera	NĀḌĪHIṄGU	469

Gentiana kurro	TRĀYAMĀṆĀ	498
Gloriosa superba	LĀṄGALĪ	569
Glycyrrhiza glabra	MADHUYAṢṬI	189
Gmelina arborea	GAMBHĀRĪ	298
Gossypium herbaceum	KĀRPĀSA	386
Grewia asiatica	PARŪṢAKA	390
Grewia hirsuta	GUḌAŚARKARĀ	392
Grewia populifolia	GĀṄGERUKĪ	391
Grewia tiliaefolia	DHANWANA	393
Gymnema sylvestre	MEṢAŚṚṄGĪ	495
Hedychium spicatum	ŚAṬĪ	554
Helicteres isora	ĀVARTANĪ	389
Hemidesmus indicus	SĀRIVĀ	268
Hibiscus abelmoschus	LATĀKASTŪRĪ	383
Holarrhena antidysentrica	KUṬAJA	261
Holoptelea integrifolia	CIRABILWA	545
Hydnocarpus wightiane	TUVARAKA	160
Hyoscyamus niger	PĀRASĪKA YAVĀNĪ	282
Hyssopus officinalis	JŪPHĀ	519
Indigofera tinctoria	NĪLĪ	422
Inula racemosa	PUṢKARAMŪLA	253
Ipomoea hederaceae	KṚṢṆABĪJA	503
Jasminum auriculatum	YŪTHIKĀ	490
Jasminum grandiflorum	JĀTĪ	489
Juglans regia	AKṢOṬA	547
Juniperus communis	HAPUṢĀ	553
Lagenaria leucantha	KAṬUTUMBĪ (IKṢVĀKU)	461
Lawsonia inermis	MADAYANTIKĀ	456
Lepidium iberis	TODARĪ	369
Lepidium sativum	CANDRAŚŪRA	367
Leptadenia reticulata	JĪVANTĪ	494
Leucas cephalotus	DROṆAPUṢPĪ	302
Linum usitatissimum	ATASĪ	394
Litsea chinensis	MEDĀSAKA	530
Luffa acutangula	KOŚĀTAKĪ	462
Luffa aegyptiaca	DHĀMĀRGAVA	464
Luffa echinata	JĪMŪTAKA	463
Madhuca longifolia	MADHŪKA	486
Mallotus philippensis	KAMPILLAKA	533
Mangifera indica	ĀMRA	413

Marsdenia tenacissima	MŪRVĀ	496
Mentha piperata	PŪTIHĀ	518
Merremia emarginata	AKHUPARṆĪ	504
Mesua ferrea	NĀGAKEŚARA	161
Michelia champaka	CAMPAKA	354
Mimosa pudica	LAJJĀLU	446
Mimusops elengi	BAKULA	487
Momordica charantia	KĀRAVELLAKA	466
Moringa oleifera	ŚIGRU	184
Morus alba	TŪDA	543
Moschus moschiferus	KASTŪRĪ	601
Mucuna prurita	KAPIKACCHŪ	199
Musa paradisiaca	KADALĪ	560
Myrica nagi	KAṬPHALA	548
Myristica fragrans	JĀTIPHALA	309
Mytilus margaritiferus	MUKTĀ	605
Nardostachys jatamansi	JAṬĀMĀṀSĪ	250
Nelumbo nucifera	KAMALA	359
Nerium indicum	KARAVĪRA	264
Nicotiana tobaccum	TĀMRAPARṆA	508
Nigella sativa	UPAKUÑCIKĀ	351
Nyctanthes arbortristis	PĀRIJĀTA	488
Nymphaea stellata	KUMUDA	361
Ochrocarpus longifolius	SURAPUNNĀGA	378
Ocimum sanctum	TULASĪ	300
Onosma bracteatum	GOJIHWĀ	500
Operculina turpethum	TRIVṚT	275
Oroxylum indicum	ŚYONĀKA	287
Ostrea edulis	ŚUKTI	608
Ougeinia dalbergioides	TINIŚA	441
Oxalis corniculata	CĀṄGERĪ	170
Paederia foetida	GANDHAPRASĀRIṆĪ	249
Pandanus tectorius	KETAKĪ	577
Papaver somniferum	AHIPHENA	158
Parmelia perlata	ŚAILEYA	591
Peganum harmala	HARAMALA	399
Phaseolus trilobus	MUDGAPARṆĪ	425
Phoenin sylvestris	KHARJŪRA	575
Phyllanthus emblica	ĀMALAKĪ	219
Phyllanthus urinaria	BHŪMYĀMALAKĪ	535

Picrorhiza kurroa	KAṬUKĪ	283
Pinus longifolia	SARALA	552
Piper chaba	CAVYA	353
Piper cubeba	KAṄKOLA	528
Piper longum	PIPPALĪ	307
Piper longum	PIPPALĪMŪLA	345
Piper nigrum	MARICA	306
Pistacia intergerrima	KARKAṬAŚṚṄGĪ	180
Pistacia lentiscus	RUMĪMASTAGĪ	418
Plantago ovata	AŚVAGOLA	521
Pluchea lanceolate	RĀSNĀ	485
Plumbago zeylanica	CITRAKA	256
Podophyllum hexandrum	GIRI PARPAṬA	358
Polyalthia longifolia	KĀṢṬHADĀRU	356
Pongamia pinnata	KARAÑJA	195
Prosopis cineraria	ŚAMĪ	432
Prunus amygdalus	VĀTĀDA	448
Prunus puddum	PADMAKA	449
Psoralea corylifolia	BĀKUCĪ	203
Pterocarpus marsupium	BĪJAKA	427
Pterocarpus santalinus	RAKTACANDANA	437
Pterospermum diversifolium/ P. acerifolium	MUCAKUNDA	387
Pueraria tuberosa	VIDĀRĪ	438
Punica granatum	DĀḌIMA	224
Putranjiva roxburghii	PUTRAJĪVAKA	534
Quercus incana	MĀYĀPHALA	549
Randia dumetorum	MADANAPHALA	247
Ranunculus sceleratus	KĀNDĪRA	352
Raphanus sativus	MŪLAKA	370
Rauwolfia serpentina	SARPAGANDHĀ	263
Rheum emodi	PĪTAMULĪ	524
Rhus parviflora	TINTIḌĪKA	415
Ricinus communis	ERAṆḌA	316
Rosa indica	TARUṆĪ	447
Rubia cordifolia	MAÑJIṢṬHĀ	245
Rumex vesicarius	CUKRIKĀ (CUKRA)	523
Ruta graveolens	SUDDĀVA	398
Saccharam munja	ŚARA	584
Saccharum spontaneum	KĀŚA	585

Salacia roxburghii	SAPTACAKRĀ	458
Salvadora persica	PĪLU	492
Santalum album	CANDANA	314
Sapindus trifoliatus	ARIṢṬAKA	411
Saraca asoca	AŚOKA	207
Saussurea lappa	KUṢṬHA	254
Schleichera trijuga	KOŚĀMRA	412
Scirpus grossus	KAŚERUKA	581
Semecarpus anacardium	BHALLĀTAKA	182
Sesamum indicum	TILA	511
Sesbania aegyptiaca	JAYANTĪ	421
Sesbania grandiflora	AGASTYA	420
Shorea robusta	ŚĀLA	162
Sida cordifolia	BALĀ	163
Sida humilis	NĀGABALĀ	165
Sisymbrium irio	KHŪBAKALĀ	368
Smilax glabra	DWIPĀNTARA VACĀ	567
Smilax zeylanica	UŚAVA	568
Solanum indicum	BṚHATĪ	278
Solanum nigrum	KĀKAMĀCĪ	506
Solanum surattense	KAṆṬAKĀRĪ	276
Soymida febrifuga	MĀṀSAROHIṆĪ	406
Spheranthus indicus	MUṆḌĪ	476
Stereospermum suaveolens	PĀṬALĀ	289
Strychnos nux-vomica	KŪPĪLU	270
Strychnos potatorum	KATAKA	497
Swertia chirata	KIRĀTATIKTA	272
Symplocos racemosa	LODHRA	259
Syzygium caryophyllum	LAVAṄGA	221
Syzygium cumini	JAMBŪ	222
Tagetus erecta	JHAṆḌU	480
Tamarindus indica	AMLIKĀ	431
Taraxacum officinale	DUGDHAPHENĪ	482
Tecoma undulata	ROHITAKA	510
Tephrosia purpurea	ŚARAPUṄKHĀ	201
Teramnus labialis	MĀṢAPARṆĪ	426
Terminalia arjuna	ARJUNA	320
Terminalia bellirica	VIBHĪTAKA	217
Terminalia chebula	HARĪTAKĪ	215
Thalictrum foliolosum	MAMĪRĀ	349

Thespesia populnea	PĀRĪṢA	384
Tinospora cordifolia	GUḌŪCĪ	153
Trapa bisponosa	SṚṄGĀṬAKA	457
Tribulus terrestris	GOKṢURA	168
Trichodesma indicum	ADHAḤPUṢPĪ	501
Trichosanthes dioica	PAṬOLA	233
Trigonella foenumgraecum	METHIKĀ	436
Turbinella rapa	ŚAṄKHA	606
Uraria picta	PṚŚNIPARṆĪ	194
Urginea indica	VANAPALĀṆḌU	566
Valeriana wallichii	TAGARA	472
Vateria indica	SARJA	380
Vernonia cinerea	SAHADEVĪ	475
Vetiveria zizanioides	UŚĪRA	344
Viola odorata	BANAPHŚĀ	375
Vitex negundo	NIRGUṆḌĪ	293
Vitis vinifere	DRĀKṢĀ	409
Viverra civetta Linn.	PŪTI (KHATTĀŚĪ)	604
Withania somnifera	AŚWAGANDHĀ	279
Woodfordia fruiticosa	DHĀTAKĪ	226
Zanthoxylum alatum	TEJOHVA	176
Zingiber officinale	ĀRDRAKA	330
Ziziphus mauritiana	BADARA	407
Zizyphus sativa	UNNĀVA	408